COVID-19 and Environment: Impacts of a Global Pandemic

COVID-19 and Environment: Impacts of a Global Pandemic

Editors

Sachiko Kodera
Essam Rashed

MDPI • Basel • Beijing • Wuhan • Barcelona • Belgrade • Manchester • Tokyo • Cluj • Tianjin

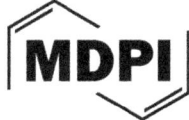

Editors
Sachiko Kodera
Department of Electrical and
Mechanical Engineering
Nagoya Institute of
Technology
Nagoya-shi
Japan

Essam Rashed
Graduate School of
Information Science
University of Hyogo
Kobe
Japan

Editorial Office
MDPI
St. Alban-Anlage 66
4052 Basel, Switzerland

This is a reprint of articles from the Special Issue published online in the open access journal *International Journal of Environmental Research and Public Health* (ISSN 1660-4601) (available at: www.mdpi.com/journal/ijerph/special_issues/COVID_Environment).

For citation purposes, cite each article independently as indicated on the article page online and as indicated below:

LastName, A.A.; LastName, B.B.; LastName, C.C. Article Title. *Journal Name* **Year**, *Volume Number*, Page Range.

ISBN 978-3-0365-5842-4 (Hbk)
ISBN 978-3-0365-5841-7 (PDF)

© 2022 by the authors. Articles in this book are Open Access and distributed under the Creative Commons Attribution (CC BY) license, which allows users to download, copy and build upon published articles, as long as the author and publisher are properly credited, which ensures maximum dissemination and a wider impact of our publications.
The book as a whole is distributed by MDPI under the terms and conditions of the Creative Commons license CC BY-NC-ND.

Contents

Preface to "COVID-19 and Environment: Impacts of a Global Pandemic" vii

Xin Dong, Shili Yang and Chunxiao Zhang
Air Pollution Increased the Demand for Gym Sports under COVID-19: Evidence from Beijing, China
Reprinted from: *Int. J. Environ. Res. Public Health* 2022, 19, 12614, doi:10.3390/ijerph191912614 . 1

Chunli Wei, Qingqing Li, Ziyi Lian, Yijun Luo, Shiqing Song and Hong Chen
Variation in Public Trust, Perceived Societal Fairness, and Well-Being before and after COVID-19 Onset—Evidence from the China Family Panel Studies
Reprinted from: *Int. J. Environ. Res. Public Health* 2022, 19, 12365, doi:10.3390/ijerph191912365 . 17

Ahmed Karam, Abdelrahman E. E. Eltoukhy, Ibrahim Abdelfadeel Shaban and El-Awady Attia
A Review of COVID-19-Related Literature on Freight Transport: Impacts, Mitigation Strategies, Recovery Measures, and Future Research Directions
Reprinted from: *Int. J. Environ. Res. Public Health* 2022, 19, 12287, doi:10.3390/ijerph191912287 . 31

Sonia Venancio-Guzmán, Alejandro Ivan Aguirre-Salado, Carlos Soubervielle-Montalvo and José del Carmen Jiménez-Hernández
Assessing the Nationwide COVID-19 Risk in Mexico through the Lens of Comorbidity by an XGBoost-Based Logistic Regression Model
Reprinted from: *Int. J. Environ. Res. Public Health* 2022, 19, 11992, doi:10.3390/ijerph191911992 . 59

Zhong Chen and Dongping Shi
The Atmospheric Environment Effects of the COVID-19 Pandemic: A Metrological Study
Reprinted from: *Int. J. Environ. Res. Public Health* 2022, 19, 11111, doi:10.3390/ijerph191711111 . 79

Fang Wang, Jin-Ming Wu, Yi-Chieh Lin, Te-Wei Ho, Hui-Lin Lin and Hsi-Yu Yu et al.
Coronavirus Disease Pandemic Effect on Medical-Seeking Behaviors Even in One Resource-Competent Community: A Case Controlled Study
Reprinted from: *Int. J. Environ. Res. Public Health* 2022, 19, 10822, doi:10.3390/ijerph191710822 . 95

Ka-Huen Yip, Yuk-Chiu Yip and Wai-King Tsui
The Lived Experiences of Women without COVID-19 in Breastfeeding Their Infants during the Pandemic: A Descriptive Phenomenological Study
Reprinted from: *Int. J. Environ. Res. Public Health* 2022, 19, 9511, doi:10.3390/ijerph19159511 . . . 105

Nobuyuki Wakui, Mayumi Kikuchi, Risa Ebizuka, Takahiro Yanagiya, Chikako Togawa and Raini Matsuoka et al.
Survey of Pharmacists' Knowledge, Attitudes, and Practices (KAP) concerning COVID-19 Infection Control after Being Involved in Vaccine Preparation: A Cross-Sectional Study
Reprinted from: *Int. J. Environ. Res. Public Health* 2022, 19, 9035, doi:10.3390/ijerph19159035 . . . 123

Biruk G. Mesfin, Daniel(Jian) Sun and Bo Peng
Impact of COVID-19 on Urban Mobility and Parking Demand Distribution: A Global Review with Case Study in Melbourne, Australia
Reprinted from: *Int. J. Environ. Res. Public Health* 2022, 19, 7665, doi:10.3390/ijerph19137665 . . . 137

Nobuyuki Wakui, Nanae Noguchi, Kotoha Ichikawa, Chikako Togawa, Raini Matsuoka and Yukiko Yoshizawa et al.
Psychological and Physical Changes Caused by COVID-19 Pandemic in Elementary and Junior High School Teachers: A Cross-Sectional Study
Reprinted from: *Int. J. Environ. Res. Public Health* **2022**, *19*, 7568, doi:10.3390/ijerph19137568 . . . **153**

Marta Baselga, Juan J. Alba and Alberto J. Schuhmacher
The Control of Metabolic CO_2 in Public Transport as a Strategy to Reduce the Transmission of Respiratory Infectious Diseases
Reprinted from: *Int. J. Environ. Res. Public Health* **2022**, *19*, 6605, doi:10.3390/ijerph19116605 . . . **167**

Jeadran Malagón-Rojas, Daniela Mendez-Molano, Julia Almentero, Yesith G. Toloza-Pérez, Eliana L. Parra-Barrera and Claudia P. Gómez-Rendón
Environmental Effects of the COVID-19 Pandemic: The Experience of Bogotá, 2020
Reprinted from: *Int. J. Environ. Res. Public Health* **2022**, *19*, 6350, doi:10.3390/ijerph19106350 . . . **187**

Zivile Pranskuniene, Rugile Grisiute, Andrius Pranskunas and Jurga Bernatoniene
Ethnopharmacology for Skin Diseases and Cosmetics during the COVID-19 Pandemic in Lithuania
Reprinted from: *Int. J. Environ. Res. Public Health* **2022**, *19*, 4054, doi:10.3390/ijerph19074054 . . . **199**

Nawfel Mosbahi, Jean-Philippe Pezy, Jean-Claude Dauvin and Lassad Neifar
COVID-19 Pandemic Lockdown: An Excellent Opportunity to Study the Effects of Trawling Disturbance on Macrobenthic Fauna in the Shallow Waters of the Gulf of Gabès (Tunisia, Central Mediterranean Sea)
Reprinted from: *Int. J. Environ. Res. Public Health* **2022**, *19*, 1282, doi:10.3390/ijerph19031282 . . . **211**

Priscilla Gomes da Silva, José Gonçalves, Ariana Isabel Brito Lopes, Nury Alves Esteves, Gustavo Emanuel Enes Bamba and Maria São José Nascimento et al.
Evidence of Air and Surface Contamination with SARS-CoV-2 in a Major Hospital in Portugal
Reprinted from: *Int. J. Environ. Res. Public Health* **2022**, *19*, 525, doi:10.3390/ijerph19010525 . . . **229**

Yuyang Zhao and Fernando Bacao
How Does Gender Moderate Customer Intention of Shopping via Live-Streaming Apps during the COVID-19 Pandemic Lockdown Period?
Reprinted from: *Int. J. Environ. Res. Public Health* **2021**, *18*, 13004, doi:10.3390/ijerph182413004 . **243**

Heesup Han, Chen Che and Sanghyeop Lee
Facilitators and Reducers of Korean Travelers' Avoidance/Hesitation Behaviors toward China in the Case of COVID-19
Reprinted from: *Int. J. Environ. Res. Public Health* **2021**, *18*, 12345, doi:10.3390/ijerph182312345 . **267**

Preface to "COVID-19 and Environment: Impacts of a Global Pandemic"

COVID-19 outbreak was first reported in China in 2019 and spread worldwide in early 2020. With the spread of COVID-19 and the corresponding negative impact on different life aspects, it has become important to understand the ways to deal with the pandemic as a part of daily life. Numerous studies on COVID-19 have investigated meteorological factors, clinical features, and public health interventions that affect infection and morbidity. However, the problems still exists and more investigation is required. Challenges are the limitation of accurate/complete data, the effect of restrictions, and variabilities of medical service quality in different countries. In addition, circumstances are dynamically changing due to policies, vaccines, and the advent of new variants all over the world. The investigation of correlation between COVID-19 and environmental factors based on long-term analysis and data curation would lead to better sustainable management of healthcare resources and government policies.

This Special Issue aims to collect articles of high academic standards investigating the links between the COVID-19 pandemic and environmental factors. We have received several manuscripts, from which 17 papers have passed the peer-review process and are presented here as a reprint.

Sachiko Kodera and Essam Rashed
Editors

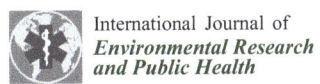

Article

Air Pollution Increased the Demand for Gym Sports under COVID-19: Evidence from Beijing, China

Xin Dong [1], Shili Yang [2] and Chunxiao Zhang [1,*]

1 School of Information Engineering, China University of Geosciences, Beijing 100083, China
2 Beijing Meteorological Observation Centre, Beijing Meteorological Bureau, Beijing 100089, China
* Correspondence: zcx@cugb.edu.cn; Tel.: +86-186-1821-9549

Abstract: Air pollution may change people's gym sports behavior. To test this claim, first, we used big data crawler technology and ordinary least square (OLS) models to investigate the effect of air pollution on people' gym visits in Beijing, China, especially under the COVID-19 pandemic of 2019–2020, and the results showed that a one-standard-deviation increase in PM2.5 concentration (fine particulate matter with diameters equal to or smaller than 2.5 μm) derived from the land use regression model (LUR) was positively associated with a 0.119 and a 0.171 standard-deviation increase in gym visits without or with consideration of the COVID-19 variable, respectively. Second, using spatial autocorrelation analysis and a series of spatial econometric models, we provided consistent evidence that the gym industry of Beijing had a strong spatial dependence, and PM2.5 and its spatial spillover effect had a positive impact on the demand for gym sports. Such a phenomenon offers us a new perspective that gym sports can be developed into an essential activity for the public due to this avoidance behavior regarding COVID-19 virus contact and pollution exposure.

Keywords: air pollution; PM2.5 concentration; gym sports; spatial econometric model; COVID-19

1. Introduction

Many Chinese megacities are extremely polluted, and the problem of serious haze has aroused widespread concern among the public [1,2]. Air pollution not only significantly causes great harm to public health [3,4], it also affects people's daily life [5,6]. Air pollution may inhibit outdoor physical activity, as people have engaged in avoidance behavior [7,8]. Some studies have demonstrated that air pollution has negative effects on the frequency of travel to indoor amenities such as restaurants, shopping areas and movie theatres [9,10] and outdoor venues such as public parks [11].

Notably, research related to indoor air pollution concentration in gyms is dominated by evidence from some developed countries, which generally show that people may inhale more pollutants while exercising in indoor gyms [12–14]. In cities of the developing world, however, the role of gym sports is under-researched. The existing literature, mainly focusing on the impact of air pollution on the frequency of gym physical activity, remains rare.

To further investigate how gym sports can be affected by air pollution and actual external environmental factors, this study focuses on the effect of air pollution under the COVID-19 pandemic. As is known, the COVID-19 pandemic is currently one of the greatest challenges to human life and health and economic development [15]. Beginning in 2020, starting in China, the coronavirus rapidly spread around the world due to globalization, which caused great harm to travel behavior [16]. The strictest social travel restrictions imposed by the Chinese government in response to the first outbreak of the pandemic included restricting all outdoor activities and closing all recreational facilities, including public indoor sports places [17,18]. Although lockdown restrictions started to lift in many cities around the world, regular pandemic prevention and control measures have remained unchanged in China, such as transport suspension [19] and 14 days of quarantine when traveling [20,21], referring to the post-pandemic era.

Recently, a significant number of studies have shown that the pandemic has reduced the frequency of people traveling to both outdoor physical activities [22,23] and indoor gym sports [24]. In addition, some scholars have found changes in air quality because of the travel restrictions during the COVID-19 pandemic [25,26]. Gym exercise behavior is affected by air pollution, and was especially affected during the COVID-19 pandemic [27]. Nevertheless, there is still a lack of studies that have analyzed the impact of air pollution on gym sports behavior under the impact of the pandemic in spatiotemporal dimensions.

The purpose of this study is to fill the gap aforementioned by examining this case in Beijing, China. Beijing, as the capital of China, with its vast territory, dense population and complex terrain, makes air pollution a serious threat [28]. Beijing was the second-largest city in China with gym exercisers in 2020, after Shanghai [29]. In this paper, we used big data crawling techniques and panel regression models to examine the effect of PM2.5 concentration conducted by land use regression (LUR) models [30,31] on gym visits during COVID-19 from 1 January 2019 to 31 December 2020. We divided 2019–2020 into five COVID-19 periods due to air pollution prevention levels published by the Chinese government, including the Pre-COVID period (the period before the pandemic, spanning from 1 January 2019 to 24 January 2020), COVID-Lock period (the period during the outbreak of the pandemic and the blockade of non-essential travel, spanning from 25 January to 25 February 2020), COVID-Recover-I period (the period during pandemic prevention and control downgrade, spanning from 26 January to 10 June 2020), Xinfadi-COVID period (the period of another outbreak of the pandemic in Xinfadi, spanning from 11 June to 6 August 2020) and COVID-Recover-II period (the period when the pandemic outbreak alert was lifted, spanning from 7 August to 31 December 2020), abbreviated as P1–P5 (Figure 1) [32]. Gym comments crawled from the platform "Meituan.com" were used to describe Beijing's gym visits in P1–P5 of the COVID-19 pandemic.

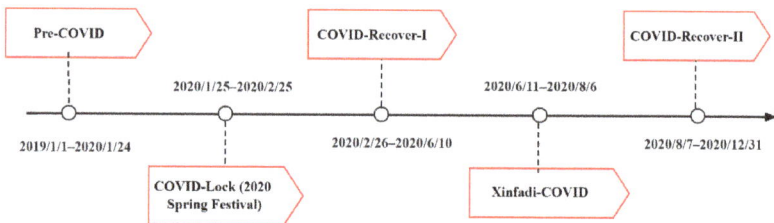

Figure 1. Timeline of five periods of the COVID-19 pandemic of Beijing, China.

In this study, we aimed to not only access the effect of air pollution on people's gym visits under five different COVID-19 periods, but also to evaluate the spatial spillover effect of air pollution on the entire development of the gym industry from the perspective of a space–time analysis. Therefore, this study was designed to examine two research questions: (1) How does air pollution affect people's demand for gym sports under COVID-19? (2) Is there a spatial spillover effect on the impact of air pollution on gym sports?

Our findings from the space–time analysis about the impact of air pollution on gym sports have contributed to the literature on air pollution and avoidance behavior. At the same time, it is necessary to pay attention to the impact of COVID-19 on people's behavior regarding gym sports, which has been well documented as a new behavioral moderator regarding avoiding outdoor exposure of the virus when exercising.

2. Materials and Methods

2.1. Gym Data

This study aimed to test daily gym activity changes in Beijing that were associated with air pollution and climate conditions under the COVID-19 period. The study area and spatial distribution of 2452 gyms are shown in Figure 2. Because a lack of direct evidence on consumer mobility limited our ability to characterize local gym consumption conditions, to a certain degree, we used online consumption recorded data, which was used to represent the actual number of gym visits according to previous studies [9,33]. Therefore, we used big data crawler technology and crawled the data from the Chinese leading local lifestyle information and trading platform "Meituan.com" to describe Beijing residents' gym activities. The information of each gym in Beijing included its precise location information and its attributes data, including users' reviews, ratings and their per capita consumption from 1 January 2019 to 31 December 2020.

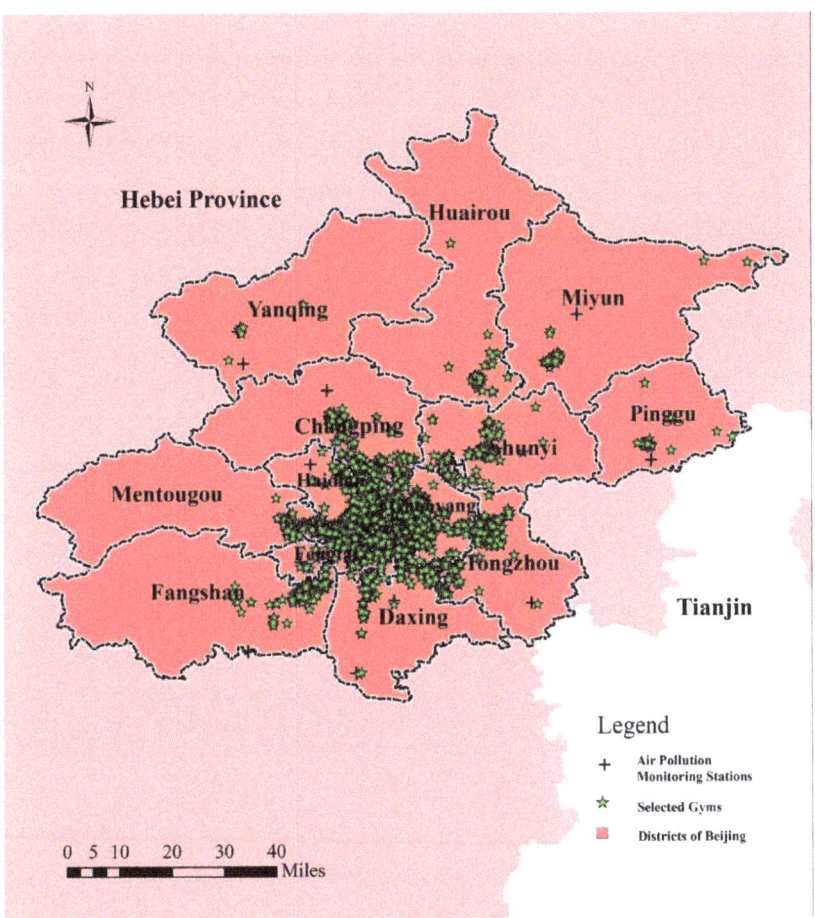

Figure 2. Study area. The spatial distribution of 2452 gyms of 16 administrative districts are indicated in Beijing, China.

Finally, our analysis data included 2452 gyms with 144,904 comments. The comments data were merged according to the timeline of five different COVID-19 periods to describe Beijing's gym visits during COVID-19. This study implicitly assumed that the probability of writing a review was not relevant to the air pollution level by using the count of reviews as a proxy for the count of gym visits.

2.2. PM2.5 Concentration Data

Hourly PM2.5 data in Beijing from 1 January 2019 to 31 December 2020 were obtained from the Beijing Municipal Environmental Monitoring Center [34]. Since 2013, there have been 35 environmental monitoring stations (EMSs) in Beijing (Figure 2). The botanical garden EMS was eliminated from the twelve urban EMSs in this study, and 34 EMSs were used to obtain hourly PM2.5 concentration in this study based on the Ambient Air Quality Standards (GB 3095-2012) [35]. We averaged the PM2.5 data based on the five different periods of the COVID-19 pandemic for the subsequent air pollution modeling.

2.3. Land Use Regression (LUR) Model

We used the LUR model to replace traditional spatial interpolation methods to obtain average PM2.5 concentrations of P1–P5 more accurately [30,31]. In our study, we divided the process into two steps as follows, including preparing predictor variables and building the LUR model.

2.3.1. Predictor Variables

We used average PM2.5 concentrations of P1–P5 and independent variables to build LUR models, including land use, digital elevation model (DEM), meteorological variables, road length, population density, remote sensing PM2.5 data, normalized difference vegetation index (NDVI), aerosol optical depth (AOD) and points of interest (POI). These nine driving factors were selected on the basis of their significant impact on PM2.5 concentrations [36,37]. Overall, this study considered a total of 29 subcategories, which included 103 independent variables within the nine major independent variable categories.

As shown in Table 1, land use data, traffic information and POI data, the three major vector predictor variables, are included in the LUR model. Land use data were derived from Esri 2020 Land Cover with a spatial resolution of 10 m (https://livingatlas.arcgis.com/landcover/, accessed on 5 May 2021). Land use type was divided into cropland, woodland, grassland, water bodies, construction land, and unused land. The specific indicator of the land factor was the ratio of land area to buffer area (area of circular buffer).

Table 1. Description of the vector predictor variables in the LUR models of P1–P5.

No.	Predictor Variables	Abbreviations	Unit	Buffer Size
Land use				
1	Cultivated land	Cul_xx	m^2	100, 300, 500, 1000, 3000, 5000
2	Forest	For_xx	m^2	100, 300, 500, 1000, 3000, 5000
3	Grass land	Gra_xx	m^2	100, 300, 500, 1000, 3000, 5000
4	Waterbody	Wat_xx	m^2	100, 300, 500, 1000, 3000, 5000
5	Built-up area	Bui_xx	m^2	100, 300, 500, 1000, 3000, 5000
6	Unused land	Unu_xx	m^2	100, 300, 500, 1000, 3000, 5000
Traffic information				
7	Trunk road length	Tru_xx	m	100, 300, 500, 1000, 3000, 5000
8	Primary road length	Pri_xx	m	100, 300, 500, 1000, 3000, 5000
9	Secondary road length	Sec_xx	m	100, 300, 500, 1000, 3000, 5000
10	Railroad length	Rai_xx	m	100, 300, 500, 1000, 3000, 5000
POI information				
11	Bus station number	POI1_xx	-	100, 300, 500, 1000, 3000, 5000, 7000
12	Gas station number	POI2_xx	-	100, 300, 500, 1000, 3000, 5000, 7000
13	Polluted enterprise number	POI3_xx	-	100, 300, 500, 1000, 3000, 5000, 7000
14	Chinese restaurant number	POI4_xx	-	100, 300, 500, 1000, 3000, 5000, 7000
15	Distance to the nearest bus station	D_bus	m	NA
16	Distance to the nearest gas station	D_gas	m	NA
17	Distance to the nearest polluted enterprise	D_pol	m	NA
18	Distance to the nearest Chinese restaurant	D_res	m	NA

Road data were obtained from OpenStreetMap (https://www.openstreetmap.org, accessed on 5 May 2021). The specific road factor indicator was the ratio of road length to buffer area.

Points of interest (POI) data were derived from Amap, by applying API based on category and keyword semantics (http://lbs.amap.com/api/webservice/guide/api/search/, accessed on 25 May 2021). Different POI categories in different buffer sizes represent different emission information with regard to PM2.5. In this study, we used four types of POI as pollutant emission sources, including bus stations, gas stations, polluted enterprises and Chinese restaurants. To reflect the impact of local emission sources and possible regional transmission, the buffer sizes for POI in this study were set from 100 to 7000 m [38].

As shown in Table 2, population data, geographical information, vegetation index, remote sensing data, meteorological data and aerosol optical depth data, the six major raster predictor variables, are included in the LUR model.

Table 2. Description of the raster predictor variables in the LUR models of P1–P5.

No.	Predictor Variables	Abbreviations	Unit	Original Spatial Resolution
Population				
1	Population density	Pop	people/m^2	1 km
Geographic information				
2	Elevation	DEM	m	30 m
Vegetation index				
3	NDVI	NDVI	-	1 km
Remote sensing data				
4	CHAP_PM2.5	CHAP	μg/m^3	1 km
Meteorological data				
5	Boundary layer height	BLH	m	0.125°
6	2 m temperature	T2M	K	0.125°
7	Total precipitation	TP	mm	0.125°
8	Surface pressure	SP	10^6 Pa	0.125°
9	10 m u-component of wind	U10m	m/s	0.125°
10	10 m v-component of wind	V10m	m/s	0.125°
Aerosol optical depth				
11	Optical_Depth_047	AOD_047	-	1 km

The population density data used in this study were based on Gridded Population of the World (GPW) from the Columbia University Socioeconomic Data and Application Center (CU2020) as raster data, with a resolution of 1 × 1 km [39].

Elevation data were obtained from the Advanced Spaceborne Thermal Emission and Reflection Radiometer Global Digital Elevation Model, version2 (ASTER GDEM v2) on the USGS Earth Explorer site, with a spatial resolution of 30 m (https://yceo.yale.edu/aster-gdem-global-elevation-data, accessed on 8 May 2021).

Normalized difference vegetation index (NDVI) data were provided by the MOD13A2 Version 6 product distributed by NASA EOSDIS Land Processes DAAC, which was a MODIS/Terra Vegetation Indices 16-Day L3 Global 1 km SIN Grid with a spatial resolution of 1 km (https://lpdaac.usgs.gov/products/mod13a2v006/, accessed on 12 May 2021). Data were calculated into mean data for the corresponding period of P1–P5 [40].

Remote sensing PM2.5 data were provided by the MODIS/Terra + Aqua Level 3 (L3) Yearly 0.01 degree gridded ground-level PM2.5 products in Eastern China (ECHAP_PM2.5_Y1K) from 2019 to 2020 (https://zenodo.org/record/4660858#.YU2JKux0IdU, accessed on 14 May 2021) [41,42].

Meteorological data were extracted from the ERA–Interim reanalysis dataset of European Centre for Medium-Range Weather Forecasts (ECMWF), with a spatial resolution of 0.125° × 0.125°. The data downloaded were daily means of 2-meter temperature data, U wind speed data, V wind speed data, boundary layer height data, surface pressure data and total precipitation data, which needed to be summed into mean data of P1–P5 by Python, prepared for later modeling [43].

Aerosol Optical Depth (AOD) data were obtained from the MCD19A2 Version 6 data product distributed by NASA EOSDIS Land Processes DAAC, which was a Moderate Resolution Imaging Spectroradiometer (MODIS) Terra and Aqua combined Multi-angle Implementation of Atmospheric Correction (MAIAC) Land Aerosol Optical Depth (AOD) gridded Level 2 product produced daily at 1 km pixel resolution. (https://lpdaac.usgs.gov/products/mcd19a2v006/, accessed on 15 May 2021) [44].

2.3.2. Building the LUR Model

A five-step backward method was adopted for fitting the LUR model [45]. For all available potential predictor variables, bivariate correlation analysis with average PM2.5 concentrations of P1–P5 were conducted first. Second, the predictor variables were sorted by adjusted R^2. Third, other variables (Pearson correlation coefficient $R \geq 0.7$) with high relevance to the highest ranked variables in each subcategory were removed. Fourth, all the remaining predictor variables and PM2.5 concentrations were entered into the stepwise linear regression model to obtain the multiple linear regression equation. Finally, the significance level (p value < 5%) and variance inflation factor (VIF < 4) of each predictor variable were checked to confirm the variables' significance levels and to ensure no issues of multicollinearity. The leave-one cross-validation (LOOCV) and 10-fold CV method were chosen to evaluate the predictive capacity of the model. From the cross-validation, the R^2 and root mean squared error (RMSE) were used to evaluate and compare the predictivity of the model [46,47].

2.4. Statistical Analysis

Figure 3 shows the overall theoretical framework used for assessing the effect of PM2.5 concentration on gym visits under COVID-19.

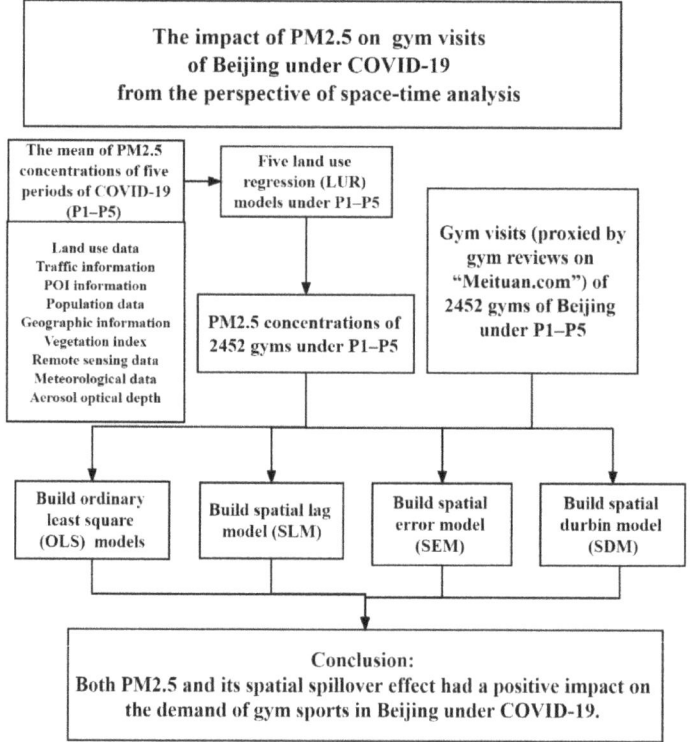

Figure 3. Theoretical framework model of this study.

2.4.1. Building Ordinary Least Squares (OLS) Model

First, we used an OLS panel regression model to test how the count of the gym visits varies as a function of air pollution and climate conditions.

$$NUM_{it} = \alpha_0 + \alpha_1 PM2.5_{it} + \alpha_2 W_{it} + \alpha_3 X_{it} + T_t + \gamma_i + \varepsilon_{it}, \tag{1}$$

where NUM_{it} and $PM2.5_{it}$ represent the comments, reviews, and PM2.5 concentrations of gym i on COVID-19 period t. W_{it} represents weather conditions, including gym mean temperature and precipitation of P1–P5. X_{it} is used as a control variable, including for residents' gym ratings and per capita consumptions. T_t and γ_i are used to control for COVID-19 wave-fixed effects and gym area-fixed effects. ε_{it} is the random error term. The standard errors are clustered by individual. To avoid collinearity with the PM2.5 data generated by the LUR model, the average temperature and precipitation data of P1–P5 used in Equation (1) are based on other meteorological data obtained from 18 standard meteorological stations at the Beijing Meteorological Informational Center, including hourly temperature and precipitation.

Second, we defined the variable COVID-19 to denote the number of confirmed cases in P1–P5 waves into Equation (1) to generate Equation (2).

$$NUM_{it} = \alpha_0 + \alpha_1 COVID\text{-}19_t + \alpha_2 PM2.5_{it} + \alpha_3 W_{it} + \alpha_4 X_{it} + T_t + \gamma_i + \varepsilon_{it}, \quad (2)$$

where $COVID\text{-}19_t$ represents the cumulative number of confirmed cases of COVID-19 in P1–P5. Coefficient α_2 reflects the effect of PM2.5 concentration on gym visits under the background of the COVID-19 pandemic, which is expected to be consistent with coefficient α_1 in Equation (1). The meanings of other characters are as the same as the above model.

Third, a robustness check was used to replace the PM2.5 variable with PM2.5 data obtained from the Kriging interpolation method of the MEP PM2.5 monitoring sites and that from the United States Embassy and Consulates to verify the association of actual PM2.5 concentration with gym visits in P1–P5 of the COVID-19 pandemic [48].

2.4.2. Building Spatial Econometric Models

To begin, we used Moran's Index to examine whether there was a spatial autocorrelation relationship or not between gym visits in P1–P5 of the COVID-19 pandemic [49] as Equation (3).

$$Moran's\ I = \frac{N}{\sum_{ij}^{N} w_{ij}} \frac{\sum_{ij}^{N} w_{ij}(x_i - \bar{x})(x_j - \bar{x})}{\sum_{i=1}^{N}(x_i - \bar{x})^2} \quad (3)$$

with $i \neq j$, where x_i is the interest variable in gym i, $\bar{x}$ is the variable mean value, N is the number of observations, and w_{ij} is the spatial weight. The Moran index varies between -1 and 1. A value close to 1 indicates the presence of clusters, and a value close to -1 indicates spatial dispersion in the data. If the value is 0, then there is no spatial autocorrelation.

If the spatial factor was ignored or classified as a random disturbance term, the results obtained by the OLS modeling would have errors. Therefore, when analyzing the impact of PM2.5 on gym visits, spatial econometric models need to be considered [50].

Then, spatial factors were taken into account in the spatial lag model (SLM), which emphasized the spatial spillover effect of the local gym visits to the number of exercisers in other nearby gyms. The SLM model is expressed formally as Equation (4):

$$NUM_{it} = \alpha + \rho \sum_{j=1}^{n} w_{ij} NUM_{jt} + \beta_1 COVID\text{-}19_t + \beta_2 PM2.5_{it} + \beta_3 W_{it} + T_t + \gamma_i + \varepsilon_{it} \quad (4)$$

where ρ is the influence degree of the explained variable with spatial lag on the explained variable, w_{ij} represents the weight matrix, β is the degree of influence of each explanatory variable (COVID-19, PM2.5 and weather situations) on gym visits, and the meanings of other characters are the same as the above models.

Furthermore, the spatial error model (SEM) measured the error impact of local influential factors on the gym visits themselves and the impact of these influential factors on other gyms in Beijing. The SEM model is expressed formally as Equation (5):

$$NUM_{it} = \alpha + \beta_1 COVID\text{-}19_t + \beta_2 PM2.5_{it} + \beta_3 W_{it} + T_t + \gamma_i + \varepsilon_{it} \quad (5)$$

$$\varepsilon_{it} = \lambda \sum_{j=1}^{n} w_{ij}\, \varepsilon_{jt} + \mu_{it}\,,\ \mu_{it} \sim N\left[0,\, \delta^2 I\right]$$

where λ represents the spatial error correlation coefficient, μ_{it} is the error term that satisfies the OLS assumption, and the meanings of other characters are the same as the above models.

Lastly, the spatial Durbin model (SDM) reflects the degree of agglomeration of gym visits in a single gym, the level of agglomeration of gym visits in adjacent gyms, and the impact of the overall gym visits on the development of the gym industry in Beijing. The SDM model is expressed formally as Equation (6)

$$NUM_{it} = \alpha + \rho \sum_{j=1}^{n} w_{ij}\, NUM_{jt} + \beta_1 \text{COVID-19}_t + \beta_2 \text{PM2.5}_{it} + \beta_3 W_{it} + \gamma\, w_{ij}\text{COVID-19}_t + \gamma\, w_{ij}\text{PM2.5}_t + \gamma\, w_{ij}W_t + T_t + \gamma_i + \varepsilon_{it} \tag{6}$$

where $w_{ij}\text{COVID-19}_t$, $w_{ij}\text{PM2.5}_t$ and $w_{ij}W_t$ represent the spatial lag COVID-19, PM2.5 and weather situations (temperature and precipitation) of the average observation value of the adjacent gyms. γ is the spatial correlation coefficient, and the meanings of other characters are the same as the above models.

3. Results

3.1. PM2.5 Concentration Estimates from the LUR Model

The results of the five LUR model simulations were strongly correlated with the independent in situ PM2.5 values based on the leave-one cross-validation (LOOCV) and 10-fold CV results on the pandemic scale of P1–P5 (Table 3). After the final regression models were obtained, regular 1 × 1 km grids were generated and predicted PM2.5 concentrations were calculated at the grid points. Then, Kriging interpolation was conducted to generate PM2.5 concentration distribution simulation maps of Beijing in P1–P5 (Figure 4). Finally, we extracted the corresponding PM2.5 concentration values of all gyms in P1–P5 as PM2.5 exposure concentrations in P1–P5 of the COVID-19 pandemic, preparing for the follow-up study of the effect of air pollution on gym visits under COVID-19.

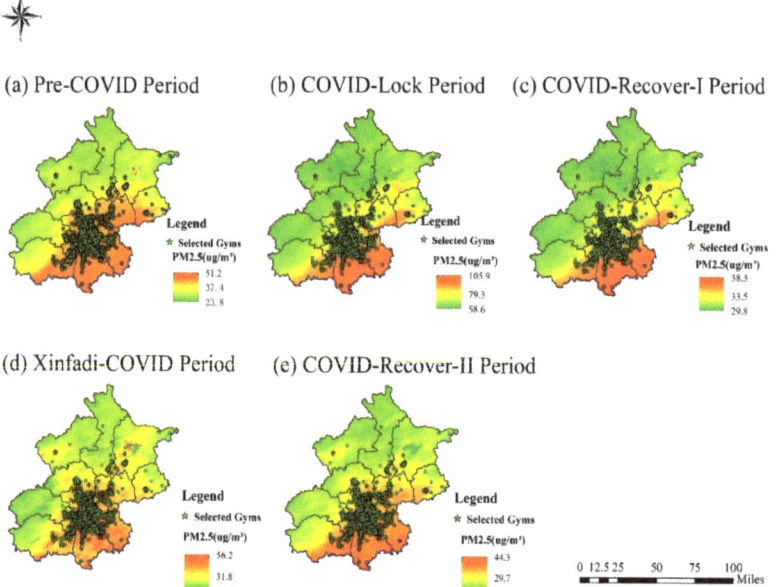

Figure 4. Spatial distribution of simulation results of PM2.5 concentrations in Beijing in P1–P5.

Table 3. Summary of the final LUR models for PM2.5 in P1–P5.

Model	Variable	Coefficient	Std. Error	T Value	p (>|t|)	VIF	Global Statistics
Pre-COVID PM2.5 ($\mu g/m^3$)	Intercept	2.34	5.552	0.421	0.676	NA	Adjusted R^2 = 0.68; LOOCV R^2 = 0.68 RMSE = 3.10 $\mu g/m^3$; 10-fold CV R^2 = 0.68; RMSE = 3.72 $\mu g/m^3$.
	CHAP	0.079	0.014	7.192	0.000	1.039	
	Cul_3000	4.174×10^{-7}	1.363×10^{-7}	3.063	0.004	1.039	
COVID-Lock PM2.5 ($\mu g/m^3$)	Intercept	5.868	8.578	0.684	0.499	NA	Adjusted R^2 = 0.73; LOOCV R^2 = 0.73 RMSE = 5.12 $\mu g/m^3$; 10-fold CV R^2 = 0.73; RMSE = 6.26 $\mu g/m^3$.
	CHAP	2.197	0.265	8.274	0.000	1.002	
	Cul_300	4.23×10^{-4}	9.5×10^{-5}	3.063	0.000	1.002	
COVID-Recover-I PM2.5 ($\mu g/m^3$)	Intercept	20.925	2.973	7.039	0.000	NA	Adjusted R^2 = 0.64; LOOCV R^2 = 0.64 RMSE = 1.95 $\mu g/m^3$; 10-fold CV R^2 = 0.64; RMSE = 2.34 $\mu g/m^3$.
	CHAP	0.398	0.093	4.297	0.000	1.048	
	Tru_500	1198.099	345.514	3.468	0.002	1.053	
	Cul_300	1.17×10^{-4}	3.3×10^{-5}	3.577	0.001	1.017	
	Gra_100	−0.001	2.52×10^{-4}	−2.545	0.017	1.033	
Xinfadi-COVID PM2.5 ($\mu g/m^3$)	Intercept	2.032	6.088	0.334	0.741	NA	Adjusted R^2 = 0.73; LOOCV R^2 = 0.73 RMSE = 3.36 $\mu g/m^3$; 10-fold CV R^2 = 0.73; RMSE = 3.97 $\mu g/m^3$.
	AOD_047	0.066	0.013	5.24	0.000	1.674	
	POI3_7000	0.215	0.046	4.723	0.000	2.854	
	Pri_500	−2640.034	445.498	−5.926	0.000	1.017	
	POI2_7000	−0.19	0.058	−3.274	0.003	3.94	
	Wat_100	−49.1	1.72×10^{-4}	−2.615	0.014	1.101	
COVID-Recover-II PM2.5 ($\mu g/m^3$)	Intercept	8.407	4.257	1.975	0.057	NA	Adjusted R^2 = 0.54; LOOCV R^2 = 0.54 RMSE = 2.89 $\mu g/m^3$; 10-fold CV R^2 = 0.542; RMSE = 3.61 $\mu g/m^3$
	AOD_047	0.079	0.014	5.505	0.000	1.044	
	Cul_1000	3.7×10^{-6}	8.407	4.257	0.045	1.044	

3.2. The Impact of PM2.5 Concentration on Gym Visits under COVID-19

As shown in Table 4, we used a series of OLS models to present specifications that include progressively more controls from Model 1 to 3. Model 1 only controls for time-fixed effects of five different COVID-19 waves, adding in area-fixed effects in Model 2, gym attributes control variables in Model 3, and finally the level and squared terms of PM2.5 in Model 4, which were used to explore the nonlinearity of the relationship between PM2.5 concentration and gym visits. The standardized coefficients of PM2.5 from Model 1 to 3 steadily decreased (0.150, 0.148 and 0.119), showing that PM2.5 was significantly positively associated with gym visits. Furthermore, precipitation was significantly negatively associated with gym visits with an effect that was 18.05 in Model 4 after controlling for time-fixed effects, area-fixed effects and gym attribute variables. Model 4 exhibits a nonlinear positive relationship between PM2.5 concentration and gym visits; thereby, our study mainly focused on the linear effect of PM2.5 on gym visits under COVID-19.

Table 4. Estimated associations between PM2.5 and gym visits from the OLS models.

Dependent Variable: Gym Comments	Model 1	Model 2	Model 3	Model 4
PM2.5	0.150 ***	0.148 ***	0.119 ***	0.366 ***
	(0.000)	(0.000)	(0.000)	(0.008)
(PM2.5)^2	-	-	-	−0.00165 *
	-	-	-	(0.065)
Precipitation	4.509	−20.01 ***	−18.05 ***	−19.17 ***
	(0.153)	(0.000)	(0.000)	(0.000)
Temperature	1.486 ***	−0.0322	0.0259	-0.0561
	(0.001)	(0.897)	(0.916)	(0.823)
Constant	11.16 *	36.81 ***	0.327	30.61 ***
	(0.075)	(0.000)	(0.939)	(0.000)
COVID-19 Wave FEs	Yes	Yes	Yes	Yes
Gym FEs	No	Yes	Yes	Yes
Gym Controls	No	No	Yes	Yes
Observations	12,260	12,260	12,260	12,260
Participant number	2452	2452	2452	2452

Note: We suppressed the coefficients on control variables to conserve space. The 95% confidence intervals are based on heteroscedastic robust standard errors. *** $p < 0.001$; * $p < 0.01$.

Moreover, the positive impact of PM2.5 grew from 0.119 in Model 3 of Table 4 to 0.171 in Model 1 of Table 5, which meant that such a positive effect increased to a 0.051 standard deviation when introducing the COVID-19 variable into Model 3. Notably, we found that COVID-19 was negatively associated with gym visits (−0.0272 in Model 1 of Table 5), which could be explained by Chinese pandemic control measures and people's high awareness of pandemic prevention under the COVID-19 pandemic.

Table 5. Estimated associations between PM2.5 and gym visits in P1–P5.

Dependent Variable: Gym Comments	Model 1	Model 2	Model 3
COVID-19	−0.0272 ***	−0.0246 ***	−0.0246 ***
	(0.000)	(0.000)	(0.000)
PM2.5	0.171 ***	-	-
	(0.000)	-	-
PM2.5 Kriging	-	0.00305	-
	-	(0.952)	-
PM2.5 US Embassy	-	-	2.341 ***
	-	-	(0.000)
Precipitation	−19.14 ***	−17.14 ***	−17.04 ***
	(0.000)	(0.000)	(0.000)
Temperature	0.116	0.0712	0.0707
	(0.626)	(0.771)	(0.773)
Constant	−2.985	4.568	−94.63 ***
	(0.479)	(0.307)	(0.000)
Gym FEs	YES	YES	YES
COVID-19 Wave FEs	YES	YES	YES
Gym Controls	YES	YES	YES
Observations	12,260	12,260	12,260
Participant Number	2452	2452	2452

Note: We included time-fixed effects of five different COVID-19 waves, area-fixed effects and gym attributes control variables in all Models. In Model 2 and 3, we replaced the PM2.5 variable with PM2.5 data obtained from the Kriging interpolation method of the MEP PM2.5 monitoring sites and that from the US Embassy and Consulates, as mentioned in Materials and Methods. The 95% confidence intervals are based on heteroscedastic robust standard errors. *** $p < 0.001$.

In our robustness check, PM2.5 from the Kriging interpolation method in Model 2 of Table 5 was not statistically significantly associated with gym visits. However, the positive impact of PM2.5 from the US Embassy and Consulates grew to almost 14 times of that in Model 3 (2.341 versus 0.171). This might be due to the fact that there is only one PM2.5 monitoring site in the US Embassy and Consulates of Beijing, leading to an overestimation of the positive impact of pollution on gym visits. The correlation between any two of the three PM2.5 indicators was as high as 0.96. We found that the coefficient of precipitation was significant and negative.

When considering the spatial autocorrelation, the z-value and p value of the overall Moran's Index for the gym visits showed that at the 1% significant level (Table 6), the number of gym exercisers had a significantly positive spatial autocorrelation among different gyms in Beijing, indicating that there was an obvious agglomeration phenomenon among the gym crowds.

Because of the spatial autocorrelation, spatial econometric models needed to be taken into account, which included the spatial lag model (SLM), spatial error model (SEM) and the spatial Durbin model (SDM).

As shown in Table 7, PM2.5 concentrations were positively associated with gym visits in the OLS model, SLM model and SEM model after controlling for both fixed effects, with coefficients of 0.171, 0.205 and 0.197, respectively, which effectively illustrated that PM2.5 had a positive effect on gym visits under COVID-19. Notably, the standardized coefficients of COVID-19 from the OLS model, SLM model, SEM model and SDM model were similar

(−0.027, −0,027, −0.028 and −0.024), which indicated that the COVID-19 variable itself inhibited people's gym sports behavior.

Table 6. Moran's Index of gym comments in P1–P5.

Dependent Variable: Gym Comments under P1–P5	I	z	p Value
Pre-COVID	0.181 ***	6.137	0.000
COVID-Lock	0.062 ***	2.159	0.015
COVID-Recover-I	0.100 ***	3.394	0.000
Xinfadi-COVID	0.102 ***	3.490	0.000
COVID-Recover-II	0.122 ***	4.229	0.000

Note: *** $p < 0.001$.

Table 7. Four regression model results in P1–P5.

Dependent Variable: Gym Comments under P1–P5	OLS	SLM	SEM	SDM
COVID-19	−0.027 ***	−0.027 ***	−0.028 ***	−0.024 ***
	(0.000)	(0.000)	(0.000)	(0.008)
PM2.5	0.171 ***	0.205 **	0.197 **	0.110
	(0.000)	(0.017)	(0.025)	(0.233)
Precipitation	−19.14 ***	−14.128	−13.897	5.397
	(0.000)	(0.223)	(0.253)	(0.757)
Temperature	0.116	0.164	0.196	0.347
	(0.626)	(0.671)	(0.614)	(0.376)
ρ	-	0.078 ***	-	-
	-	(0.000)	-	-
λ	-	-	0.078 ***	0.076 ***
	-	-	(0.000)	(0.000)
Gym FEs	YES	YES	YES	YES
COVID-19 Wave FEs	YES	YES	YES	YES
Observations	12,260	12,260	12,260	12,260
Participant Number	2452	2452	2452	2452

Note: *** $p < 0.001$; ** $p < 0.05$.

In addition, the spatial autocorrelation coefficients ρ of both the SLM model and the SDM model and the spatial autoregressive coefficient λ of the error term in the SEM model were all significantly positive (0.078, 0.076 and 0.078), indicating that gyms with large gym visits could increase the number of exercisers of surrounding gyms and drive the development of the gym industry of Beijing, which was consistent with the previous analysis of the Moran's Index.

Compared with the SLM model and SEM model, we adopted the SDM model to carry out the following analysis due to LR test rejecting the null hypothesis, which showed that the SDM model was more reliable and stable. In order to analyze the spatial effect of each influencing factor more concretely, we decomposed the SDM model to obtain the direct effect (the influence of PM2.5 on local gyms), indirect effect (the impact of PM2.5 on other adjacent gyms), and total effect (the impact of PM2.5 on all gyms of Beijing). The specific results are listed in Table 8.

As shown in Table 8, the direct effect of PM2.5 was not significant, while the indirect and total effects of PM2.5 were both significantly positive. It was proven that every 1% increase in PM2.5 promoted an increase in gym visits at adjacent gyms by 0.394%, and an increase in gym visits in all of Beijing by 0.512%. This phenomenon could be explained because the air pollution had a spatial heterogeneity, that was to say, people with exposure to higher pollution concentrations would refuse to go outside for exercise, while people with relatively lower exposure to pollution nearby were more willing to travel to gyms. This phenomenon needs to be discussed in future studies.

Table 8. Direct effect, indirect effect and total effect of the SDM model.

Dependent Variable: Gym Comments under P1–P5	Direct	Indirect	Total
COVID-19	−0.024 ***	−0.003	−0.027 ***
	(0.006)	(0.788)	(0.001)
PM2.5	0.118	0.394 ***	0.512 ***
	(0.210)	(0.003)	(0.000)
Precipitation	4.025	−45.799 **	−41.773 ***
	(0.810)	(0.028)	(0.007)
Temperature	0.367	−1.412 *	-1.045
	(0.328)	(0.065)	(0.215)
Gym FEs	YES	YES	YES
COVID-19 Wave FEs	YES	YES	YES
Observations	12,260	12,260	12,260
Participant Number	2452	2452	2452

Note: *** $p < 0.001$; ** $p < 0.05$; * $p < 0.01$.

Furthermore, the direct effect and the total effect of COVID-19 on fitness were significantly negative, while the indirect effect was not significant. In reality, there was a negative impact on gym fitness for all people when the pandemic was severe enough.

4. Discussion

4.1. Discussion of Main Findings

Given the high level of air pollution in Beijing, China, its air pollution dynamics offered the opportunity to test how the demand for gym sports for this consumer city was affected by pollution in the context of the intertwined impact of air pollution and the COVID-19 pandemic.

Our study chose Beijing as the case to investigate how air pollution influenced people's demand for gym sports, focusing on the effect of PM2.5 on the frequency of traveling to gyms during the COVID-19 pandemic. Our OLS model results showed that PM2.5 was positively associated with gym visits, which was opposite of previous research studies showing that air pollution was negatively associated with both outdoor physical activity [51,52] and indoor leisure places such as restaurants and shopping areas [9,10]. Such a positive impact was larger when considering the influence of the COVID-19 pandemic. One reason to explain this result was that people could not wait to exercise and participate in recreational activities after the strict travel mandates of the COVID-19 pandemic [16,18]. Therefore, gym indoor physical activity gave them a chance to ignore the harmful effects of both air pollution and COVID-19 virus contact when exercising. We also observed that COVID-19 reduced the demand for gym sports, which was consistent with our expected results [24]. Whether the accelerating effect of the COVID-19 pandemic on the positive impact of air pollution on gym sports could trade off its own negative impact on gym sports or not still needs more research and exploration. Future research should explore the interweaving effects of the climate and social environment on people's sports behavior.

Furthermore, in the section about measuring PM2.5 concentrations in the P1–P5 periods under COVID-19, five LUR models were constructed to accurately evaluate the long-term exposure of gym crowds while traveling to the gym. Seasonality (i.e., spring, summer, autumn and winter) was not included as a variable in the analysis of this section because collinearity existed between season and ambient temperature after we controlled for seasonality in this study. In the following robust check, we replaced the PM2.5 data from the LUR models with that obtained through the Kriging interpolation method of the MEP PM2.5 monitoring sites and that from the US Embassy and Consulates [48]. When taken together, the reported positive effects of air pollution on gym visits derived from OLS models in our study may be pronounced and solid.

Lastly, our study employed spatial econometric models, including SLM, SEM and SDM to explore the spatial pattern of the gym visits in Beijing. We concluded that there was an obvious agglomeration phenomenon among the gym crowds, in other words, the increase in gym visits at local gyms would lead to an increase in gym visits at other nearby gyms, thereby making it possible to facilitate rapid development of the entire gym industry of Beijing. Furthermore, we used the SDM model to obtain the direct effect, indirect effect and total effect to verify the spatial spillover influence of PM2.5 on gym visits in Beijing under COVID-19. The results showed that PM2.5 had a positive spatial spillover effect on gyms visits of nearby gyms and on the all gyms in Beijing. COVID-19 was negatively associated with gyms visits of all gyms, which was consistent with the above OLS models.

4.2. Implications for Pollution Health and Gym Sports Research

To the best of our knowledge, the present study provides evidence of the relationship between air pollution and gym sports under COVID-19. Gyms, as a combination of sports and indoor leisure consumption activity, are becoming relatively safe and comfortable places for people to exercise and avoid pollution exposure. Furthermore, gym exercise played an important role in improving people's fitness and enriching their daily life under the rigorous pandemic prevention and control measures. This phenomenon offers us a new perspective that promoting gym use can produce considerable health benefits mainly from less outdoor pollution and from COVID-19 virus exposure, as well as from increased levels of physical activity.

Constructing more public indoor fitness facilities can be a good option to promote the vigorous development of mass sports. However, the local government and companies should consider the unintended impacts that constructing and operating new gyms may have on local air pollution, for example emissions from construction activities [53], onsite energy generators or increased demand for electricity from local power plants [54]. Furthermore, previous research has shown that people are more willing to pay for greenspace under air pollution [55]. It is essential to ensure that enough greenspace is provided in indoor fitness facilities to prevent each individual from pollution exposure and to create a comfortable and fresh exercise environment, which are beneficial for human mental health [56].

Taking into account the situation of the COVID-19 pandemic and its prevention, the government also needs to guarantee enough personal exercise space and avoid dangerous problems caused by big occupancy on the basis of increasing indoor gym infrastructure. For the issue of charging for private or public gyms, the government should improve the free or low-cost opening subsidy policy for public sports facilities and promote the opening of facilities to all groups of people.

Therefore, the local government should encourage gym sports and promote the benefits of indoor fitness after the comprehensive consideration of the impact of various influencing factors on people's indoor fitness, especially under the COVID-19 pandemic. As a result, more and more citizens are aware of the importance of physical activity under the intertwined influences of both the pandemic and air pollution, which will continuously improve the participation rate of national fitness in the future.

4.3. Research Limitations and Future Research Agenda

Our study has important limitations. First, given the high level of air pollution in Beijing, China, our data come from 2452 gyms in Beijing, which may lead to possible selection bias, and we need to be careful in generalizing this bias to other contexts. Further research in other cities and countries is needed to cross-validate the external validity of our quantitative findings. Second, we consider PM2.5 as the main source of pollutants in this study, ignoring other urban pollutants, such as PM_{10}, NO_2 and SO_2 [57]. Third, we used PM2.5 generated from LUR models under five COVID-19 periods to represent the pollution exposure concentration of gym crowds. However, this lacks measurements of the specific time of their gym visits and their personalized pollution exposure risk from different commutes to the gym, which are expected to be resolved in follow-up research. Finally, it is unclear whether exercise in a gym produce similar health benefits as outdoor sports. We need to consider multifaceted environmental attributes to possibly exert the health effects at different spatial scales of gyms, which requires further research.

5. Conclusions

Using big gym datasets of Beijing in 2019–2020, we documented that air pollution had a positive impact on residents' gym visits (proxied by gym reviews on "Meituan.com") under COVID-19. Such a positive impact was larger when considering the influence of the COVID-19 pandemic. From the perspective of space analysis, PM2.5 had a positive spatial spillover effect on the development of the whole gym industry in Beijing under COVID-19.

Overall, this study offers us a new perspective that gym sports can be developed into an essential activity for the public due to the avoidance of COVID-19 virus contact and pollution exposure. Furthermore, this study may provide useful information for a number of relevant stakeholders and policymakers and may be informative for city and gym infrastructure planning that aims to promote better public health outcomes.

In the future, we need to consider the health hazards caused by large gatherings of gym crowds and make some reasonable suggestions about gym management, for example, making sure there are enough greenhouses in gyms and increasing gym facilities on the basis of causing as little air pollution as possible and ensuring enough personal exercise space under a pandemic prevention environment. In addition, due to the lack of direct evidence on people's movement, we had to use online consumption data to replace the original activity track data. In follow-up research, we need to measure personalized exposure pollution, such as different levels of air pollution exposure by different commutes to gyms and real-time indoor pollution concentration of indoor gyms.

Author Contributions: Conceptualization, X.D. and C.Z.; methodology, X.D.; software, X.D.; validation, X.D., S.Y. and C.Z.; formal analysis, X.D.; investigation, X.D.; resources, S.Y. and C.Z.; data curation, X.D. and S.Y.; writing—original draft preparation, X.D.; writing—review and editing, X.D., S.Y. and C.Z.; visualization, X.D.; supervision, S.Y. and C.Z.; project administration, C.Z.; funding acquisition, S.Y. All authors have read and agreed to the published version of the manuscript.

Funding: This study was funded by National Natural Science Foundation of China (grant no. 42075044).

Institutional Review Board Statement: Not applicable.

Informed Consent Statement: Not applicable.

Data Availability Statement: The data that support the findings of this study are available from the corresponding author upon reasonable request.

Acknowledgments: We thank Beijing Meteorological Informational Center for help with meteorological data from Beijing Meteorological Monitoring Stations.

Conflicts of Interest: The authors declare no conflict of interest.

References

1. Zheng, S.; Kahn, M.E. Understanding China's urban pollution dynamics. *J. Econ. Abstr.* **2013**, *51*, 731–772. [CrossRef]
2. Xu, B.; Lin, B. Regional differences of pollution emissions in China: Contributing factors and mitigation strategies. *J. Clean. Prod.* **2016**, *112*, 1454–1463. [CrossRef]
3. Graff-Zivin, J.; Neidell, M. Environment, health, and human capital. *J. Econ. Lit.* **2013**, *51*, 689–730. [CrossRef]
4. Li, L.; Yang, J.; Song, Y.F.; Chen, P.Y.; Ou, C.Q. The burden of COPD mortality due to ambient air pollution in Guangzhou, China. *Sci. Rep.* **2016**, *6*, 25900. [CrossRef]
5. Ebenstein, A.; Fan, M.; Greenstone, M.; He, G.; Zhou, M. New evidence on the impact of sustained exposure to air pollution on life expectancy from China's Huai River Policy. *Proc. Natl. Acad. Sci. USA* **2017**, *114*, 10384–10389. [CrossRef]
6. Zheng, S.; Wang, J.; Sun, C.; Zhang, X.; Kahn, M.E. Air pollution lowers Chinese urbanites' expressed happiness on social media. *Nat. Hum. Behav.* **2019**, *3*, 237–243. [CrossRef]
7. Graff-Zivin, J.; Neidell, M. Days of haze: Environmental information disclosure and intertemporal avoidance behavior. *J. Environ. Econ. Manag.* **2009**, *58*, 119–128. [CrossRef]
8. Neidell, M. Information, avoidance behavior, and health the effect of ozone on asthma hospitalizations. *J. Hum. Resour.* **2009**, *44*, 450–478. [CrossRef]

9. Sun, C.; Zheng, S.; Wang, J.; Kahn, M.E. Does Clean air increase the demand for the consumer city? Evidence from Beijing. *J. Reg. Sci.* **2019**, *59*, 184. [CrossRef]
10. He, X.; Luo, Z.; Zhang, J. The impact of air pollution on movie theater admissions. *J. Environ. Econ. Manag.* **2022**, *112*, 102626. [CrossRef]
11. Chen, C.M.; Lin, Y.L.; Hsu, C.L. Does air pollution drive away tourists? A case study of the sun moon lake national scenic area, Taiwan. *Transp. Res. Part D Transp. Environ.* **2017**, *53*, 398–402. [CrossRef]
12. Andrade, A.; Dominski, F.; Bio, H.; Coimbra, D.R. Scientific production on indoor air quality of environments used for physical exercise and sport practice: Bibliometric analysis. *J. Environ. Manag.* **2017**, *196*, 188–200. [CrossRef] [PubMed]
13. Slezakova, K.; Peixoto, C.; Oliveira, M.; Delerue-Matos, C.; Pereira, M.D.C.; Morais, S. Indoor particulate pollution in fitness centres with emphasis on ultrafine particles. *Environ. Pollut.* **2018**, *233*, 180–193. [CrossRef] [PubMed]
14. Salonen, H.; Salthammer, T.; Morawska, L. Human exposure to air contaminants in sport environments. *Indoor Air* **2020**, *30*, 1109–1129. [CrossRef]
15. Kummitha, R.K.R. Smart technologies for fighting Pandemics: The techno and human driven approaches in controlling the virus transmission. *Gov. Inf. Q.* **2020**, *37*, 101481. [CrossRef]
16. De Vos, J. The effect of COVID-19 and subsequent social distancing on travel behavior. *Transp. Res. Interdiscip. Perspect.* **2020**, *5*, 100121. [CrossRef]
17. Jiang, L.; Wang, B.; Qu, T.; Liao, J. Thirty Provinces Activated First-Level Public Health Emergency Response. Xinhua News. Available online: http://www.xinhuanet.com/politics/2020-01/25/c_1125502232.htm (accessed on 25 January 2020).
18. Tian, H.; Liu, Y.; Li, Y.; Wu, C.; Chen, B.; Kraemer, M.U.G.; Li, B.; Cai, J.; Xu, B.; Yang, Q.; et al. An investigation of transmission control measures during the first 50 days of the COVID-19 epidemic in China. *Science* **2020**, *368*, 638–642. [CrossRef]
19. Li, T.; Rong, L.; Zhang, A. Assessing regional risk of COVID-19 infection from Wuhan via high-speed rail. *Transp. Policy* **2021**, *106*, 226–238. [CrossRef]
20. Zhu, P.; Guo, Y. The Role of High-speed Rail and Air Travel in the Spread of COVID-19 in China. *Travel Med. Infect. Dis.* **2021**, *42*, 102097. [CrossRef]
21. Kapser, S.; Abdelrahman, M.; Bernecker, T. Autonomous delivery vehicles to fight the spread of COVID-19—How do men and women differ in their acceptance? *Transp. Res. Part A Policy Pract.* **2021**, *148*, 183–198. [CrossRef]
22. Guo, Y.; Liao, M.; Cai, W.; Yu, X.; Li, S.; Ke, X.; Tan, S.; Luo, Z.; Cui, Y.; Wang, Q.; et al. Physical activity, screen exposure and sleep among students during the pandemic of COVID-19. *Sci. Rep.* **2021**, *11*, 8529. [CrossRef] [PubMed]
23. Raiola, G.; Domenico, F.D. Physical and sports activity during the COVID-19 pandemic. *J. Phys. Educ. Sport* **2021**, *21*, 477–482. [CrossRef]
24. Levy, J.J.; Tarver, T.L.; Douglas, H.R. Examining the impact of gym closures due to the COVID-19 pandemic on combat sport athletes' mental health. *J. Clin. Sport Psychol.* **2021**, *15*, 289–305. [CrossRef]
25. Shen, H.; Shen, G.; Chen, Y.; Russell, A.G.; Hu, Y.; Duan, X.; Meng, W.; Xu, Y.; Yun, X.; Lyu, B.; et al. Increased air pollution exposure among the Chinese population during the national quarantine in 2020. *Nat. Hum. Behav.* **2021**, *5*, 239–246. [CrossRef] [PubMed]
26. Tian, J.; Wang, Q.; Zhang, Y.; Yan, M.; Liu, H.; Zhang, N.; Ran, W.; Cao, J. Impacts of primary emissions and secondary aerosol formation on air pollution in an urban area of China during the COVID-19 lockdown. *Environ. Int.* **2021**, *150*, 106426. [CrossRef]
27. Blocken, B.; Druenen, T.; Ricci, A.; Kang, L.; Hooff, T.; Qin, P.; Xia, L.; Ruiz, C.A.; Arts, J.H.; Diepens, J.F.L.; et al. Ventilation and air cleaning to limit aerosol particle concentrations in a gym during the COVID-19 pandemic. *Build. Environ.* **2021**, *193*, 107659. [CrossRef]
28. Kahn, M.E.; Zheng, S. Blue skies over Beijing: Economic growth and the environment in China. *J. Chin. Political Sci.* **2016**, *23*, 141–142. [CrossRef]
29. Wei, X.; Chen, Y.; An, J.; Xu, X.; Yu, S.; Xu, C.; Yu, H.; Li, A. *2020 China Fitness Industry Statistics Report*; SAAS Data Center: Shanghai, China, 2020; pp. 17–27.
30. Briggs, D.J.; Susan Collins, S.; Elliott, P.; Fisher, P.; Kingham, S.; Lebret, E.; Pryl, K.; Hans Van Reeuwijk, H.V.; Smallbone, K.; Veen, A.V.D. Mapping urban air pollution using GIS: A regression-based approach. *Int. J. Geogr. Inf. Sci.* **1997**, *11*, 699–718. [CrossRef]
31. Shi, T.; Hu, Y.; Liu, M.; Li, C.; Zhang, C.; Liu, C. Land use regression modelling of PM2.5 spatial variations in different seasons in urban areas. *Sci. Total Environ.* **2020**, *743*, 140744. [CrossRef]
32. Yuan, Q.; Qi, B.; Hu, D.; Wang, J.; Zhang, J.; Yang, H.; Zhang, S.; Liu, L.; Xu, L.; Li, W. Spatiotemporal variations and reduction of air pollutants during the COVID-19 pandemic in a megacity of Yangtze River Delta in China. *Sci. Total Environ.* **2021**, *751*, 14182. [CrossRef]
33. Agarwal, S.; Jensen, J.B.; Monte, F. *Consumer Mobility and the Local Structure of Consumption Industries*; NBER Working Paper No. 23616; National Bureau of Economic Research: Cambridge, MA, USA, 2017. [CrossRef]
34. Beijing Air Quality of Beijing Municipal Environmental Monitoring Center (BMEMC), China. Available online: http://zx.bjmemc.com.cn/ (accessed on 3 August 2021).
35. *GB 3095-2012*; Ambient Air Quality Standards. China Environmental Science Press: Beijing, China, 2012.
36. Tai, A.P.K.; Mickley, L.J.; Jacob, D.J. Correlations between fine particulate matter (PM2.5) and meteorological variables in the United States: Implications for the sensitivity of PM2.5 to climate change. *Atmos. Environ.* **2010**, *44*, 3976–3984. [CrossRef]

37. Nyhan, M.M.; Kloog, I.; Britter, R.; Ratti, C.; Koutrakis, P. Quantifying population exposure to air pollution using individual mobility patterns inferred from mobile phone data. *J. Expo. Sci. Environ. Epidemiol.* **2019**, *29*, 238–247. [CrossRef] [PubMed]
38. Zhang, Y.; Cheng, H.; Huang, D.; Fu, C. High Temporal Resolution Land Use Regression Models with POI Characteristics of the PM2.5 Distribution in Beijing, China. *Int. J. Environ. Res. Public Health* **2020**, *18*, 6143. [CrossRef]
39. Columbia University (CU). Socio-Economic Data and Applications Center. Available online: http://beta.sedac.ciesin.columbia.edu/ (accessed on 5 August 2021).
40. Lyapustin, A.; Wang, Y. MCD19A2 MODIS/Terra+Aqua Land Aerosol Optical Depth Daily L2G Global 1 km SIN Grid V006. NASA EOSDIS Land Processes DAAC. Available online: https://lpdaac.usgs.gov/products/mcd19a2v006/ (accessed on 12 May 2021).
41. Wei, J.; Li, Z.; Cribb, M.; Huang, W.; Xue, W. Improved 1 km resolution PM2.5 estimates across China using enhanced space-time extremely randomized trees. *Atmos. Chem. Phys.* **2020**, *20*, 3273–3289. [CrossRef]
42. Wei, J.; Li, Z.; Lyapustin, A.; Peng, Y.; Xue, W.; Su, T.; Cribb, M. Reconstructing 1-km-resolution high-quality PM2.5 data records from 2000 to 2018 in China: Spatiotemporal variations and policy implications. *Remote Sens. Environ.* **2021**, *252*, 112136. [CrossRef]
43. Dee, D.P.; Uppala, S.M.; Simmons, A.J.; Berrisford, P.; Poli, P.; Kobayashi, S.; Andrae, U.; Balmaseda, M.A.; Balsamo, G.; Bauer, P.; et al. The ERA-Interim reanalysis: Configuration and performance of the data assimilation system. *Q. J. R. Meteorol. Soc.* **2011**, *137*, 553–597. [CrossRef]
44. Lyapustin, A.; Wang, Y.; Laszlo, I.; Kahn, R.; Korkin, S.; Remer, L.; Levy, R.; Reid, J.S. Multiangle implementation of atmospheric correction (MAIAC): 2. Aerosol algorithm. *J. Geophys. Res. Atmos.* **2011**, *116*, D03211. [CrossRef]
45. Hoek, G.; Beelen, R.; Hoogh, K.D.; Vienneau, D.; Gulliver, J.; Fischer, P.; Briggset, D. A review of land-use regression models to assess spatial variation of outdoor air pollution. *Atmos. Environ.* **2008**, *42*, 7561–7578. [CrossRef]
46. Henderson, S.B.; Beckerman, B.; Jerrett, M.; Brauer, M. Application of land use regression to estimate long-term concentrations of traffic-related nitrogen oxides and fine particulate matter. *Environ. Sci. Technol.* **2007**, *41*, 2422–2428. [CrossRef]
47. Ryan, P.H.; LeMasters, G.K. A review of land-use regression models for characterizing Intraurban air pollution exposure. *Inhal. Toxicol.* **2007**, *19*, 127–133. [CrossRef]
48. Sellier, Y.; Galineau, J.; Hulin, A.; Caini, F.; Marquis, N.; Navel, V.; Bottagisi, S.; Giorgis-Allemand, L.; Jacquier, C.; Slama, R.; et al. Health effects of ambient air pollution: Do different methods for estimating exposure lead to different results? *Environ. Int.* **2014**, *66*, 165–173. [CrossRef] [PubMed]
49. Bohórquez, I.A.; Ceballos, H.V. Algunos conceptos de la econometría espacial y el análisis exploratorio de datos espaciales. *Ecos. Econ. Lat. Am. J. Appl. Econ.* **2008**, *12*, 9–12.
50. Anselin, L. Spatial Effects in Econometric Practice in Environmental and Resource Economics. *Am. J. Agric. Econ.* **2001**, *83*, 705–710. [CrossRef]
51. Tainio, M.; Jovanovic Andersen, Z.; Nieuwenhuijsen, M.J.; Hu, L.; de Nazelle, A.; An, R.; Garcia, L.M.T.; Goenka, S.; Zapata-Diomedi, B.; Bull, F.; et al. Air pollution, physical activity and health: A mapping review of the evidence. *Env. Int.* **2021**, *147*, 105954. [CrossRef] [PubMed]
52. Yu, H.; Yu, M.; Gordon, S.P.; Zhang, R. The association between ambient fine particulate air pollution and physical activity: A cohort study of university students living in Beijing. *Int. J. Behav. Nutr. Phys. Act.* **2017**, *14*, 136. [CrossRef]
53. Xue, Y.; Liu, X.; Cui, Y.; Shen, Y.; Wu, T.; Wu, B.; Yang, X. Characterization of air pollutant emissions from construction machinery in Beijing and evaluation of the effectiveness of control measures based on information code registration data. *Chemosphere* **2022**, *103*, 135064. [CrossRef]
54. Jiang, P.; Khishgee, S.; Alimujiang, A.; Dong, H. Cost-effective approaches for reducing carbon and air pollution emissions in the power industry in China. *J. Environ. Manag.* **2020**, *264*, 110452. [CrossRef]
55. Liu, Z.; Hanley, N.; Campbell, D. Linking urban air pollution with residents' willingness to pay for greenspace: A choice experiment study in Beijing. *J. Environ. Econ. Manag.* **2020**, *104*, 102383. [CrossRef]
56. Boudier, A.; Iana Markevych, I.; Jacquemin, B.; Abramson, M.J.; Accordini, S.; Forsberg, B.; Elaine Fuertes, E.; Garcia-Aymerich, J.; Joachim Heinrich, J.; Johannessen, A.; et al. Long-term air pollution exposure, greenspace and health-related quality of life in the ECRHS study. *Sci. Total Environ.* **2022**, *849*, 157693. [CrossRef]
57. Shen, F.; Zhang, L.; Jiang, L.; Tang, M.; Gai, X.; Chen, M.; Ge, X. Temporal variations of six ambient criteria air pollutants from 2015 to 2018, their spatial distributions, health risks and relationships with socioeconomic factors during 2018 in China. *Environ. Int.* **2020**, *137*, 105556. [CrossRef]

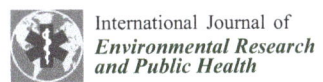

Article

Variation in Public Trust, Perceived Societal Fairness, and Well-Being before and after COVID-19 Onset—Evidence from the China Family Panel Studies

Chunli Wei [1,2], Qingqing Li [3], Ziyi Lian [4], Yijun Luo [4], Shiqing Song [5] and Hong Chen [4,6,7,*]

1. Center for Studies of Education and Psychology of Ethnic Minorities in Southwest China, Southwest University, Chongqing 400715, China
2. Psychological Development Guidance Center, Guangxi University, Nanning 530004, China
3. School of Psychology, Central China Normal University, Wuhan 430079, China
4. Faculty of Psychology, Southwest University, Chongqing 400715, China
5. School of Psychology, Shaanxi Normal University, Xi'an 710062, China
6. Key Laboratory of Cognition and Personality of Ministry of Education, Southwest University, Chongqing 400715, China
7. Chongqing Key Research Bases in Humanities and Social Sciences, Chongqing 400715, China
* Correspondence: chenhg@swu.edu.cn; Tel.: +86-23-6836-7975

Abstract: The sudden onset of the COVID-19 pandemic had a significant impact on all aspects of people's lives, including their attitudes toward society and psychological well-being. This study aimed to analyze the variation in public trust, perceived societal fairness, and well-being before and after the outbreak of the coronavirus disease 2019 (COVID-19). This study used two-wave longitudinal data of 15,487 residents (2018, T1; 2020, T2) derived from the Chinese Family Panel Studies (CFPS). A repeated measures analysis of variance showed that (a) public trust, perceived societal fairness, and subjective well-being significantly improved and (b) depression significantly increased. Linear regression analysis showed that education and socioeconomic status had a significant predictive effect on public trust, perceived societal fairness, and depression; socioeconomic status had a significant predictive effect on subjective well-being. This study provides evidence and direction for current social governance, namely, policy implementation and pandemic response.

Keywords: COVID-19; public trust; perceived societal fairness; mental health

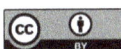

1. Introduction

The sudden onset of the COVID-19 pandemic has had a major impact on economic activities and social functioning. Several pandemic prevention and control measures have been implemented such as halting certain work operations, enforcing home quarantine, as well as travel restrictions. However, these measures have had a significant impact on all aspects of people's lives, including their attitudes toward society and psychological well-being [1–3]. Public trust and perceived societal fairness form the foundation of attitudes toward society and play a pivotal role in mental health, human survival, and development [4,5]. Depression and subjective well-being are a direct reflection of an individual's mental health, especially during the COVID-19 crisis. Therefore, public trust, perceived societal fairness, depression, and subjective well-being have been described to function as a social "barometer", which provides tools and indicators for analyzing and measuring the trend of social development, contributing significantly to policy implementation, exploring social operation mechanisms, grasping social thought dynamics, and promoting long-term social governance [6].

To assess the variation in public trust, perceived societal fairness, and well-being before and after the COVID-19 onset, this study used two-wave longitudinal data of 15,487 residents (2018, T1; 2020, T2) derived from the Chinese Family Panel Studies (CFPS).

Comparing the responses of those who completed the CFPS from June 2018 to March 2019, (prior to the pandemic) to those who completed the CFPS from July 2020 to December 2020 offered the setting for a natural experiment to compare how participants' perceptions of the country, the government, and their lives changed after COVID-19 began. Most relevant studies conducted in China have been cross-sectional, and thus do not highlight the changes in public trust, perceived societal fairness, and well-being [3,7–10]. This study aimed to explore the changes in public trust, perceived societal fairness, and well-being, and verify the predictive role of education and socioeconomic status during the COVID-19 crisis. Furthermore, this study provides a basis and direction for current social governance, such as the implementation of policies and laws, as well as pandemic response.

1.1. Public Trust and Perceived Societal Fairness

Trust is a psychological state of willingness to take risks based on positive expectations of external intentions or behaviors [11]. The COVID-19 pandemic has highlighted the vital role that trust plays in producing and maintaining compliance with public health instructions during times of crisis [12]. It has emphasized the several varieties of trust that influence behavior when public health is at risk. People are expected to trust public health professionals to identify hazards to the public's health with accuracy and to suggest appropriate mitigation measures. They are expected to trust officials to faithfully and rapidly implement those policies. Specifically, citizens and communities need to trust and adhere to advice from government officials and doctors. Recent studies indicate that trust in government and public health guidelines have a close relationship [13–16]. Local government officials may communicate information to ensure that citizens are aware of new public health regulations [12]. Furthermore, during the pandemic, because the effort to increase public awareness has the effect of reducing negative emotions and engaging in rescue activities, interpersonal trust is an invisible force that reduces social dangers [17]. In order to deal with COVID-19, many people are required to work with strangers. These acts come at a cost to the individual (e.g., social isolation), but are beneficial to the group as a whole (e.g., safeguarding vulnerable groups; i.e., a societal conundrum) [18]. A recent study revealed that educating individuals about the dangers the pandemic poses to their health significantly increased their trust in strangers [19].

The pandemic can influence individual trust in the government, doctors, and strangers [20]. A study found that trust in the government among Chinese residents was at an overall high level during the COVID-19 pandemic [21], as individuals were required to trust and comply with the recommendations provided by government officials and doctors to mitigate the pandemic. Trust in institutions may be enhanced instinctively among individuals in the context of a common external threat owing to limitations imposed on choices [22]. In accordance with the source model of group threat, perceptions of intergroup threat will strengthen (in)group identification processes and relations because the perceived source of a threat is crucial in forecasting its repercussions [23]. According to the source model of group threat, groups such as nations confronting external threats react by strengthening their intragroup connections [23]. Particularly, the emotional connections of individuals are strengthened through both location and national identity, developing a strong sense of community [23,24]. Thus, public trust increases after natural disasters, possibly as a result of the need for everyone to work collaboratively to overcome the tragedy [25]. Based on research conducted in the United States during the H1N1 epidemic, individuals exhibited substantial trust in public health officials [26]. Furthermore, longitudinal data analyzed in Switzerland showed that individuals initially had high levels of trust in government and public health officials. However, that trust gradually declined as the H1N1 pandemic progressed [27].

In the present study, several indices of public trust relevant to the COVID-19 pandemic were included: trust in local government officials, doctors, and strangers [12,18,19]. Local government officials and doctors are cooperating to initiate response and communicate the corresponding reasons to the public [12]. Trust and cooperation among strangers may be the key to understanding how societies are dealing with the COVID-19 pandemic [18]. These indicators cannot cover all aspects of public trust, but are representative, and the content and orientations involved are the focal issues deeply felt by the general public in a sudden pandemic [6]. Most research demonstrates that being exposed to natural disasters like earthquakes, typhoons, and volcanic eruptions strengthens relationships of trust and collaboration [25,28–31]. We, therefore, assumed that trust in local government officials, doctors, and strangers would increase after the outbreak.

Perceived societal fairness was also considered. Perceived societal fairness is the ability of an individual to perceive and judge the extent of social fairness and includes three types, namely, distributive, procedural, and interactional fairness [32,33]. An imbalance in perceived societal fairness can lead to the accentuation of social conflicts and contradictions, affecting social harmony and stability [34–36]. Maintaining societal cohesion by dealing with injustices would be critical in improving well-being post-pandemic [37]. The Chinese government adopted three measures, including increasing the construction of the public health system, improving the capacity of large-scale nucleic acid testing, and fully covering the cost of treating patients with coronary pneumonia, in order to maintain social harmony and stability [38]. Therefore, it was assumed that residents would experience more perceived societal fairness. Coordinated efforts among individuals, communities, and governments to combat a pandemic indicate a strong signal of cooperation, facilitating the reorganization of external and internal groups into communities of purpose. Moreover, the renewed social identity can help to coordinate and manage responses to threats while promoting adherence to commitments and norms among group members, thus facilitating national leadership behaviors [20]. An individual sense of common fate, which involves identification and positive feelings about the nation, may have also increased with the COVID-19 outbreak [23,24]. Similarly, patriotism and identification with fellow citizens increased among Americans following the 9/11 incident [39]. Thus, social identity during the COVID-19 pandemic can enhance group relations and enhance perceived societal fairness [37].

1.2. Depression and Subjective Well-Being

People's mental health is likely to be impacted by the lived experience of witnessing the pandemic unfold, in addition to the social isolation and financial uncertainty brought on by the pandemic [22]. Relevant studies demonstrate that experiencing widespread calamities (e.g., natural disasters and war) instantly puts people's mental health at risk [40,41]. First, anxiety, panic, depression, and other negative emotions may be exacerbated among individuals during the pandemic, as well as profound changes to their mental health [42,43]. Furthermore, studies found that people experienced relatively high levels of anxiety and depression after the outbreak [7,8], which is consistent with the findings underscoring high levels of fear and anxiety following the global SARS outbreak in 2003 [44,45]. Second, pandemics are considered a social threat as they reduce offline interpersonal and social contact, which undermines the subjective well-being of individuals [46], causing a specific decline in life satisfaction, future confidence, and interpersonal relationships. However, social threats also provide opportunities to enhance social cohesion and bonding [40,47], which can mitigate the negative effects of the pandemic.

To assess pre- and post-pandemic mental health, we took depression and subjective well-being as the mental health index, which reflect people's psychological state from different aspects [48]. Subjective well-being refers to the overall judgment of an individual's life state based on personal criteria. Furthermore, it provides a subjective, holistic, and relatively stable perspective, serving as a comprehensive psychological indicator outlining the quality of an individual's life [49,50]. Moreover, subjective well-being emphasizes a comprehensive subjective evaluation that includes pleasurable experiences of the individual's body and mind, emotional feelings, and satisfaction. Furthermore, two indicators of subjective well-being were examined [22,51,52]: satisfaction with life and personal well-being (future security, personal relationships, and impact of happy event). Diener et al. [51] proposed that subjective well-being includes an indicator of life satisfaction. Moreover, Cummins et al. [52] proposed a Theory of Subjective Wellbeing Homeostasis, which proposes that subjective well-being includes indicators of personal well-being, involving satisfaction with standard of living, future security, personal relationships, impact of happy/sad event, and health. Therefore, this study used life satisfaction, future confidence, interpersonal relationships, and experience of happiness to measure subjective well-being. The outbreak of the COVID-19 pandemic is likely to lead to changes in the mental health of residents. Therefore, we assumed that increased depression would be associated with decreased subjective well-being after the outbreak of COVID-19.

1.3. Education and Socioeconomic Status

Education is associated with public trust, perceived societal fairness, and depression. A recent study found that a higher level of education is associated with higher government trust during COVID-19 [53]. Furthermore, education has a profound impact on shaping the public's perceived societal fairness [54]. A follow-up study found that education had a protective effect against an increase in depressive symptoms [55]. Socioeconomic status is a social classification that reflects an individual's position in the social hierarchy, which comprises subjectively perceived social status and objective material resources measured by income, education level, and occupational status [56,57]. Socioeconomic status has an impact on all parts of an individual's life [58], including public trust, perceived societal fairness, and well-being. The positive predictive effect of socioeconomic status on interpersonal trust has been confirmed by many cross-cultural studies [59]. Moreover, socioeconomic status affects individuals' perceived societal fairness [60]. Some research indicated that individuals with a higher socio-economic status had greater advantages in personal health [61,62]. Evidence-based studies have shown that those with a lower socioeconomic status experienced higher rates of depressive symptoms [63], and had lower satisfaction with life [64]. In response to the COVID-19 crisis, we envision to verify the predictive role of education and socioeconomic status based on these studies.

2. Materials and Methods

2.1. Data and Study Population

The data were derived from the China Family Panel Studies (CFPS), which is a project financed by Peking University and the National Natural Science Foundation of China. The CFPS was first conducted in 2010 by its affiliate, the Institute of Social Science Survey, with a goal sample size of 16,000 homes. Furthermore, the CFPS is a multidisciplinary, national, large-scale social tracking survey including 25 autonomous regions [65]. This study linked a sample of 37,354 data points from Wave 4 of the survey, which was from June 2018 to March 2019 (hereafter referred to as T1 or 2018) with 28,590 data points from Wave 5 of the survey, which was from July 2020 to December 2020 (hereafter referred to as T2 or 2020), and 15,487 valid questionnaires were finally collected. The 15,487 participants were the same in both waves. Data were screened according to the following conditions: (1) complete data were available for the fourth and fifth waves on the measures of public trust, perceived societal fairness, depression, and subjective well-being; and (2) samples with missing values for the variables in this study were excluded. Listwise deletion was used in all analyses owing to low levels of missing data (5% on any variable) [19]. Consequently, a total of 15,487 valid data points were obtained, which consisted of 7801 men, 7686 women, 8158 living in urban areas, and 7329 living in rural areas. Their ages ranged from 16 to 90 years old (M = 45.49 years, SD = 15.22) in the fourth wave of the survey and from 18 to 92 years old (M = 47.48 years, SD = 15.22) in the fifth wave of the survey. Education levels ranged from illiterate and semi-literate (2739), elementary (2882), middle school (4786), high school (2632), college (1310), bachelor's degree (1037), master's degree (96), to doctoral degree (5), with values from 1 to 8.

2.2. Measures

2.2.1. Public Trust and Perceived Societal Fairness

Participants were asked about their trust in local government officials, doctors, and strangers [12,18,19], which were scored between 0 and 10. The composite reliability coefficients were 0.77 at T1 and 0.76 at T2, which indicated acceptable reliability [66]. The factor analysis revealed that the inequality scale included two factors, one of which is five positive scoring questions and the other is three reverse scoring questions [67]. In this study, the five positively scored items, related to life during the pandemic, were used to measure individual perceptions of social justice, which were shown to be valid and reliable in previous studies [67,68]. Respondents indicate the extent of their agreement with the items using a five-point scale (strongly disagree, disagree, neither agree nor disagree, agree, and strongly agree). An example item is "There is equality in harmonious interpersonal relationships". Higher scores indicate a stronger sense of social justice [68,69]. In this study, the composite reliability coefficients were 0.76 at T1 and 0.76 at T2.

2.2.2. Depression and Subjective Well-Being

Measures included the eight-item Center for Epidemiologic Studies Depression Scale (CES-D) used to assess depressive symptoms. Participants were asked to rate the frequency of each symptom experienced throughout the previous week on a scale from 1 ("rarely or none of the time (<1 day)") to 4 ("most or all of the time (5–7 days)"). Furthermore, previous studies showed that the eight-item CES-D scale was a valid and reliable screening measure of depressive symptoms [48,70]. In this study, the Cronbach's alpha coefficients at T1 and T2 were 0.76 and 0.77, respectively; the composite reliability coefficients at T1 and T2 were 0.79 and 0.79, respectively. Participants' subjective well-being was also assessed, which included life satisfaction, future confidence, interpersonal relationships, and experience of happiness [22,51,52]. Consequently, four items were selected: "satisfaction with your life" (scored between 1 and 5), "confidence in your future" (scored between 1 and 5), "the quality of your relationships" (scored between 0 and 10), and "how happy are you" (scored between 0 and 10). In order to better reflect the meaning of subjective well-being, we transformed 0 points into 1 point for "the quality of your relationships" and "how happy are you", and performed a two-fold weighting for the points of "satisfaction with your life" and "confidence in your future". The composite reliability coefficients at T1 and T2 were 0.82 and 0.83, respectively.

2.2.3. Socioeconomic Status

Socioeconomic status was measured by two items "What is your personal income here?" and "What is your social status here?" [58]. Participants were asked about their current situation on a scale from 1 to 5 (1 = very low, 5 = very high). The two indicators were converted into standard scores according to Tan and Kraus [71] before being added. A higher level of socioeconomic status was reflected by higher scores. Socioeconomic status ranged from -1.96 to 1.89 (M = 0.00, SD = 0.88).

2.3. Data Analysis

SPSS software version 26 (IBM, Armonk, NY, USA) was used to manage and analyze the data. First, the existence of a common method bias was examined using Harman's single-factor test. Thereafter, a one-way repeated measures ANOVA was conducted to explore the variation in public trust, perceived societal fairness, and well-being before and after the COVID-19 outbreak. Finally, linear regression analysis was used to examine the predictive effects of education and socioeconomic status on public trust, perceived societal fairness, depression, and subjective well-being.

3. Results

Harman's single-factor test was used to assess the common method bias based on the self-reported data used. According to the exploratory factor analysis, the first factor accounted for 14.17%, which was 40% below the critical value [72], indicating that there was no significant common method bias in this study.

3.1. The One-Way Repeated Measures ANOVA of Public Trust and Perceived Societal Fairness

A one-way repeated measures ANOVA was conducted on public trust and perceived societal fairness, with gender, urban/rural, and age as covariates. The one-way repeated measures ANOVA results for public trust and perceived societal fairness are shown in Table 1. We chose η^2_p as the effect size for the ANOVA, which can respond to the size of the difference. Notably, the value of η^2_p is less than 0.04, which indicated a very small effect [73–75].

Table 1. Repeated measures ANOVA of public trust, perceived societal fairness, depression, and subjective well-being (the main effect of time).

Variables	T1 (M ± SD)	T2 (M ± SD)	F	p	η^2_p	90% CI [Lower, Upper]
Public trust	14.03 ± 5.27	15.17 ± 5.08	111.66	0.000	0.007	[0.005, 0.01]
Perceived societal fairness	19.07 ± 2.64	19.15 ± 2.56	4.50	0.034	0.000	[0.000, 0.001]
Depression	13.46 ± 3.85	13.55 ± 4.06	4.27	0.039	0.000	[0.000, 0.001]
Subjective well-being	30.95 ± 5.63	30.98 ± 5.65	14.87	0.000	0.001	[0.000, 0.002]

For public trust, the main effect of time was significant, $F(1, 15,483) = 111.66$, $p = 0.000$, $\eta^2_p = 0.007$, 90% confidence interval; CI [76]: [0.005, 0.01], and T2 was significantly higher than T1. In terms of societal fairness, the main effect of time was significant, $F(1, 15,483) = 4.50$, $p = 0.034$, $\eta^2_p = 0.000$, 90% CI: [0.000, 0.001], and T2 was significantly higher than T1.

3.2. The One-Way Repeated Measures ANOVA of Depression and Subjective Well-Being

A one-way repeated measures ANOVA was conducted on depression and subjective well-being, with gender, urban/rural, and age as covariates. The one-way repeated measures ANOVA results for depression and subjective well-being are shown in Table 1.

For depression, the main effect of time was significant, $F(1, 15,483) = 4.27$, $p = 0.039$, $\eta^2_p = 0.000$, 90% CI: [0.000, 0.001], and T2 was significantly higher than T1. With regard to subjective well-being, the main effect of time was significant, $F(1, 15,483) = 14.87$, $p = 0.000$, $\eta^2_p = 0.001$, 90% CI: [0.000, 0.002], and T2 was significantly higher than T1.

3.3. Linear Regression Analysis with Public Trust, Perceived Societal Fairness, Depression, and Subjective Well-Being as the Dependent Variables

Hierarchical multiple regression analysis was used to examine the predictive effects of education level and socioeconomic status on T2 public trust, with T1 public trust, gender, urban/rural, and age as control variables. We use the same approach to analyze perceived societal fairness, depression, and subjective well-being, with the dependent variable at T1, and gender, urban/rural, and age as control variables. As indicated in Table 2, results showed that education ($\beta = 0.17$, $p < 0.001$) and socioeconomic status ($\beta = 0.91$, $p < 0.001$) had a significant predictive effect on T2 public trust. As indicated in Table 3, the results showed that education ($\beta = -0.08$, $p < 0.001$) and socioeconomic status ($\beta = 0.48$, $p < 0.001$) had a significant predictive effect on T2 perceived societal fairness. As indicated in Table 4, the results showed that education ($\beta = -0.22$, $p < 0.001$) and socioeconomic status ($\beta = -0.45$, $p < 0.001$) had a significant predictive effect on T2 depression. As indicated in Table 5, the results showed that socioeconomic status ($\beta = 1.99$, $p < 0.001$) had a significant predictive effect on T2 subjective well-being.

Table 2. Public trust as the dependent variable.

Variables	First Level		Second Level	
	β	t	β	t
Constant	9.30 ***		9.47 ***	
T1 Public trust	0.45 ***	66.43	0.43 ***	61.92
Gender	0.27 ***	3.79	0.24 **	3.30
Urban/rural	0.01	0.18	0.02	0.20
Age	−0.01 ***	−5.69	−0.02 ***	−6.99
Education			0.17 ***	5.74
Socioeconomic status			0.91 ***	21.58
R^2	0.22		0.25	
ΔR^2	0.22 ***		0.02 ***	
F	1118.42 ***		849.82 ***	

Note: ** $p < 0.01$, *** $p < 0.001$.

Table 3. Perceived societal fairness as the dependent variable.

Variables	First Level		Second Level	
	β	t	β	t
Constant	13.11 ***		14.25 ***	
T1 Perceived societal fairness	0.31 ***	42.43	0.29 ***	39.00
Gender	0.22 ***	5.59	0.25 ***	6.61
Urban/rural	−0.31 ***	−8.00	−0.17 ***	−4.16
Age	0.00	1.95	−0.01 ***	−5.29
Education			−0.08 ***	−5.29
Socioeconomic status			0.48 ***	21.42
R^2	0.12		0.14	
ΔR^2	0.12 ***		0.03 ***	
F	509.15 ***		432.81 ***	

Note: *** $p < 0.001$.

Table 4. Depression as the dependent variable.

Variables	First Level		Second Level	
	β	t	β	t
Constant	7.26 ***		8.27 ***	
T1 Depression	0.50 ***	66.85	0.48 ***	63.66
Gender	−0.37 ***	−6.43	−0.32 ***	−5.64
Urban/rural	−0.42 ***	−7.32	−0.33 ***	−5.40
Age	−0.00	−0.32	−0.00	−1.69
Education			−0.22 ***	−9.28
Socioeconomic status			−0.45 ***	−13.37
R^2	0.24		0.25	
ΔR^2	0.24 ***		0.01 ***	
F	1216.65 ***		865.99 ***	

Note: *** $p < 0.001$.

Table 5. Subjective well-being as the dependent variable.

Variables	First Level		Second Level	
	β	t	β	t
Constant	13.54 ***		17.25 ***	
T1 Subjective well-being	0.52 ***	76.00	0.43 ***	63.74
Gender	0.11	1.48	0.12	1.58
Urban/rural	−0.32 ***	−4.18	0.02	0.21
Age	0.03 ***	11.95	0.01 *	2.17

Table 5. Cont.

Variables	First Level		Second Level	
	β	t	β	t
Education			0.02	0.61
Socioeconomic status			1.99 ***	44.71
R^2	0.28		0.37	
ΔR^2	0.28 ***		0.08 ***	
F	1532.81 ***		1487.42 ***	

Note: * $p < 0.05$, *** $p < 0.001$.

4. Discussion

Globally, countries are taking action against COVID-19. The present study analyzed the variation in public trust, perceived societal fairness, and well-being before and after the outbreak of the COVID-19 and verified the predictive role of education and socioeconomic status. In addition to theoretical and scientific implications, these findings provide valuable information to governments, which must rapidly develop and alter COVID-19 management plans, as well as to the global population, who are confronted with this dilemma [22].

4.1. Variation in Public Trust and Perceived Societal Fairness

The present study found that public trust and perceived societal fairness significantly improved, which was supported by previous studies [21,25,26]. Firstly, consistent with group threat theory that perceptions of intergroup threat will strengthen (in)group identification processes and relations, a significant increase in public trust was observed in this study because external threats motivate people to unite and trust each other [23]. Secondly, the bold and decisive actions of the Chinese government, including the shutdown of the economy, have the potential to unite people in the fight against the pandemic. A recent study indicated that individuals' trust is a critical factor at various stages of a complicated causal chain of pandemic response, such as diagnosis, regulation, promulgation, and enforcement [12]. Furthermore, public trust facilitates the implementation of pandemic prevention and control measures [20]. Studies have found that the implementation of official recommendations for preventive behaviors occurs most likely when trust in the government is high and negative feelings are low [77]. Several findings suggest that trust in local governments contributes to lower infection rates [78]. Similarly, a Dutch follow-up study found that pandemic lockdown measures increased residents' trust in the government and science [79]. Perceived societal fairness is related to the residents' social identities [37]. The COVID-19 pandemic outbreak has facilitated the international recognition and validation of China's rapid response, efficient strategy, and successful experience in mitigating the pandemic. Moreover, China's response to the outbreak has enhanced the pride of the nation. The Chinese government has created new norms within existing groups to address societal inequalities by prioritizing the safety and health of its people, thereby underscoring the concept of "life first, people first" [38]. Therefore, this may result in a very stable perceived societal fairness for residents.

4.2. Variation in Depression and Subjective Well-Being

The present study found that depression significantly increased among residents, which is supported by previous empirical studies [7,8]. Another surprising finding was that subjective well-being has also increased. Notably, both depression and subjective well-being had low effect sizes. First, this result may be related to the time period. In February 2020, the development trend of the pandemic was very alarming, with the most serious period in the Chinese mainland. During this stage, the negative impact of the pandemic was the most representative and intense. By April 2020, the Chinese government had curbed the development trend of the pandemic through a series of measures, with people in most areas gradually returning to work and school. As a result, the negative effects may have decreased. Data from the survey were collected from July to December

2020; therefore, individuals' depression and subjective well-being during this period did not change significantly [42]. Second, public trust may have contributed to the stability in mood (i.e., level of depressive symptoms) and subjective well-being. A large survey conducted across several countries, including China, found that social trust was positively associated with life satisfaction [80]. Furthermore, our study found that people's public trust and perceived societal fairness significantly improved, which may contribute to the stability in their mental health. Moreover, the improvement in subjective well-being may be impacted significantly by the positive effects of the increased public trust and perceived societal fairness. However, the adverse short-term effects of the pandemic on depression and subjective well-being were limited, which may partly be due to an increase in public trust and perceived societal fairness. Nevertheless, depressive symptoms increased after the pandemic, which is consistent with previous research showing that social threats have a negative effect on mental health [81,82]. Overall, the individuals showed resilience in mental health.

4.3. Predictive Role of Education and Socioeconomic Status

The present study verified the predictive role of education and socioeconomic status. Education and socio-economic status are important factors in determining public trust, perceived societal fairness, and well-being [83]. The subjective evaluation of the COVID-19 crisis responsiveness varies depending on the individual. To establish an opinion, one must have the ability and motivations to look for and analyze relevant information. Education is an essential source of information [53]. Socioeconomic status reflects an individual's objective social resources and subjective perceptions of social status [56,57]. It is thus crucial to develop measures that correspond to the educational and socioeconomic status of individuals. The predictive role of education and socioeconomic status contributes to understanding the factors of public trust, perceived societal fairness, and well-being in crisis management. Furthermore, offering insightful information about how individuals respond to government action may be helpful in future instances.

4.4. Limitations and Future Research Directions

This study used public trust, perceived societal fairness, and well-being data of 15,487 residents from 2018 (T1) to 2020 (T2) from the CFPS. Overall, the residents in this study showed resilience, which is consistent with previous findings. For example, Zhou [84] underscored that the improvement in psychosocial resilience is the future direction for the social mindset of Chinese people. However, this study has several limitations. First, the data from the CFPS conducted in 2018 and 2020 were secondary. As a result, it is possible that the variables chosen for measurement did not accurately capture the concept's meaning. Future research should employ specific subjective well-being and public trust research methods. Second, although we found a significant effect of public trust, perceived societal fairness, and well-being, the effect size was small. Future studies should concentrate on other variables that affect public trust and subjective well-being. The effects on public trust, perceived societal fairness, depression, and subjective well-being are ongoing as a result of economic, political, and social development, as well as the repeated adverse effects of the pandemic. Thus, future in-depth studies regarding this topic still need to be conducted.

First, the proportion of depressed people may increase with the recurrence of the pandemic imposed by the impact of various management policies on interpersonal socialization, such as pandemic prevention and control, and constraints on economic development [22]. Simultaneously, an immediate increase in public trust may decline over time. A follow-up study of the pandemic in Italy found that people's sense of social responsibility increased. However, trust in the government remained largely unchanged over time owing to the impact on economic development, while trust in science and health participation decreased [85].

Second, there should be an increased focus on the differences in the ability of various groups to cope with the pandemic, focusing on assessing protective and risk factors for different groups to cope with the pandemic. For example, groups lacking social support and pre-existing underlying problems that pose a greater risk during a pandemic should be included in future research [82,86]. Furthermore, combined stressors such as unemployment or relationship instability can exacerbate the impact of a pandemic [22]. Longitudinal studies conducted in the United States after 9/11 found that most people were resilient, despite a significant proportion who developed post-traumatic stress disorder [86]. Thus, future studies should prioritize exploring approaches to help different groups cope with a pandemic [20].

Finally, the results of this study highlight the need for a unified response to the pandemic amidst adversity and the importance of gaining social acceptance for pandemic control initiatives [20,87]. This study shows that the strong response to the pandemic in China could contribute significantly to the increased public trust among the population. Furthermore, China has always adhered to the concept of building a community of human purpose. Moreover, China has been responsible for life safety and physical health within its population, which has implications for global public health and has gained widespread acceptance, most likely increasing trust in the government among residents [38].

5. Conclusions

The current study analyzed the variation in public trust, perceived societal fairness, and well-being before and after the outbreak of COVID-19 based on two-wave longitudinal data of 15,487 residents (2018, T1; 2020, T2) derived from the CFPS. The results showed that public trust, perceived societal fairness, and subjective well-being significantly improved and depression significantly increased. Linear regression analysis showed that education and socioeconomic status had a significant predictive effect on public trust, perceived societal fairness, and depression; socioeconomic status had a significant predictive effect on subjective well-being. Thus, this research provides evidence and direction for current social governance, with implications for policy implementation and effective pandemic response methods.

Author Contributions: Conceptualization, C.W., Q.L. and S.S.; methodology, C.W. and Y.L.; data curation, C.W. and Z.L.; writing—original draft preparation, C.W.; writing—review and editing, C.W. and Q.L.; supervision, H.C.; project administration, H.C. All authors have read and agreed to the published version of the manuscript.

Funding: This research was funded by the National Nature Science Foundation of China (NO.32271087), Collaborative Innovation Team Project for Philosophy and Social Sciences in Chongqing Universities (NO.7110200530), and Key research topics on the theory and practice of ideological and political education for college students in Guangxi higher education institutions (NO.2020MSZ038).

Institutional Review Board Statement: Ethical review and approval were waived for this study due to publicly open data from the China Family Panel Survey.

Informed Consent Statement: All the participants in CFPS survey were required to sign an informed consent form (http://www.isss.pku.edu.cn/cfps/docs/20200615141215123435.pdf, accessed on 11 May 2021) before interview, and all the obtained information from participants was handled voluntarily, confidentially, and anonymously.

Data Availability Statement: Original data in this study are obtained from the Institute of Social Science Survey of Peking University and are available at http://www.isss.pku.edu.cn/cfps/index.htm (registration and approval needed, accessed on 8 January 2022).

Acknowledgments: We gratefully acknowledge Peking University for giving us the permission to use the data of the China Family Panel Studies conducted in 2018 and 2020.

Conflicts of Interest: The authors declare that they have no known competing financial interests or personal relationships that could have appeared to influence the work reported in this paper.

References

1. Wu, Z.; McGoogan, J.M. Characteristics of and Important Lessons from the Coronavirus Disease 2019 (COVID-19) Outbreak in China: Summary of a Report of 72 314 Cases from the Chinese Center for Disease Control and Prevention. *JAMA* **2020**, *323*, 1239–1242. [CrossRef] [PubMed]
2. Brooks, S.K.; Webster, R.K.; Smith, L.E.; Woodland, L.; Wessely, S.; Greenberg, N.; Rubin, G.J. The psychological impact of quarantine and how to reduce it: Rapid review of the evidence. *Lancet* **2020**, *395*, 912–920. [CrossRef]
3. Xiang, Y.-T.; Yang, Y.; Li, W.; Zhang, L.; Zhang, Q.; Cheung, T.; Ng, C.H. Timely mental health care for the 2019 novel coronavirus outbreak is urgently needed. *Lancet Psychiatry* **2020**, *7*, 228–229. [CrossRef]
4. Zhou, T.M.; Yin, G.E. Adolescent mental health diathesis: A study of mental health- related self development in Chinese adolescent. *Psychol. Res. Behav. Manag.* **2007**, *5*, 252–253.
5. Wu, J.; Wang, Y.; Chen, H.; Huang, J. From Self to Social Cognition: The Default Mode Network and Mirror-Neuron System. *Adv. Psychol. Sci.* **2015**, *23*, 1808. [CrossRef]
6. Li, L.L.; Wang, P. Changing Social Attitudes in China in Transition (2005–2015). *Soc. Sci. Chin.* **2018**, *3*, 83–101.
7. Qiu, J.; Shen, B.; Zhao, M.; Wang, Z.; Xie, B.; Xu, Y. A nationwide survey of psychological distress among Chinese people in the COVID-19 epidemic: Implications and policy recommendations. *Gen. Psychiatry* **2020**, *33*, e100213. [CrossRef]
8. Wang, C.; Pan, R.; Wan, X.; Tan, Y.; Xu, L.; Ho, C.S.; Ho, R.C. Immediate Psychological Responses and Associated Factors during the Initial Stage of the 2019 Coronavirus Disease (COVID-19) Epidemic among the General Population in China. *Int. J. Environ. Res. Public Health* **2020**, *17*, 1729. [CrossRef]
9. Xinhua News Agency. New Edelman Survey: China Government Trust Rating Rises to 95%. Available online: http://xhpfmapi.zhongguowangshi.com/vh512/share/9279491 (accessed on 27 July 2022).
10. Wang, J.X.; Chen, M.Q. *Blue Book of Social Mentality: Annual Report on Social Mentality of China (2020)*; Social Sciences Academic Press: Beijing, China, 2021.
11. Zhang, N.; Zhang, Y.Q.; Wu, K.K. Psychological and Neurophysiologic Mechanisms of Trust. *J. Psychol. Sci.* **2011**, *34*, 1137–1143. [CrossRef]
12. Blair, R.A.; Curtice, T.; Dow, D.; Grossman, G. Public trust, policing, and the COVID-19 pandemic: Evidence from an electoral authoritarian regime. *Soc. Sci. Med.* **2022**, *305*, 115045. [CrossRef]
13. Lalot, F.; Heering, M.S.; Rullo, M.; Travaglino, G.A.; Abrams, D. The dangers of distrustful complacency: Low concern and low political trust combine to undermine compliance with governmental restrictions in the emerging Covid-19 pandemic. *Group Process. Intergroup Relat.* **2022**, *25*, 106–121. [CrossRef]
14. Pagliaro, S.; Sacchi, S.; Pacilli, M.G.; Brambilla, M.; Lionetti, F.; Bettache, K.; Bianchi, M.; Biella, M.; Bonnot, V.; Boza, M.; et al. Trust predicts COVID-19 prescribed and discretionary behavioral intentions in 23 countries. *PLoS ONE* **2021**, *16*, e0248334. [CrossRef]
15. Brodeur, A.; Grigoryeva, I.; Kattan, L. Stay-at-home orders, social distancing, and trust. *J. Popul. Econ.* **2021**, *34*, 1321–1354. [CrossRef]
16. Oksanen, A.; Kaakinen, M.; Latikka, R.; Savolainen, I.; Savela, N.; Koivula, A. Regulation and Trust: 3-Month Follow-up Study on COVID-19 Mortality in 25 European Countries. *JMIR Public Health Surveill.* **2020**, *6*, e19218. [CrossRef]
17. Chan, R.K. Tackling COVID-19 risk in Hong Kong: Examining distrust, compliance and risk management. *Curr. Sociol.* **2021**, *69*, 547–565. [CrossRef]
18. Romano, A.; Spadaro, G.; Balliet, D.; Joireman, J.; Van Lissa, C.; Jin, S.; Agostini, M.; Bélanger, J.J.; Gützkow, B.; Kreienkamp, J.; et al. Cooperation and Trust Across Societies During the COVID-19 Pandemic. *J. Cross-Cultural Psychol.* **2021**, *52*, 622–642. [CrossRef]
19. Gambetta, D.; Morisi, D. COVID-19 infection induces higher trust in strangers. *Proc. Natl. Acad. Sci. USA* **2022**, *119*, e2116818119. [CrossRef]
20. Van Bavel, J.J.; Baicker, K.; Boggio, P.S.; Capraro, V.; Cichocka, A.; Cikara, M.; Crockett, M.J.; Crum, A.J.; Douglas, K.M.; Druckman, J.N.; et al. Using social and behavioural science to support COVID-19 pandemic response. *Nat. Hum. Behav.* **2020**, *4*, 460–471. [CrossRef]
21. Cao, N.M.; Sun, B.H.; Yue, G.A.; Li, W.J. Development Characteristics and Cause Analysed of People's Trust in Current Chinese Government from the Perspective of Social Psychology. *J. Southwest Univ.* **2022**, *2*, 184–191. [CrossRef]
22. Sibley, C.G.; Greaves, L.M.; Satherley, N.; Wilson, M.S.; Overall, N.C.; Lee, C.H.J.; Milojev, P.; Bulbulia, J.; Osborne, D.; Milfont, T.L.; et al. Effects of the COVID-19 pandemic and nationwide lockdown on trust, attitudes toward government, and well-being. *Am. Psychol.* **2020**, *75*, 618–630. [CrossRef]
23. Greenaway, K.H.; Cruwys, T. The source model of group threat: Responding to internal and external threats. *Am. Psychol.* **2019**, *74*, 218–231. [CrossRef] [PubMed]
24. Li, Q.; Brewer, M.B. What Does It Mean to Be an American? Patriotism, Nationalism, and American Identity After 9/11. *Politi-Psychol.* **2004**, *25*, 727–739. [CrossRef]
25. Toya, H.; Skidmore, M. Do Natural Disasters Enhance Societal Trust? *Kyklos* **2014**, *67*, 255–279. [CrossRef]

26. Quinn, S.C.; Parmer, J.; Freimuth, V.S.; Hilyard, K.M.; Musa, D.; Kim, K.H. Exploring Communication, Trust in Government, and Vaccination Intention Later in the 2009 H1N1 Pandemic: Results of a National Survey. *Biosecurity Bioterrorism* **2013**, *11*, 96–106. [CrossRef]
27. Ibuka, Y.; Chapman, G.B.; Meyers, L.A.; Li, M.; Galvani, A.P. The dynamics of risk perceptions and precautionary behavior in response to 2009 (H1N1) pandemic influenza. *BMC Infect. Dis.* **2010**, *10*, 296. [CrossRef]
28. Cassar, A.; Healy, A.; von Kessler, C. Trust, Risk, and Time Preferences After a Natural Disaster: Experimental Evidence from Thailand. *World Dev.* **2017**, *94*, 90–105. [CrossRef]
29. Rodríguez, H.; Trainor, J.; Quarantelli, E.L. Rising to the Challenges of a Catastrophe: The Emergent and Prosocial Behavior following Hurricane Katrina. *Ann. Am. Acad. Politi- Soc. Sci.* **2006**, *604*, 82–101. [CrossRef]
30. Veszteg, R.F.; Funaki, Y.; Tanaka, A. The impact of the Tohoku earthquake and tsunami on social capital in Japan: Trust before and after the disaster. *Int. Politi- Sci. Rev.* **2015**, *36*, 119–138. [CrossRef]
31. Calo-Blanco, A.; Kovářík, J.; Mengel, F.; Romero, J.G. Natural disasters and indicators of social cohesion. *PLoS ONE* **2017**, *12*, e0176885. [CrossRef]
32. Zhang, S.W. Social justice, institutional trust and public cooperation intention. *Acta Psychol. Sin.* **2017**, *49*, 794–813. [CrossRef]
33. Hu, X.Y.; Guo, Y.Y.; Li, J.; Yang, S.L. Perceived societal fairness and goal attainment: The differnet effects of social class and their mechanism. *Acta Psychol. Sin.* **2016**, *48*, 271–289. [CrossRef]
34. Tao, S.; Xu, Y.; Yuan, C.C. The activation effect of complementary stereotypes on justice perception. *China J. Soc. Dev.* **2015**, *4*, 647–650.
35. Wei, Q.G.; Zhang, Y.; Li, H. Double impression in process of social development: Research on people's attitude towards income distribution and inequality in urban China. *J. Soc. Dev.* **2014**, *3*, 240.
36. Li, L.L.; Tang, L.N.; Qin, G.Q. Fear of inequality, but more fear of unfairness: Sense of fairness and consciousness of conflict in the period of social transformation. *J. Renmin Univ. China* **2012**, *26*, 80–90.
37. Templeton, A.; Guven, S.T.; Hoerst, C.; Vestergren, S.; Davidson, L.; Ballentyne, S.; Madsen, H.; Choudhury, S. Inequalities and identity processes in crises: Recommendations for facilitating safe response to the COVID-19 pandemic. *Br. J. Soc. Psychol.* **2020**, *59*, 674–685. [CrossRef]
38. Guowuyuan. State Council Government Work Report. Available online: http://www.gov.cn/guowuyuan/zfgzbg.htm (accessed on 5 March 2022).
39. Skitka, L.J. Patriotism or Nationalism? Understanding Post-September 11, 2001, Flag-Display Behavior1. *J. Appl. Soc. Psychol.* **2005**, *35*, 1995–2011. [CrossRef]
40. Bonanno, G.A.; Brewin, C.R.; Kaniasty, K.; La Greca, A.M. Weighing the Costs of Disaster: Consequences, risks, and resilience in individuals, families, and communities. *Psychol. Sci. Public Interes.* **2010**, *11*, 1–49. [CrossRef]
41. Norris, F.H.; Friedman, M.J.; Watson, P.J. The summary and implications of the disaster mental health research. 60,000 Disaster Victims Speak: Part II. Summary and Implications of the Disaster Mental Health Research. *Psychiatry* **2002**, *65*, 240–260. [CrossRef]
42. Li, Q.; Xiang, J.; Song, S.; Li, X.; Liu, Y.; Wang, Y.; Luo, Y.; Xiao, M.; Chen, H. Trait self-control and disinhibited eating in COVID-19: The mediating role of perceived mortality threat and negative affect. *Appetite* **2021**, *167*, 105660. [CrossRef]
43. Li, S.; Wu, Y.; Zhang, F.; Xu, Q.; Zhou, A. Self-affirmation buffering by the general public reduces anxiety levels during the COVID-19 epidemic. *Acta Psychol. Sin.* **2020**, *52*, 886–894. [CrossRef]
44. Shi, K.; Fan, H.; Jia, J.; Li, W.; Song, Z.; Gao, J.; Chen, X.; Lu, J.; Hu, W. The risk perceptions of SARS and sociopsychological behaviors of urban people in China. *Acta Psychol. Sin.* **2003**, *35*, 546–554.
45. Yu, H.Y.R.; Ho, S.C.; So, K.F.E.; Lo, Y.L. The psychological burden experienced by Hong Kong midlife women during the SARS epidemic. *Stress Health* **2005**, *21*, 177–184. [CrossRef]
46. Kaniasty, K.; Norris, F.H. A test of the social support deterioration model in the context of natural disaster. *J. Pers. Soc. Psychol.* **1993**, *64*, 395–408. [CrossRef]
47. Kessler, R.; Kessler, R.C.; Galea, S.; Jones, R.T.; Parker, H.A.; Hurricane Katrina Community Advisory Group. Mental illness and suicidality after Hurricane Katrina. *Bull. World Health Organ.* **2006**, *84*, 930–939. [CrossRef]
48. Cai, Y.; Kong, W.; Lian, Y.; Jin, X. Depressive Symptoms among Chinese Informal Employees in the Digital Era. *Int. J. Environ. Res. Public Health* **2021**, *18*, 5211. [CrossRef]
49. Xin, S.F.; Liang, X.; Sheng, L.; Zhao, Z.R. Changes of Teachers' Subjective Well-being in Mainland Chinese (2002~2019): The Perspective of Cross-temporal Meta-analysis. *Acta Psychol. Sin.* **2021**, *8*, 875–889. [CrossRef]
50. Diener, E.; Oishi, S.; Tay, L. Advances in subjective well-being research. *Nat. Hum. Behav.* **2018**, *2*, 253–260. [CrossRef]
51. Diener, E.; Emmons, R.A.; Larsen, R.J.; Griffin, S. The satisfaction with life scale. *J. Pers. Assess.* **1985**, *49*, 71–75. [CrossRef]
52. Cummins, R.A.; Eckersley, R.; Pallant, J.; Van Vugt, J.; Misajon, R. Developing a National Index of Subjective Wellbeing: The Australian Unity Wellbeing Index. *Soc. Indic. Res.* **2003**, *64*, 159–190. [CrossRef]
53. Rieger, M.O.; Wang, M. Trust in Government Actions During the COVID-19 Crisis. *Soc. Indic. Res.* **2021**, *159*, 967–989. [CrossRef]
54. Lu, C.T.; Zhao, Y.Z.; Zhang, Z.J. On the Shaping of perceived societal fairness by Educational Attainment and Media Connotation. *Modern Communication. J. Commun. Univ. China* **2017**, *39*, 149–155.

55. Assari, S. Combined Racial and Gender Differences in the Long-Term Predictive Role of Education on Depressive Symptoms and Chronic Medical Conditions. *J. Racial Ethn. Health Disparities* **2016**, *4*, 385–396. [CrossRef] [PubMed]
56. Kraus, M.W.; Piff, P.K.; Mendoza-Denton, R.; Rheinschmidt, M.L.; Keltner, D. Social class, solipsism, and contextualism: How the rich are different from the poor. *Psychol. Rev.* **2012**, *119*, 546–572. [CrossRef] [PubMed]
57. Kraus, M.W.; Tan, J.J.X.; Tannenbaum, M.B. The Social Ladder: A Rank-Based Perspective on Social Class. *Psychol. Inq.* **2013**, *24*, 81–96. [CrossRef]
58. Wang, Y.; Yang, C.; Hu, X.; Chen, H. The Mediating Effect of Community Identity between Socioeconomic Status and Sense of Gain in Chinese Adults. *Int. J. Environ. Res. Public Health* **2020**, *17*, 1553. [CrossRef]
59. Alesina, A.; La Ferrara, E. Who trusts others? *J. Public Econ.* **2002**, *85*, 207–234. [CrossRef]
60. Zhao, Q.; Psychological and Social Factors Affecting the Perceived Societal Fairness. Guangming Daily. Available online: https://www.gmw.cn/01gmrb/2005-05/10/content_229635.htm (accessed on 10 May 2005).
61. Hu, X.; Yang, S.; Zhong, Q.; Yu, F.; Chen, H. The relationship between social class and health: Their "social-psychological-physiological" mechanism. *Chin. Sci. Bull.* **2019**, *64*, 194–205. [CrossRef]
62. Wang, F.Q. Socioeconomic status, lifestyle and health inequality (in Chinese). *Society* **2012**, *2*, 125–143.
63. Bromberger, J.T.; Schott, L.L.; Avis, N.E.; Crawford, S.L.; Harlow, S.D.; Joffe, H.; Kravitz, H.M.; Matthews, K.A. Psychosocial and health-related risk factors for depressive symptom trajectories among midlife women over 15 years: Study of Women's Health Across the Nation (SWAN). *Psychol. Med.* **2019**, *49*, 250–259. [CrossRef]
64. Xu, W.; Sun, H.; Zhu, B.; Bai, W.; Yu, X.; Duan, R.; Kou, C.; Li, W. Analysis of Factors Affecting the High Subjective Well-Being of Chinese Residents Based on the 2014 China Family Panel Study. *Int. J. Environ. Res. Public Health* **2019**, *16*, 2566. [CrossRef]
65. Xie, Y.; Hu, J.W.; Zhang, C.N. The China Family Panel Studies: Design and Practice. *Chin. J. Sociol.* **2014**, *34*, 1–32.
66. Wen, Z.L.; Ye, B.J. Evaluating Test Reliability: From Coefficient Alpha to Internal Consistency Reliability. *Acta Psychol. Sin.* **2011**, *43*, 821–829. [CrossRef]
67. Xie, Y.; Zhang, X.B.; Tu, P.; Ren, Q.; Sun, Y.; Lv, P.; Ding, H.; Hu, J.W.; Wu, Q. China Family Panel Studies (2017) User's Manual (3rd Edition). Available online: http://www.isss.pku.edu.cn/cfps/wdzx/yhsc/index.htm (accessed on 30 July 2017).
68. Li, Q.R.; Yang, Y.Y.; Li, C.X.; Gong, S.Y. A latent transition analysis of depressive symptoms in self-employed workers. *Chin. Ment. Health J.* **2021**, *35*, 856–862.
69. Du, H.; King, R.B. What predicts perceived economic inequality? The roles of actual inequality, system justification, and fairness considerations. *Br. J. Soc. Psychol.* **2022**, *61*, 19–36. [CrossRef]
70. Chen, W.; Huang, Y.; Riad, A. Gender Differences in Depressive Traits among Rural and Urban Chinese Adolescent Students: Secondary Data Analysis of Nationwide Survey CFPS. *Int. J. Environ. Res. Public Health* **2021**, *18*, 9124. [CrossRef]
71. Tan, J.J.X.; Kraus, M.W. Lay Theories About Social Class Buffer Lower-Class Individuals Against Poor Self-Rated Health and Negative Affect. *Pers. Soc. Psychol. Bull.* **2015**, *41*, 446–461. [CrossRef]
72. Zhou, H.; Long, L.R. Statistical Remedies for Common Method Biases. *Adv. Psychol. Sci.* **2004**, *12*, 942–950.
73. Ferguson, C.J. An effect size primer: A guide for clinicians and researchers. *Prof. Psychol. Res. Pract.* **2009**, *40*, 532–538. [CrossRef]
74. Zheng, H.M.; Wen, Z.L.; Wu, Y. The appropriate effect sizes and their calculations in psychological research. *Adv. Psychol. Sci.* **2011**, *12*, 1868–1878. [CrossRef]
75. Lu, X.F.; Tang, Y.H.; Zeng, F.M. Effect size: Estimation, reporting and interpretation. *Phychol. Explor.* **2011**, *3*, 260–264.
76. Steiger, J.H. Paul Meehl and the evolution of statistical methods in psychology. *Appl. Prev. Psychol.* **2004**, *11*, 69–72. [CrossRef]
77. Min, C.; Shen, F.; Yu, W.; Chu, Y. The relationship between government trust and preventive behaviors during the COVID-19 pandemic in China: Exploring the roles of knowledge and negative emotion. *Prev. Med.* **2020**, *141*, 106288. [CrossRef]
78. Ye, M.; Lyu, Z. Trust, risk perception, and COVID-19 infections: Evidence from multilevel analyses of combined original dataset in China. *Soc. Sci. Med.* **2020**, *265*, 113517. [CrossRef]
79. Groeniger, J.O.; Noordzij, K.; van der Waal, J.; de Koster, W. Dutch COVID-19 lockdown measures increased trust in government and trust in science: A difference-in-differences analysis. *Soc. Sci. Med.* **2021**, *275*, 113819. [CrossRef]
80. Zhang, R.J. Social trust and satisfaction with life: A cross-lagged panel analysis based on representative samples from 18 societies. *Soc. Sci. Med.* **2020**, *251*, 112901. [CrossRef]
81. Bolin, B.; Kurtz, L.C. Race, Class, Ethnicity, and Disaster Vulnerability. In *Handbook of Disaster Research*; Springer International: Berlin/Heidelberg, Germany, 2018; pp. 181–203.
82. Jetten, J.; Haslam, C.; Haslam, S.A. *The Social Cure: Identity, Health and Wellbeing*; Taylor and Francis: Oxford, UK, 2011; p. 2. [CrossRef]
83. Hu, X.Y.; Li, L.Y.; Du, T.Y.; Wang, T.T.; Yang, J. The protective effects of the "shift-and-persist" strategy on the health of the lower class and their mechanisms. *Adv. Psychol. Sci.* **2022**, *30*, 2088. [CrossRef]
84. Zhou, X.H. Social Transformation and Historical Mission of the Chinese Social Sciences. *Nanjing J. Soc. Sci.* **2014**, *1*, 1–10. [CrossRef]
85. Graffigna, G.; Palamenghi, L.; Savarese, M.; Castellini, G.; Barello, S. Effects of the COVID-19 Emergency and National Lockdown on Italian Citizens' Economic Concerns, Government Trust, and Health Engagement: Evidence from a Two-Wave Panel Study. *Milbank Q.* **2021**, *99*, 369–392. [CrossRef]

86. Bonanno, G.A.; Galea, S.; Bucciarelli, A.; Vlahov, D. What predicts psychological resilience after disaster? The role of demographics, resources, and life stress. *J. Consult. Clin. Psychol.* **2007**, *75*, 671–682. [CrossRef]
87. Haslam, S.A.; Reicher, S.D. 50 years of "obedience to authority": From blind conformity to engaged followership. Annual review of law and social science. *Annu. Rev. Law Soc. Sci.* **2017**, *13*, 59–78. [CrossRef]

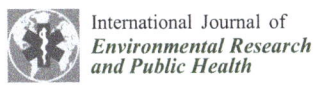

Review

A Review of COVID-19-Related Literature on Freight Transport: Impacts, Mitigation Strategies, Recovery Measures, and Future Research Directions

Ahmed Karam [1,2,*], Abdelrahman E. E. Eltoukhy [3], Ibrahim Abdelfadeel Shaban [4] and El-Awady Attia [5]

1 Department of the Built Environment, Aalborg University, 9220 Aalborg, Denmark
2 Department of Mechanical Engineering (Shoubra), Benha University, Benha 11672, Egypt
3 Department of Industrial and Systems Engineering, The Hong Kong Polytechnic University, Hong Kong SAR, China
4 Mechanical and Aerospace Engineering Department, UAE University, Al-Ain P.O. Box 111, United Arab Emirates
5 Department of Industrial Engineering, College of Engineering, Prince Sattam bin Abdulaziz University, Al Kharj 11942, Saudi Arabia
* Correspondence: akam@build.aau.dk

Citation: Karam, A.; Eltoukhy, A.E.E.; Shaban, I.A.; Attia, E.-A. A Review of COVID-19-Related Literature on Freight Transport: Impacts, Mitigation Strategies, Recovery Measures, and Future Research Directions. *Int. J. Environ. Res. Public Health* **2022**, *19*, 12287. https://doi.org/10.3390/ijerph191912287

Academic Editors: Sachiko Kodera and Essam A. Rashed

Received: 4 August 2022
Accepted: 20 September 2022
Published: 27 September 2022

Publisher's Note: MDPI stays neutral with regard to jurisdictional claims in published maps and institutional affiliations.

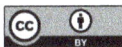

Copyright: © 2022 by the authors. Licensee MDPI, Basel, Switzerland. This article is an open access article distributed under the terms and conditions of the Creative Commons Attribution (CC BY) license (https://creativecommons.org/licenses/by/4.0/).

Abstract: The COVID-19 pandemic has caused significant disruptions in the freight transport sector. The number of studies on the impact of COVID-19 on freight transport and possible mitigation strategies are growing. However, a systematic and comprehensive review highlighting the research themes, main findings, research methods, and future research directions of these studies remains scarce. Therefore, this study presents a mixed review comprising scientometric and systematic reviews to cover these research gaps. Results show that 68 studies have been published on this topic since the beginning of 2020 and that they cover three main themes: the impacts of COVID-19 on freight transport, mitigation strategies, and recovery during and after COVID-19. In addition, we describe the research methods, main findings, and possible research directions in each of them. Thus, the findings of our work present both theoretical and practical analyses of COVID-19-related research on freight transport and provide important future research directions in this domain.

Keywords: freight transport; COVID-19; air freight; sea shipping; road transport; recovery measures; strategies

1. Introduction

In December 2019, China announced the first case of the novel coronavirus disease, called "SARS-CoV2". Since then, the virus has spread over the world, infecting and killing people. By March 2020, the World Health Organization (WHO) had declared it a pandemic and officially named it "COVID-19". By the end of 2020, the virus had infected more than 82 million people and killed over 1.8 million. Therefore, the pandemic may be referred to as the most disastrous black swan event in 2020. To curb the spread of COVID-19, travel restrictions were firmly implemented by governments worldwide. As a result, these restrictions have significantly affected all modes of freight transport and caused severe disruptions. As of April 2020, global demand for air freight has dramatically declined by approximately 27.7% compared to 2019 [1], while air freight capacity shrank by 42% compared to 2019 [2]. This dire situation has also been observed in global road freight, with an estimated loss of EUR 550 billion due to movement restrictions imposed by governments [3]. Similarly, sea freight transport was not spared, as container ship mobility reduced by approximately 14% in June 2020 [4].

Freight transport has always been an important aspect of the supply chain. Therefore, since 2020, many studies have studied the impact of COVID-19 on freight transport logistics and possible mitigation strategies. Examples of these impacts include shortage of transport resources [5,6], higher operating costs [7,8], and fluctuations in demand for transport services [6,9]. The identification of appropriate strategies for managing such impacts has been addressed in some studies [10,11]. Given the significance of this topic, it is valuable to report the up-to-date status of research regarding freight transport during COVID-19 and outline some future research directions. It is worth noting that some previous studies have addressed the impact of other types of pandemics, e.g., influenza [12], cholera [13], Ebola [14], and malaria [15]. In addition, some scholars have published review papers on the impacts and response strategies to these disease outbreaks [16,17]. However, these review papers are focused on the pre-COVID 19 pandemics with emphasis on logistics [16], supply chains [17], and buying behaviors of customers due to pandemic outbreaks [18]. Compared to the previous pandemics, COVID-19 stands out with extraordinary impacts on virtually all human activities. Unlike the previous pandemics, that disrupt activities in some locales, COVID-19 affects businesses around the globe. Furthermore, to curb the spread of the disease, many countries implement lockdowns that halt all industrial and social activities with attendant disruptions to most global and local supply chains [19]. Although the COVID-related literature on freight transport is constantly growing, the findings from these studies are still scattered across several sources and rather unsystematized. More specifically, the literature reporting COVID-19-pandemic-related freight transport studies in a systematic approach remains scarce. In this regard, there are only two relevant review papers [19,20]. Chowdhury, Paul, Kaisar and Moktadir [19] conduct a review study on the impacts of the COVID-19 pandemic on eight supply chain-related areas including transportation and logistics. Despite the significance of this review study, it considers only a small set of the COVID-19-related freight transport studies, i.e., 12 studies. Borca, Putz and Hofbauer [20] review the literature on the different crises that hit Europe in the previous 20 years and their effects on freight transport modes. Although the authors list COVID-19 as one of the crises, only three studies related to the impact of COVID-19 on freight transport are covered.

Unlike the previous studies, this current work analyzes 57 COVID-19-related studies on freight transport. In particular, this work seeks to answer the following three main research questions (RQ):

RQ1: What are the research themes and main findings of the literature on freight transport during COVID-19?

RQ2: What are the main research methods used in the COVID-19-related literature on freight transport?

RQ3: What are the future research directions in the freight transport sectors with respect to the COVID-19 pandemic?

To answer these three research questions, the present study uses a mixed review method that combines scientometric and systematic review methods. A scientometric analysis is conducted to identify the major research scopes, linkage of researchers, countries, and others on research articles related to COVID-19 and freight transport. Next, a systematic review of these articles is undertaken to summarize the main research themes in this domain. The findings of this work will be of immense benefits to researchers and forestall duplication of research efforts at this stage of the pandemic. Additionally, researchers can take cues from the identified future research avenues to enrich the existing body of knowledge in the domain of freight transport. Furthermore, practitioners will gain deep insight into the main themes of freight transport and how scholars have addressed them. This will help bring more innovation and performance improvement in this field.

The remainder of this paper is organized as follows. Section 2 presents the review methodology for scientometric analysis and systematic review. In Section 3, results of the scientometric analysis are presented, whereas Section 4 discusses the systematic literature review. Lastly, Section 5 concludes the study.

2. Review Methodology

Figure 1 summarizes the methodology of the review process, which combined bibliometric analysis, scientometric analysis, and systematic review. Note that the bibliometric analysis was conducted before the scientometric analysis and systematic review, to ensure that the collected bibliographic data were representative of the proposed review topic. The following sub-sections expatiate on the details of each process.

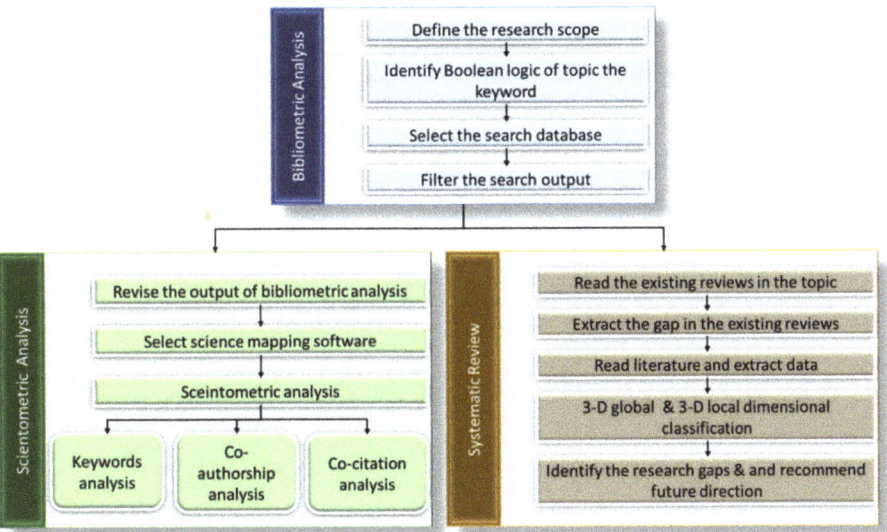

Figure 1. Summary of the review methodology.

2.1. Bibliometric Analysis

The bibliometric analysis started with the definition of the scope, which was freight transport amid the outbreak of COVID-19. Next, based on this scope, combinations of three keywords and their related synonyms were used to search for the related literature in a scientific database. These keywords, "COVID-19, coronavirus, and SARS-CoV-2", "transport", and "freight, cargo, and goods", were combined by using Boolean logic, as shown in Figure 2. After generating the combination of keywords, the SCOPUS database was selected due to its updated and wide coverage of existing literature on the proposed topic [21]. The search results gave 101 research documents, which further dropped to 57 articles when only English language documents were extracted. Note, the search results were downloaded in a CSV file, which included each article's title, abstract, author list, funding details, etc. The bibliometric analysis ended with the filtering process, which comprised screening the articles' titles and reading their abstracts to eliminate irrelevant research papers.

2.2. Scientometric Analysis

Scientometric analysis is a data and text mining technique that uses the filtered data from the bibliometric study to visualize the relationships between keywords, citations, authors, and others. This analysis reduces the subjectivity associated with the findings of narrative reviews [22]. Thus, this analysis is adopted in several studies in different research fields, including transportation [23], construction management [21], and healthcare management [24]. As shown in Figure 1, the first step in conducting the scientometric analysis was to revise the results of the bibliometric analysis and then select a suitable software to perform the scientometric analysis. In this study, VOSviewer [25] was utilized for the scientometric analysis, including analysis of keyword co-occurrence, co-citation, and co-authorship.

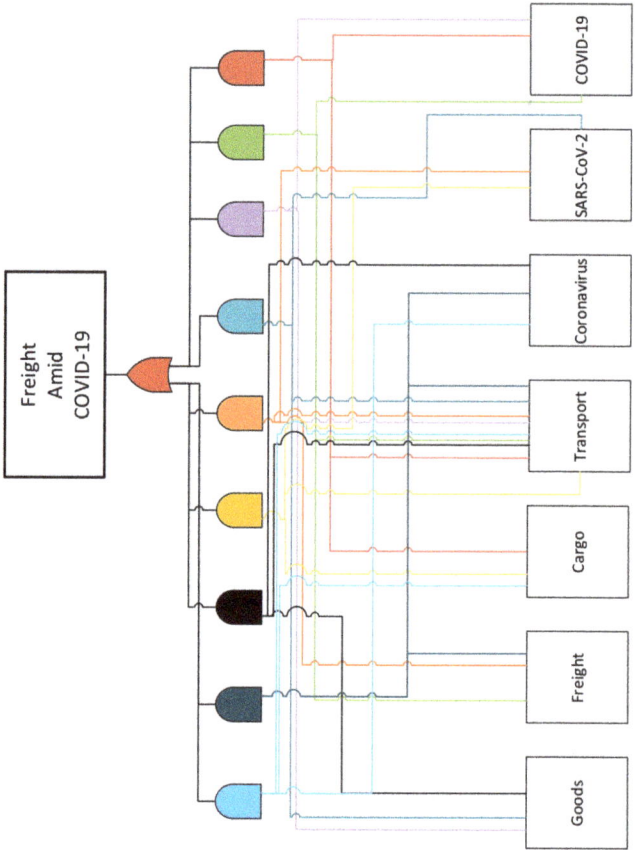

Figure 2. Keywords combination through Boolean logic gates.

2.3. Systematic Review

Despite the advantages of the scientometric analysis, it is still insufficient to provide a comprehensive understanding of the bibliometric results. Therefore, a systematic review can be deployed to organize the extracted articles based on a number of research themes. As shown in Figure 3, we identified three broad research themes in the existing studies. These included the impact of COVID-19 on freight transport, the mitigation strategies that were adopted, and the ability to recover during and after COVID-19. At the early stage of the pandemic, countries of the world proposed several measures to fight the spread of infection, which in turn influenced freight transport systems in several ways, as reported by researchers and governmental reports. We identified these studies and categorized them under five main impacts. During the pandemic or what is now called the new norm, maintaining food and medical supplies was dependent on creating robust freight transport systems. To this end, practitioners paid great attention to risk mitigation programs, researchers proposed novel mitigation strategies based on state-of-the-art technologies, and additionally, some regulations on freight transport were relaxed in many countries. Some of these mitigation strategies are expected to lead to rethinking the future of freight transport in the post-pandemic era. We categorized these mitigation strategies into five, which included (1) usage of autonomous delivery vehicles (ADVs), (2) drone delivery,

(3) deployment of mobile warehouses, (4) engagement of large ships, and (5) application of quantity discounts. In addition to adopting risk mitigation strategies, the evaluation of the recoverability of freight transport systems was tackled through several measures, such as system recovery rates, quality, demand recovery, and efficiency.

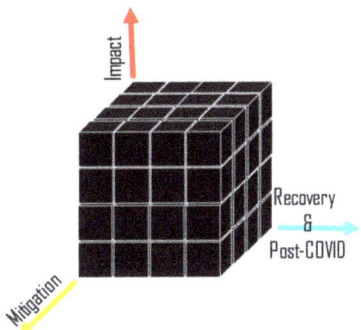

Figure 3. Schematic diagram illustrating the 3-D matrix research themes, including impact, mitigation, and recoverability.

3. Results and Discussion of the Scientometric Analysis

Table 1 summarizes the selected scientometric analysis performed in this study, including keyword co-occurrence, co-authorship, and citation analysis. For each analysis, its related criteria are fixed, as shown in Table 1. Based on the search output from the SCOPUS database, the 57 documents that cover the research scope contain 604 keywords. To study the most co-used keywords in these documents, a threshold criterion of three is applied (i.e., the minimum occurrence of a keyword is set to three). Forty-two keywords meet the threshold criterion, and all of them are connected. In analyzing co-authorship between 40 countries of the authors who have published on freight transport during COVID-19, two thresholds are applied: one for the minimum number of documents (i.e., 2) per country and another for the minimum citations (i.e., 0) of countries. Eighteen countries meet the threshold criteria, and only fourteen of them are connected. In the following sub-sections, the results of these analyses are discussed. Similarly, in the citation analysis of the sources, 36 sources meet the threshold criteria, but only 13 are connected.

Table 1. Summary of results of some selected scientometric analyses.

Analysis	Total Number of (---)	Threshold Criteria Minimum Number of			Number of (---) Meet the Threshold	Number of Connected (---)
		Occurrence	Documents	Citation		
Co-occurrence of (keywords)	604	3	–	–	42	42
Co-authorship between (countries)	40	–	2	0	18	14
Citation of (sources)	36	–	1	0	36	13

3.1. Keyword Analysis

Keyword analysis is used to generate the keywords mapping network shown in Figure 4. The mapping network consists of nodes connected by lines. Keywords with bigger nodes mean they are more frequently used than others with smaller nodes. Similarly, a thicker connecting line between two keywords indicates the frequency of their occurrence in multiple articles. Therefore, the keyword "COVID-19" is the most frequently used. Meanwhile, it co-occurs most with the keywords "Airline industry", "Maritime trade", "Transportation policy", etc. This implies that most of the research in this domain focuses on policies aimed at mitigating the impact of the COVID-19 pandemic on freight transportation.

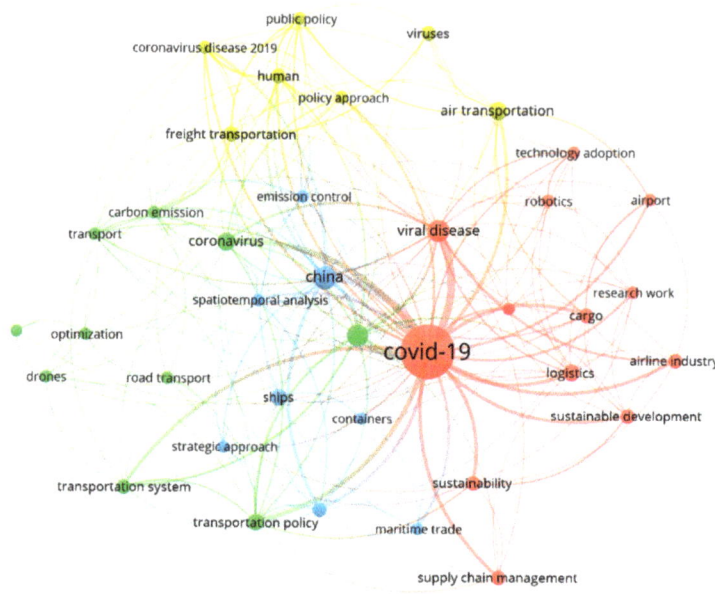

Figure 4. Keyword mapping network.

Table 2 shows the top 15 keywords used in freight transport studies amid COVID-19, while others are shown in the keyword mapping network in Figure 4. For instance, "drones" can be regarded as one of the most important mitigation strategies, though further investigations into their use are required. This is because of the legal differences to fly them in different countries [26]. Additionally, COVID-19 can be deemed as one of the long-term disruptions. For example, flight schedules are interrupted, borders are closed, and work modes have changed. However, the word "optimization" is not used sufficiently to cope with the disruption in the three modes of freight transport.

Table 2. Top used keywords.

	Keyword	Links	Occurrences
1	COVID-19	38	52
2	Freight transport	20	14
3	Supply chains	8	10
4	China	25	9
5	Epidemic	19	8
6	Viral disease	26	8
7	Sustainability	10	8
8	Air transportation	15	6
9	Logistics	14	5
10	Ships	9	5
11	Transportation policy	15	5
12	Airline industry	9	4
13	Cargo	12	4
14	Human	15	4
15	Transportation system	9	4

3.2. Co-Authorship Analysis

As COVID-19 has spread worldwide, it is interesting to see how different countries cooperate in the research on freight transport. For this purpose, a co-authorship analysis is conducted, as shown in Figure 5. Figure 5a shows that the highest co-authorship in terms of the number of published research works is found in the cluster comprising China, Hong Kong, and India. However, in Figure 5b, the cluster of the most cited authors includes Canada and the United States. This means that there is no direct correspondence between citation and number of publications.

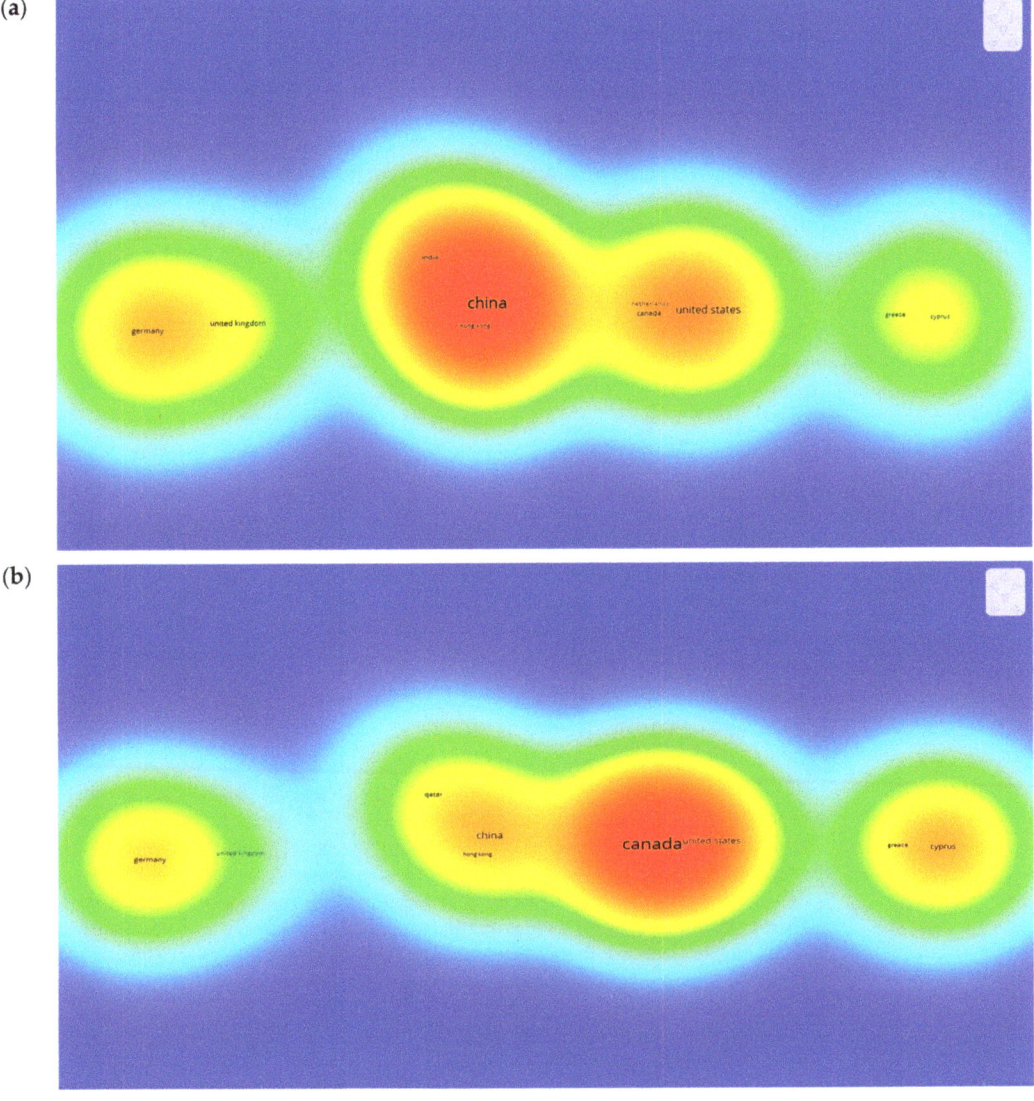

Figure 5. Density visualization of the co-authorship between countries based on (**a**) total published documents, and (**b**) number of citations.

3.3. Source Citation Analysis

The number of citations of an article does not only reflect its impact but also affects the impact of the publishing source. Thus, the analysis of citation is necessary to identify the most impactful research works, sources, and authors [22]. However, Table 3 shows that the journal sources with a high number of research articles do not necessarily publish high impact research articles with high citation counts. For more detail, until the time of our research (the last update of these scientometric data was on 11 December 2021), *Sustainability* (Switzerland) and *Science of Total Environment* (SOTE) have received 39 and 37 citations, respectively. However, these citation counts do not reflect the exact impact of these two journals, because the number of documents published by *Sustainability* and SOTE are 10 and 1, respectively. This means that the average citation for *Sustainability* does not exceed 4 compared to 37 in SOTE. Moreover, normalization of citation counts is a metric that can be used to eliminate the effect of time on source citation (i.e., the propensity that an older document is more likely to get higher citations than a newer one). For example, the average number of citations for *Transportation Research Interdisciplinary Perspectives* (TRIP) is 30, while it is 79 for the *International Journal of Advanced Manufacturing Technology* (IJAMT). However, the normalized citation of TRIP is 3.7687, which is almost three times the normalized citation of IJAMT. To conclude, the most impactful journal within the period under review is the *Canadian Journal of Agricultural Economics*, because it has the highest average citations and the highest normalized citation.

Table 3. Top cited sources.

	Source	Documents	Citations	Normalized Citations	Avg. Citations
1	Canadian Journal of Agricultural Economics	2	367	9.1039	183.5
2	Transportation Research Interdisciplinary Perspectives	3	90	3.7687	30
3	International Journal of Advanced Manufacturing Technology	1	79	1	79
4	Transport Policy	7	49	8.7427	7
5	Sustainability (Switzerland)	10	39	5.4223	3.9
6	Science of the Total Environment	1	37	6.6017	37
7	IEEE Engineering Management Review	1	30	0.7442	30
8	International Journal of Logistics Research and Applications	1	20	0.4961	20
9	Ocean and Coastal Management	1	10	1.7842	10

4. Results and Discussion of the Systematic Review

4.1. COVID-19-Related Impact

Our review shows that 36 out of the identified studies investigate different impacts of COVID-19 on the freight transport industry. These 36 studies are carefully analyzed to identify and group the different impacts of COVID-19 on freight transport. There are five categories of these impacts, including impact on: (1) transport demand, (2) transport capacity, (3) operational transport cost, (4) delivery performance, and (5) carbon emissions, as shown in Table 4. It should be noted that a study may report more than one impact; therefore, the sum of all entries under 'studies per impact' is not necessarily 36. In the following subsections, these 36 articles are classified and thoroughly analyzed based on the reported impacts, transport mode, and research methodology.

Table 4. Categorization of different impacts of COVID-19 on freight transport.

Impacts of COVID-19	Studies per Impact	References
Demand for freight transport services	24	[5–9,11,27–43]
Capacity shortage	10	[5,6,32,34,35,44–48]
Operating transport cost	13	[5–8,20,27,31,32,34,35,49–52]
Delivery performance	9	[8,9,32,47,48,53–55]
CO_2 emissions	4	[5,28,38,56]

4.1.1. Impacts of COVID-19

- Demand for freight transport services:

Twenty-four studies report the impact of the COVID pandemic on the demand for different freight transport modes, i.e., air, maritime, rail, and road. Six studies examine the impact of COVID-19 on the demand for seaports and waterways transport [6,7,9,37,39–43]. Tianming, Erokhin, Arskiy and Khudzhatov [9] show that the pandemic breaks the connectivity among seaports in China, Norway, Iceland, Russia, South Korea, and Sweden. In Australia, Munawar, Khan, Qadir, Kouzani and Mahmud [6] report that during the initial stage of the pandemic, the demand for water freight transport declines by 9.5%. Michail and Melas [7] indicate that the daily number of calls of dry bulk and clean tankers in ports is highly affected by the pandemic, while the pandemic has no impact on the calls for crude oil vessels. Narasimha, Jena and Majhi [37] confirm that the overall demand for major Indian seaports declines by 4.59% for 2020 compared to 2019. A case study of a maritime transport service provider shows that the transshipments of cargo decreases by approximately 32%, whereas the urgent supplies of medical equipment increase [39]. Further, five studies examine the impact of the COVID-19 pandemic on the demand for airfreight transport [5,6,34,36,38]. For example, in Australia, the demand for airfreight transport decreases significantly from 84.8 million kilograms in January 2020 to 54.5 million kilograms in April 2020 [6].

Nine studies examine the impact of the COVID-19 pandemic on the demand for road freight transport [6,8,11,20,27–30,33]. For example, Arellana, Márquez and Cantillo [28] show that freight trips in Colombia reduce by around 38% due to a low demand for non-essential products. Due to the lockdown and travel restrictions, people shift from in-store shopping to online shopping and demands for last-mile deliveries increase [6,8,11,27]. From January 2020 to June 2020, global retail platforms witness a 26.9% increase in online-shopping orders [57]. In Europe, online shopping sales in April 2020 increase by 30% compared to April 2019 [58]. Due to the panic buying behavior of people during the pandemic and the sharp fall in oil prices, Ho, Xing, Wu and Lee [33] report a positive correlation between road freight transport turnover and the number of confirmed cases of COVID-19 in China. In Portugal, Cruz and Sarmento [30] state that during the peak of COVID-19 in April 2020, the traffic volume of light commercial vehicles reduces by an average of 44.5%, while the traffic of heavy trucks reduces by 24%. Bartuska and Masek [29] conclude that the traffic volumes of trucks and trailers are not significantly affected on the major roads of South Bohemia (Czech Republic). Borca, Putz and Hofbauer [20] investigate road transportation in the USA at the beginning of the pandemic. They report that despite an unprecedented 46% reduction in the traffic volume of private cars, freight traffic volume reduces by a mere 13%. These values of commercial traffic volumes indicate that the supply of essential products is not significantly disrupted, especially to supermarkets and pharmacies during the pandemic. Additionally, this also implies that many companies, even if closed, increase their inventories to be safe against future uncertainties and to start production again once the lockdown ends. Although the previous studies focus on a single freight mode, some studies investigate multiple freight modes. For example, Cui, He, Liu, Zheng, Wei, Yang and Zhou [31] study the impacts of the COVID-19 pandemic on China's transport sectors. Their results show a reduction in the outputs of households and production sectors; thus, there is a reduction in the demand for transportation in these sectors. For example, aviation freight transportation reduces by 2.81%, while road freight transportation, railway freight transportation, and waterway freight transportation are down by 2.20%, 1.84%, and 1.04%, respectively. Gray [32] reports an increasing demand in the agriculture sector for different transportation services, e.g., bulk ocean freight, rail movement, and road trucks. Li, Bai, Hu, Yu and Yan [42] present equations to evaluate the traffic variations of overall provincewide traffic and tested the hypotheses for traffic recovery analysis. The results show that truck traffic dropped by 68.19% during the outbreak and found that the higher the GDP per capita the region has, the more the traffic in the region was affected by the pandemic. It is also found that truck traffic had a rapid recovery period compared to that of passenger traffic.

- Capacity shortage

Ten studies report the impact of the COVID pandemic on the transport capacity of the different freight transport modes. The imposed epidemic control requirements lead to a shortage of transport capacity, e.g., driver shortage, belly-hold shortage in airfreight transport, and shortage of empty containers. In April 2020, passenger flights decrease by approximately 95% compared to the previous year [45]. Similarly, belly capacity for international air cargo drops by 75% in April 2020, compared to the previous year. Meanwhile, at the peak of COVID-19, the demand for medical and personal protective equipment significantly increases worldwide. On the other hand, air freight capacity is severely limited due to the shutdown of passenger flights [5,6,34,48] and the available cargo aircraft cannot resolve the shortage in airfreight capacity. To resolve this, passenger aircraft are granted exemptions from July 2020 to July 2021 to carry freight in the main cabin when no passengers are being carried [59].

Workforce capacity of the transport sector has also been shown to be vulnerable to shortage because of mobility restrictions and sickness [45]. For instance, truck drivers cannot access many toilets at rest areas since they are closed. Therefore, mobile toilets are provided for truck drivers in Canada [32]. In China, the beginning of the pandemic coincides with the holiday season, when most logistics laborers have travelled to their hometowns. Subsequent restrictions on people's mobility result in a severe workforce shortage in the logistics industry [35]. On the bright side, quarantine obligations lead to the high availability of some categories of the workforce, e.g., truck drivers, in freight transportation [46]. For example, most truck drivers working in Western European countries, e.g., France, Denmark, and Germany, are from Eastern European countries, e.g., Poland and Romania. To avoid workforce shortages during the holiday periods, logistic companies request their drivers to postpone their holidays to avoid the mandatory 14-day quarantine.

Containerized trade represents 90% of the global trade volume. Therefore, containers are essential resources to transport different products between countries. In the container supply chain, containers are frequently returned empty to the exporting country. The COVID-19-related shutdown of many production facilities worldwide and the subsequent reduction in demand result in a shortage of empty containers [47]. Some food products, transported in containers, are delayed due to lack of empty containers in North America [32]. In addition, shortage of truck drivers, stringent inspection protocols, and requirement for quarantine delay the delivery of maritime freight [48]. Compared to sea and road transport, rail transport is less labor-intensive since the rail transport sector relies on a small size of very specialized crews to operate large trains. However, rail transport may have been impacted by COVID-19 if a significant proportion of the very specialized workforce is infected [32].

- Operating cost and prices of transport services

Thirteen studies report the impact of the COVID-19 pandemic on the operating costs of freight vehicles. The reviewed literature identifies three reasons responsible for the increase in operating costs of the logistics industry in China. Firstly, restriction on people's mobility cause a shortage in workforce capacity, leading to higher labor costs and freight rates [5,32,35,49]. Secondly, long-term infection prevention, e.g., disinfecting parcels and contactless delivery facilities, attract extra cost [31,34,35]. Thirdly, uncertainties in labor availability, traffic restrictions, and status of pandemic outbreaks incur extra costs in planning transportation routes [7,27,35]. Gray [32] reports that COVID-19 prevention and protective measures (e.g., multiple drivers are prevented from using the same truck) have led to increased transport costs of agricultural products in Canada. To support companies in applying such measures, Canadian transport authorities increase the maximum hours of service for drivers [60]. Some logistics enterprises adopt new modes of logistics services to fight the COVID-19 pandemic through the use of contactless delivery. This has also increased their operating costs, since contactless delivery needs extra investment cost in contactless facilities [8]. Michail and Melas [7] show that an increase of 1% in the global COVID-19 infection cases decrease the freight rates of Baltic dry and dirty Tankers by 0.03% and 0.046%, respectively. Bartle, Lutte and Leuenberger [5] report that the airfreight rates increase during the pandemic due to limited air cargo capacity. For example, in June 2020, the airfreight rates from China to Europe are 254% higher than those of June 2019 [50]. By using a multi-sectoral computable general equilibrium model of China, Cui, He, Liu, Zheng, Wei, Yang and Zhou [31] estimate that the cost of protective measures (e.g., disinfection, quarantine, and parking inspection) lead to a 1.5% reduction in the production efficiency of the freight transport sector. Grzelakowski [52] found that during the first months of 2020, the global maritime shipping sector, and specifically container transport, was affected by the lockdown and the resulting congestion in port terminals because of the inability of carriers to pick up freight from seaports and, thus, cargo ships became floating warehouses. In the middle of the third quarter of 2020, the supply chains become more stabilized, the demand on freight transport increased and, consequently, the spot freight rates also increased significantly. This was apparent in container shipping at the Far East–USA trade lane, as well as the routes towards South America or West Africa and the Middle East–Western Europe trade lanes.

On the bright side, COVID-19-related restrictions have led to a reduction in fuel prices. On 20 April 20 2020, the price of West Texas Intermediate crude oil dropped by 42.5% [61]. Fuel price accounts for approximately 15 to 20% of the total operating cost of the transport industry. The IATA reports that in July 2020, fuel prices are 45% lower than the price during the same period in 2019, resulting in a saving of nearly USD 70 billion for the airline industry [51]. Regardless of the drop in oil prices, travel restrictions and low demand for transport services result in a marginal profit for freight transport providers [6]. Some countries adopt policies, e.g., tax reduction, to reduce the operating costs of logistics companies. For example, China exempted logistics enterprises from vehicle tolls and value-added taxes on income due to delivering essential living supplies [8].

- Delivery performance

Nine studies report the impact of the COVID pandemic on the delivery performance of different freight transport modes. COVID-related restrictions exert the most impact on the delivery performance of maritime and air transport sectors. This is because these two sectors apply some quarantine virus containment measures to shipments, vessels, and crew. Several importing countries impose a 14-day quarantine for containers upon arrival at the port, resulting in a lengthy cycle times of containers [32]. In addition, COVID-19-related shortage of transport capacities, e.g., workforce, vehicle capacity, and empty containers, increase the delay in freight delivery [47,48]. Koyuncu, Tavacioğlu, Gökmen and Arican [54] suggest that the COVID-related restrictions on production and trade may break the interconnected supply chain; thereby, serious losses might be faced in some container lines.

Due to restricting people's mobility, several cities worldwide witness reduced road traffic. Therefore, some studies report positive effects on road freight transport, such as fewer traffic jams, increased efficiency, and fewer emissions [20]. For example, until the so-called "new normal" (11/05/2020), road traffic drops, on average, down to 76.28% in Madrid [27], 73% in UK [62], Sanpaolo (−55%), New York (−74%), Milan (−74%), Barcelona (−73%), Stockholm (−48%) [40]. The reduced road traffic causes delivery times to be much shorter [6]. Since the pandemic reduces demand for all nonessential products, access of essential products to seaports, rails, and trucks has generally improved [32]. However, finding truck parking is more difficult, especially for a large fleet [53]. This is because most employees are working from home and their private cars are occupying the parking slots in the streets. During the pandemic, many shops, e.g., pharmacies, grocery stores, and bakeries, start pickup and home delivery options in an attempt to stay in business. Thus, the efficiency and quality of last-mile logistics services are impaired [8,55].

- Emissions

Four studies report the impact of COVID-19 on the emissions from different freight transport modes. The COVID-19 pandemic creates an opportunity for achieving some temporary sustainability gains in the transport sector. This is mainly due to the reduction in carbon emissions, mainly because of mobility restrictions. However, this might be offset by increasing demand for cargo transport [5]. Few studies report the reduction in CO_2 emissions from freight transport during the pandemic [5,28,38,56]. In China, COVID-19 significantly reduces industrial and transport activities, resulting in lower CO_2 emissions. During the first quarter of 2020, freight transport has a 22.3% reduction in CO_2 emissions, while passenger transport is 59.1% compared with the same period of 2019 [56]. In Columbia, mobility restrictions have created positive side effects regarding externalities of transport, such as less traffic safety issues, noise, and pollution [28]. In Croatia, some airports have an average reduction of 96% in flights in April 2020 compared to April 2019. This directly affects the reduction in CO_2 emissions by a factor of 1.81 for the commercial airport and 3.49 for the seasonal airport [38].

4.1.2. Transport Mode

Table 5 classifies the 32 studies based on transport mode. Table 5 shows the studies that investigate the COVID-related impacts on only one individual transport mode, i.e., road (10 studies), air (7 studies), and seaport (9 studies). In addition, three studies address the impacts on two or more transport modes, while six studies discuss the impacts on the four modes or from a general perspective without focusing on a specific transport mode. It can be noted from Table 5 that road freight transport is the most studied mode, while rail freight transport is rarely studied. This may be because road freight transport is the dominant transport mode in most countries compared to other freight transport modes.

Table 5. Classification of COVID-19-related impact studies based on transport mode.

Transport Mode (s)	Number of Studies per Transport Mode (s)	References
Road	10	[11,27,29,30,35,41–43,46,56]
Air	5	[5,6,34,36,38]
Seaport	8	[7,9,33,37,39,40,52,54]
Air and road	1	[28]
Road and rail	1	[45]
Road, sea, and rail	1	[20]
All modes (General)	6	[31,32,44,48,49,55]

4.1.3. Research Methods

Regarding the research methods, the identified literature employs different methods to study the COVID-related impacts. These methods are grouped into four method categories: (1) empirical, (2) quantitative, (3) literature review, and (4) mixed methods. In addition, each method category includes a number of specific methods, as shown in Table 6. The most frequently used method category is the quantitative method (secondary data analysis and regression, forecasting, and mathematical models), followed by empirical methods (case studies, questionnaires, and interviews). Only one study conducts a systematic literature review on the types of crises that affect Europe in the previous 20 years [20]. Some studies employ mixed methods by merging two different methods to improve and validate the overall results [37,48]. For example, Narasimha, Jena and Majhi [37] demonstrate the negative impact of COVID-19 on four Indian seaports using sets of secondary data, i.e., cargo transshipment data of the year 2020. To obtain more insights into the results, they collect the opinions of some experts on the results.

Table 6. Classification of studies on the impact of COVID-19 based on research method.

Main Method Category	Number of Studies per Main Method Category	Specific Method	Number of Studies per Specific Method	References
Empirical methods	8	Case studies	3	[30,34,44]
		Questionnaires and interviews	5	[32,35,44,49,53]
Quantitative methods	21	Secondary data analysis	15	[5,6,27–29,38,40,41,43,45,47,50–52,56]
		Regression models	4	[7–9,33]
		Forecasting models	3	[36,39,54]
		Analytical models	4	[11,31,42,55]
Literature review methods	1	Systematic review	1	[20]
Mixed methods	2	Questionnaires and second data analysis	1	[37]
		Review and second data analysis	1	[48]

4.1.4. Research Gaps and Trends for Future Research

Reviewing the 36 studies shows a variety of interesting paths for future research as follows:

- Since most reviewed studies focus on the peak period of the COVID-19 pandemic (January–June 2020), more research is needed to analyze the impacts of COVID-19 on each transport mode, starting from the beginning of the so-called "new norm" (July 2020). This will identify the strengths and weaknesses of each transport mode under the different "new norm" policies adopted to reopen society. It is also of great importance to qualify the analysis with some statistics showing how different "new norm" policies affect the KPIs of the individual transport modes. This will support policymakers and practitioners in learning from past events and in formulating better policies for unexpected future pandemics.
- There is a lack of studies investigating the impacts of COVID-19 on freight transport in developing countries. Therefore, further research may evaluate the impacts of COVID-19 on freight transport in developing countries and compare them with those in developed countries. Additionally, it may be relevant to compare different control measures implemented by these countries and to assess the impacts of these measures on the performances of freight transport.
- Many studies report severe pressure exerted by the pandemic on city logistics [6,8,11,27]. Therefore, future research may examine the resilience of specific city logistics initiatives, e.g., smart lockers, collection points, etc., during the early and "new norm" periods of the pandemic, where new buying habits of consumers emerge and will need more resilient and efficient urban logistics. This will help policymakers and practitioners in defining better initiatives and relaxing resisting regulations for possibly occurring waves of the pandemic.
- Some studies propose prediction models for evaluating the impacts of COVID-19 on freight transport performances during 2020 [36,39,54]. Future research may extend these studies by comparing the predicted results with the actual results. Furthermore, it is relevant to develop a better understanding of the main factors that may lead to any deviations between both results. This is expected to guide researchers in developing more robust prediction models for future unexpected pandemics.
- Most studies evaluate the economic impact of the pandemic on freight transport while very few studies study the social and environmental impacts [5,28,38,56]. Therefore, future research may be directed at measuring the social and environmental impacts of the pandemic on individual freight transport modes in general, and urban freight deliveries in particular. Furthermore, existing studies use only traffic data in estimating the carbon emissions from freight transport during the pandemic. Hence, future research may give a complete picture by calculating the reduction in CO_2 emissions concerned with the utilization of different transport facilities and infrastructure.

- Most studies provide pieces of evidence of the impacts of COVID-19 based on data analysis from a macro perspective [5,6,27–29,38,45,56]. Therefore, future research may adopt various methods based on empirical data analysis from a micro perspective to develop more managerial insights by answering several questions of interest, for example:
    1. What are the short- and long-term impacts of the pandemic on different KPIs of logistics companies?
    2. What are the causal relationships among the various impacts of the COVID-19 pandemic?
    3. How do the impacts of the COVID-19 pandemic vary among logistics companies handling different freight or serving different industrial sectors?
    4. How can logistics companies deal with the pandemic and to what extent do support policies from the governments help them to alleviate the impact of COVID-19?
- Further avenues for future research may address developing simulation models to evaluate the long-term effects of different pandemic control policies on freight transport modes. This can have a significant value for policymakers, since the pandemic is still ongoing and will probably have multiple waves caused by new virus variants. In developing models, researchers can greatly benefit from the findings of the literature on the early stage of the pandemic.

4.2. COVID-19-Related Mitigation Strategies

In response to the current pandemic, some studies propose various mitigation strategies to minimize the impact of COVID-19 on the different modes of freight transport. By accurately investigating existing literature, we notice a limited number of studies, around 20 studies, discussing mitigation strategies. These strategies include (1) usage of autonomous delivery vehicles (ADVs), (2) deployment of drone delivery, (3) relaxing existing regulations, (4) utilization of mobile warehouses, (5) engagement of large ships, (6) applying quantity discounts, (7) capacity augmentation, and (8) mixed strategies. Table 7 summarizes the mitigation strategies discussed in the literature, and the impacts to be mitigated. As in the previous section, the studies identified here are classified according to the mitigation strategy, transport mode, and the research methodology. In the last subsection, the research gaps, along with future research directions, are elaborated.

Table 7. Mitigation strategies for minimizing the impact of COVID-19.

COVID-19-Related Mitigation Strategies	Impact to Be Mitigated	Studies per Strategy	References
Usage of autonomous delivery vehicles	Driver capacity shortage, emissions	6	[10,63–67]
Deployment of drone delivery	Driver capacity shortage, delivery performance, emissions	5	[68–72]
Relaxing existing regulations	Capacity shortage and operating cost	3	[8,59,60]
Utilization of mobile warehouses	Delivery performance	1	[11]
Engagement of large ships	Container capacity shortage	1	[73]
Application of quantity discounts	Demand for freight transport service	1	[74]
Capacity augmentation	Driver capacity shortage, delivery performance	2	[75,76]
Mixed strategies	Driver capacity shortage, delivery performance, emissions	1	[77]

4.2.1. Mitigation Strategies

- Usage of autonomous delivery vehicles (ADVs):

ADVs are self-driving electric ground vehicles that travel at a restricted speed, around 5–10 km/h on roadways or sidewalks. Using ADVs as a mitigation strategy can reduce the impact of driver capacity shortage, as ADVs are self-driving vehicles, and enhance the positive impact of emission reduction, as ADVs move at a low speed releasing a small amount of CO_2. There are six studies that focus on ADVs as a mitigation strategy on road freight transport. Kapser, Abdelrahman and Bernecker [63] investigate user acceptance of ADVs during COVID-19 through the acceptance unified theory. This study is conducted based on real data collected from Germany using online questionnaires. Findings reveal that the user acceptance rate is slightly low, due to a high shipment cost resulting from the expensive technology used in ADVs. Similar to Kapser, Abdelrahman and Bernecker [63], Pani, Mishra, Golias and Figliozzi [67] study the public acceptance of ADVs, but in Portland, USA. Based on a sample of 483 consumers, results indicate that the majority of US consumers, around 61.28%, are willing to pay extra to receive their goods using ADVs. Chen, Demir, Huang and Qiu [10] discuss the idea of food delivery using a traditional vehicle along with robots to serve customers in the last miles. This study shows the efficiency of using these robots in minimizing the contact between the customers and drivers. Besides delivering food products, as shown in the previous studies, Ozkan and Atli [66] present the usage of ADVs in transporting PCR testing samples between hospitals and laboratories. To this end, a mathematical model is presented as a mixed-integer linear programming model (MILP), considering the payload of the ADVs. Using a real case in Istanbul, including 219 hospitals and 23 laboratories, the proposed model shows its efficiency in transporting around 25,000 samples.

Although some studies focus on the usage of ADVs to mitigate the impact of driver shortage capacity, other studies evaluated the usage of ADVs to mitigate the impact of gas emission of traditional vehicles. Li, He, Keoleian, Kim, De Kleine, Wallington and Kemp [64] study the greenhouse gas emission of automated vehicles (last mile) assisted with robots (last 50 feet) used for last-mile delivery. Their results show the outperformance of the automated vehicles with robots over the traditional option (traditional vehicle with human for final delivery) in minimizing the gas emissions.

ADVs are also technically discussed, especially the hardware design. Liu, Liao, Gan, Ma, Cheng, Xie, Wang, Chen, Zhu, Zhang, Chen, Liu, Xie, Yu, Guo, Li, Yuan, Han, Chen, Ye, Jiao, Yun, Xu, Wang, Huang, Wang, Cai, Sun, Liu, Wang and Liu [65] assess the design of the hardware of ADVs, particularly the chassis and autonomous driving-related devices. Based on a real case study containing 25 ADVs, these ADVs are successful to run a total distance of 2500 km, satisfying 676 delivery tasks.

- Deployment of drone delivery

Technically, drones are teleoperated flying machines that do not need continual operator control. In real practice, drones often fly using batteries, which help in carrying goods. These features have attracted the attention of some companies such as UPS and AMAZON to use drones for delivery [78]. This inspires the usage of drones as a mitigation strategy to reduce the impact of driver capacity shortage, improve the impact of delivery performance, as drones are fast transport means, and enhance the positive impact of emission reduction, as drones do not emit CO_2. Four studies in the literature report the usage of drone delivery as an alternative to road freight transport. Kunovjanek and Wankmüller [69] study the viability of using existing drone infrastructure to deliver COVID-19 viral test to infected people in Australia. This study reveals the viability of using the drone in terms of time and financial measures. However, transport policy needs to be relaxed to permit widespread usage of this service. It is somewhat challenging to establish a legal framework for this service. Alsamhi, Lee, Guizani, Kumar, Qiao and Liu [68] introduce a conceptual framework of integrating blockchain with drone delivery. With the help of a consensus algorithm, the blockchain is fruitful in easing the collaboration among multi-drones by sharing the delivery information among them. Thus, the delivery time is reduced, resulting in an improvement in delivery service. Yakushiji, Fujita, Murata, Hiroi, Hamabe and Yakushiji [71] assess the usage of drones to transport medical supplies in Japan during traffic blockages. Similarly, Quintanilla García, Vera Vélez, Alcaraz Martínez, Vidal Ull and Fernández Gallo [70] investigate the efficiency of using drones as extra support for healthcare logistics in Valencia, Spain. These studies indicate a successful application of drones in transporting medical goods without needing a dedicated infrastructure. Bathke,

C, x00Fc, nch, Gracht and Hartmann [72] assess some resilience strategies in the domain of maritime container shipping with the help of 51 maritime experts. The results indicate that picking the low-hanging fruit requires the deployment of drones to improve resilience in the maritime container shipping domain.

- Relaxing existing regulations

COVID-19 prevention and protective measures (e.g., multiple drivers are prevented from using the same truck) increased transport costs. Some countries, such as Canada, increased the maximum hours of service for drivers [60]. In response to air freight capacity shortages, passenger aircraft are granted exemptions from July 2020 to July 2021 to carry freight in the main cabin when no passengers are being carried [59]. To reduce the operating costs of logistics companies, some companies, e.g., in China, exempt logistics enterprises from vehicle tolls and value-added taxes on income due to delivering essential living supplies [8]. The European Union relaxed some rules of the competition law to allow competing companies to cooperate, which might help them overcome capacity shortages or better respond to disrupted supply channels [79].

- Utilization of mobile warehouse

The mobile warehouse is simply a truck that covers a specific geographical location, carrying an inventory of some products to be sold to the customers according to the demand of these products. Utilization of the mobile warehouse as a mitigation strategy mitigates the impact of delivery performance as the mobile warehouse reaches near the customers' locations. This strategy has not received much attention from researchers, with a single study reported in road freight transport. Srivatsa Srinivas and Marathe [11] are among the first to propose the utilization of mobile warehouses during COVID-19. Using such means can aid B2C e-commerce, which can minimize store congestion during COVID-19.

- Usage of large ships

The main rationale of using this strategy is to satisfy the high demand for goods with a fewer number of ship trips, limiting human movement, and, therefore, control the spread of COVID-19. In addition, using large ships as a mitigation strategy can reduce the impact of container capacity shortage, as using large ships can fix the problem of returning empty containers to the importing companies. This strategy is discussed in the study by Pasha, Dulebenets, Fathollahi-Fard, Tian, Lau, Singh and Liang [73], who develop a mathematical model to determine the service frequency and ship sailing speed and schedules. By using 10 real cases, the proposed strategy demonstrates its efficiency in satisfying food demand while improving the total turnaround profit by approximately 22.94%.

- Application of quantity discount

Due to COVID-19, cargo demand in some routes is disrupted (e.g., demand in some routes exceeds the capacity of the aircraft (hot selling), whereas the demand in other routes is not sufficient to fill the aircraft capacity (underutilized)). This disruption results in a problem, called demand imbalance, or demand shortage for air freight transport. Shaban, Chan and Chung [74] propose a game-theoretic model to make a balance between the hot-selling and underutilized routes. The balance can be achieved by applying a quantity discount in the underutilized routes to attract some demand from hot-selling routes, ultimately leading to fixing the imbalance. To summarize, using this strategy can help to mitigate the impact of demand shortage for air freight transport.

- Capacity augmentation

The main concept of this strategy is that, instead of reserving the normal capacity of the product, the logistics facilities temporarily increase their reserved capacity. This extra reserved capacity will help face disruptions that happen during COVID-19. Aloui, Hamani and Delahoche [75] study this strategy by proposing a two-stage stochastic mixed-integer programming model that helps make some decisions related to location-allocation, inventory, and routing planning. Schofer, Mahmassani and Ng [76] conduct in-depth interviews with Rail Intermodal Freight leaders to figure out how to efficiently enhance the resilience of the U.S. rail industry. The results of these interviews reveal the importance of capacity augmentation in improving the overall freight system performance.

- Mixed strategies

In the previous sub-sections, all the studies focus on applying a single strategy. However, some studies focus on studying more than one strategy. Simić, Lazarević and Dobrodolac [77] apply a fuzzy method to select the best transportation means among drones, ADVs, cargo bicycles, and Postmates for the last-mile delivery during COVID-19. By presenting a real case in Belgrade, results indicate that "postmates" is the best mode, followed by drones and ADVs.

4.2.2. Transport Mode and Research Methods

In this subsection, we classify the studies on mitigation strategies based on transport modes. Table 8 indicates that "road" has been extensively investigated by scholars in 14 studies. On the contrary, "air" and "seaport" modes are barely discussed in the literature, as they only appear in four studies. The road is the most commonly used mode of transport worldwide. Therefore, it is frequently investigated, which is also observed in the COVID-19 impact studies.

Table 8. Classification of COVID-19-related strategies studies based on transport mode.

Transport Mode (s)	Number of Studies per Transport Mode (s)	References
Road	14	[8,10,11,60,63–71,75–77]
Air	2	[59,74]
Seaport and waterways	2	[72,73]

The research methods used in the studies of mitigation strategies are also reviewed. For this purpose, these studies are divided into two categories: empirical and quantitative, such that each category is further sub-categorized to other methods, as shown in Table 9.

Table 9. Classification of studies on COVID-19-related strategies based on research method.

Main Method Category	Number of Studies per Main Method Category	Specific Method	Number of Studies per Specific Method	References
Empirical methods	10	Case studies	4	[59,64,70,71]
		Questionnaires and interviews	6	[8,60,63,67,72,76]
Quantitative methods	10	Optimization	5	[10,65,66,68,73]
		Simulation optimization	2	[69,75]
		Analytical model	1	[11]
		Fuzzy method	1	[77]
		Game theory	1	[74]

Table 9 reveals that both the quantitative method and empirical methods are equally used research methods, each one appearing in ten of the 20 studies. Indeed, for quantitative methods, five articles focus on optimization methods using different approaches such as two-stage meta-heuristics algorithm [10], CPLEX [66], deep-learning-based algorithms [65], and recursive route re-composition heuristic [73]. The remaining quantitative methods, including simulation optimization, analytical model, fuzzy method, and game theory, are explored in the rest of studies.

Empirical methods are discussed in 10 out of 17 articles. In particular, four studies use the case studies method. For instance, Li, He, Keoleian, Kim, De Kleine, Wallington and Kemp [64] present a case study to assess greenhouse gas emissions of automated vehicles. In addition, Yakushiji et al. [10] assess a real case study on flying drones to transport medical supplies. The other six studies rely on questionnaires and interviews to investigate user acceptance of ADVs [63,67] and assess the technologies that help increase resilience efficiency at maritime container shipping companies [72]. The limited number of empirical studies indicates that scholars are still faced with the challenges of acquiring and investigating real data. However, the existing empirical studies help to understand the attitudes of people towards the usage of new transportation tools such as ADVs and drones [63,67,71].

4.2.3. Research Gaps and Trends for Future Research Directions

After investigating the 20 articles, which focus on the mitigation strategies, some research gaps along with future research directions are identified as follows:

- There is a low user acceptance of ADVs in Germany [63]. Indeed, ADVs are still immature; therefore, the results presented in these studies are largely premature. Accordingly, more research is required to check the user acceptance of ADVs after the maturation phase. In addition, limited factors, such as age, gender, and citizen income, are considered in evaluating the user acceptance of ADVs [63]. To generalize these findings, more factors, such as delivery distance and time, need to be investigated. Besides Germany, user acceptance of ADVs has only been evaluated in Portland, USA [67]. The investigation is limited to a metropolitan area with small data size, restricting the knowledge of public acceptance of ADVs. In this connection, considering multiple US states with larger data set is imperative to test the public acceptance of ADVs. In addition, making the comparison between ADVs and drones is suggested to see the advantages and disadvantages of each transportation means.
- Robots have been shown to help in minimizing the contact between customers and drivers of traditional vehicles [10]. Here, the only drawback may include overlooking some features of the robots, such as energy consumption and operational cost, which are likely to limit a large-scale deployment of robots. Accordingly, these features should be incorporated in future research to arrive at a better assessment of the applicability of robots.
- Utilization of ADVs with robots is also asserted to minimize greenhouse gas emissions [64]. However, some considerations which are known to affect gas emissions, such as traffic and weather conditions, should be incorporated into future studies to accurately determine greenhouse gas emissions.
- The viability of using existing drone infrastructure, based on time and cost measures, has been verified in Australia [69]. However, many factors, such as legal visibility and opinion of policymakers, have not been considered. For a better verification process, these factors should be investigated in future research.
- Although drones have been used to transport medical supplies in Japan during traffic blockages, it has only been during favorable weather conditions, such as low wind speed and no rain [71]. Therefore, it is imperative to investigate the usage of drones in different weather conditions to further evaluate their applicability.
- Similarly, drones can successfully transport medical goods without the need of specialized infrastructure in Spain [70]. However, this application is accomplished only on a small scale. To enable a large-scale deployment, more investigation is needed.
- The deployment of mobile warehouses has been evaluated by Srivatsa Srinivas and Marathe [11]. Indeed, this study lacks an accurate estimation of product demand. For this purpose, we suggest using data analytic techniques to accurately estimate the product demand. In addition, this study overlooks the dynamic routing and parking optimization of the mobile warehouse. Therefore, investigating this overlooked optimization problem during COVID-19 could be another research direction.
- The deployment of large ships is efficient in satisfying food demand [73]. The main pitfalls of the study include ignoring fluctuations in demand, sea weather conditions, and sailing time of ships, that are typically experienced in real practice. In this connection, it is suggested to develop a stochastic model while considering all uncertain factors to accurately capture this reality.

- Applying quantity discounts appears in the study by Shaban, Chan and Chung [74] while considering deterministic demand. Since demand usually fluctuates, it will be more reliable to consider the stochastic demand while investigating quantity discounts. The planning horizon of the study is quite limited, around one month, which limits the generalization of the gained results. To avoid this situation, it is recommended to study a longer planning horizon (i.e., one year).
- Most studies have presented mitigation strategies for "road" mode, overlooking air and sea modes. Accordingly, more research is required to develop different mitigation strategies for air and sea modes.

4.3. Recoverability Measures Related to COVID-19

As stated earlier, the COVID-19 outbreak has had a great impact on freight transport. Therefore, a research stream has studied and evaluated this impact. Then, another search stream has studied measures aimed at counteracting the impact of COVID-19. So, several strategies and policies have been developed to mitigate these impacts. In addition, it is necessary to study the ability of freight transport to recover from the disruption of COVID-19. In this regard, this section summarizes the literature which have studied the measures of recovery of freight transport, during or after COVID-19. Although this stream is still limited and needs further work, there are 15 articles in the existing literature that have assessed various recovery measures using several research methodologies.

4.3.1. Recovery Measures

Few studies tackle the ability to recover in freight transport. However, they adopt different measures of recovery for freight transport, as shown in Table 10. These measures include quality, efficiency, sustainability, capacity, and rate of recovery. The quality as a recovery measure is investigated by Gnap, et al. [80], who consider the quality of transportation infrastructure as fundamental to strengthening the recovery of road traffic and high-speed trains after COVID-19. Likewise, Tardivo, et al. [81] conclude that the quality of the management system is the most important measure for recovery. However, both studies have not given numerical recovery solutions which can be used in the future to judge the resilience of freight transport. van Tatenhove [82] and Munawar, Khan, Qadir, Kouzani and Mahmud [6] adopt the efficiency measure to study the recovery of freight transport in Europe and Australia. Moreover, sustainability measures are used to study the recoverability of freight transport during COVID-19. Guo, et al. [83] adopt performance measurement techniques to study the recoverability of the aviation industry. Four studies have used at least one sustainability aspect. For example, the socioeconomic aspects are used to study the long-term impact and government role to contribute to the recovery from COVID-19 [84]. Additionally, the economic and environmental aspects are adopted to evaluate the recovery of road transport after the usage of plug-in electric vehicles [85]. Bartle, Lutte and Leuenberger [5] and Akyurek and Bolat [86] add the social measure to economic and environmental aspects to study the recovery in air transport. However, very limited research has tackled the capacity and the recovery rates as measures of recovery. Notteboom, et al. [87] study the adaptive capacity of container shipping lines. The authors compare the capacity of the sea shipping transportation to recover in the era of COVID-19 with the capacity used to recover during the economic crisis of 2008 to 2009. They claim that sea shipping is stable during COVID-19 because the shipping liners adjust their fleets when demand drops. Gudmundsson, et al. [88] and Cheong, et al. [89] evaluate the recovery rates of the air transportation profits and demand, respectively. However, using only one single measure to study the recovery is not enough to address the recoverability of any industry. A generic study used an integrated grey decision-making trial to rank the recovery-based sustainability measures for the freight industry regardless of transportation modes

Table 10. Summary of recovery measures.

Recovery Measure	Study per Measure	References
Quality	2	[80,81]
Efficiency	3	[6,82,90]
Performance	1	[83]
Sustainability	5	[5,84–86,91]
Capacity	2	[87,90,92]
Recovery rate	3	[88–90]

4.3.2. Research Methods and Transport Modes

This subsection discusses the research methods which have been used to study the recoverability of different transportation modes amid COVID-19. As shown in Table 11, 11 studies have adopted several research methods to explore the recoverability of different transport modes for freight transport. Although the number of articles is very limited on this topic, several methods, including empirical, quantitative, and mixed methods, have been used. For example, three empirical methods are adopted: one to create a framework for the future of a freight transport mode [5], one used a scenario-based approach [82], and another one used index-based evaluation techniques to measure the resilience of transportation mode(s) [90]. As for the quantitative methods, comparative analysis [86], forecasting the recovery of demand [88,92] and profit [89], have also been evaluated. The rest of the studies use mixed methods, such as simple data acquisition and experts' opinions, to assess the current status and comment on the possibility of recovery [84,87]. Nevertheless, data acquisition is not the only mixed method used; the analytical hierarchy process has also been used to integrate the economic and environmental criteria to evaluate public transportation systems [5,85].

Table 11. Classification of research methods based on the transportation mode.

Main Method Category	Number of Studies per Main Method Category	Specific Method	Transportation Mode			References
			Road and Railways	Seaports and Waterways	Air	
Empirical methods	3	Framework study			✓	[5]
		Scenario-based research		✓		[82]
		Index-based evaluation	✓			[90]
Quantitative methods	5	Forecasting	✓	✓	✓	[88,89,92]
		Comparative analysis	✓	✓	✓	[86,91]
Mixed methods	8	AHP multi-criteria decision making	✓		✓	[83,85]
		Correlation analysis	✓			[80]
		Data acquisition	✓	✓	✓	[5,6,81,84,87]

On the focus of transport modes, Table 11 shows that all the transport modes are almost equally studied, as each transport mode is studied by around three to four studies. This observation is contrary to the observation noticed in the impact and mitigation parts.

4.3.3. Research Gaps and Trends for Future Research

Although the COVID-19 pandemic has caused severe disruptions to the freight transport sector, the number of articles does not reflect the criticality of these disruptions. Additionally, the 11 studies examined here can be considered as an initial step towards the recoverability of freight transport, and some future directions can be recommended as follows:

Although there is no numerical evidence that the air transport mode is the most affected amongst the other modes, lockdown of international borders has significantly affected air transport. Most of the studies have focused on the amount of impact, but not many studies tackled the ways to recover after the lockdown. Therefore, more future work is still needed to enhance the recoverability of the air freight transport mode, not only for the post-COVID era but also for any unexpected long-term disruptions.

The continuous mutation of COVID-19 causes huge disruption in freight transport domestically and internationally. Therefore, further studies are suggested to study the recoverability of freight transportation and the way to improve the resilience of each mode is a great challenge to be considered.

Despite the fact that the existing studies have suggested different measures for recovery, a recovery index that uses multiple measures is required to evaluate the recoverability of freight transport. The recovery index may be developed either by freight transport modes in total or for each mode separately.

5. Conclusions

The existing review studies lacked a detailed analysis regarding freight transport during COVID-19. Therefore, this study contributed by conducting a comprehensive review in the domain of freight transport to identify some research gaps and propose future research directions. To do so, 68 studies were collected and analyzed using scientometric and systematic review approaches.

The scientometric analysis revealed that: (1) the combination of China, Hong Kong, and India published the highest number of papers on freight transport during COVID-19, whereas authors from Canada and the United States had the highest citations worldwide; (2) *Sustainability* (Switzerland) and *Science of Total Environment* were the top-cited journals, while the *Canadian Journal of Agricultural Economics* was the most influential journal in this research area. Lastly, the analysis of the keywords showed that "COVID-19", and "Freight transport" appeared frequently, reflecting the focus of researchers on these areas. Meanwhile, some keywords such as "Airline industry" and "Cargo" were rarely used, indicating the need for future research in these areas. The systematic review was carried out by categorizing the studies into three main themes, including impact-related studies, mitigation strategy-related studies, recoverability-related studies. The results reveal that the most studied theme was related to the impacts of COVID-19, followed by mitigation strategies, and then recoverability. Each theme was discussed alongside types and different transportation modes (i.e., road, air, and sea) and solution methods adopted.

Our review showed that 36 studies reported several impacts of the COVID-19 pandemic on freight transport. These impacts were categorized into five main groups, which included demand for freight transport services, transport capacity, operating cost, delivery performances, and carbon emissions. Surprisingly, not all reported impacts were negative. Negative impacts included, for example, reduced demand for transport services, higher operating costs, transport capacity shortages, delayed delivery, and difficulties in finding parking areas. On the contrary, some studies reported some positive impacts, such as increased availability of truck drivers and lower operating costs, increased demand for transport services, tax reductions on the service of logistics companies, fewer traffic jams, increased efficiency, and fewer emissions. Most of these studies discussed the demand-related impact, followed by impacts on operating transport, transport capacity, delivery performance, and carbon emissions. Regarding the transport mode, road freight transport and seaports were the most evaluated modes, followed by airfreight transport, while rail freight transport was rarely addressed. Regarding the employed research methodologies, the most frequently used methods were secondary data analysis, followed by questionnaires and interviews.

After reviewing 20 studies focusing on mitigation strategies, we observed eight types of mitigation strategies, including (1) usage of autonomous delivery vehicles (ADVs), (2) deployment of drone delivery, (3) relaxing existing regulations, (4) utilization of mobile warehouses, (5) engagement of large ships, (6) applying quantity discounts, (7) capacity augmentation, and (8) mixed strategies. It was noticed that the most studied strategy was the usage of ADVs with six studies, whereas the least studied strategies were strategies 4 to 8, with each strategy appearing in one or two studies. After that, the studies were classified based on the transport mode, with the most frequent transport mode in 14 studies being the road. The least frequent modes were air and seaport, each mode occurred in one or two studies. The last classification was based on the research method, such as empirical methods and quantitative methods. This classification indicated that both quantitative methods and empirical methods were equally used, such that each one appeared in ten studies.

In light of the undesirable impacts of pandemics and the mitigation strategies to overcome these impacts, it was necessary to study the recoverability of freight transport in its three modes. Nevertheless, only 15 studies covered the recoverability topic, discussing six recovery measures, such as quality, efficiency, sustainability, performance, capacity, and rate of recovery. Most of these studies, 5 out of 15 studies, focused on sustainability as a recovery measure, while little attention was paid to the rest of the recovery measures. In addition, the recoverability studies discussed all the transport modes with the same attention, as each transport mode was studied by an average of six studies. The recoverability studies were discussed using different research methods, such as empirical methods, quantitative methods, and mixed methods. It was observed that the most studied method was the mixed method (i.e., correlation analysis and data acquisition), which comprised approximately 8 out of 15 studies, while the rest of the methods received almost the same attention from scholars, from two to four studies for each method.

After reviewing the studies on the different themes, some future research directions were highlighted. Regarding the impact theme, studying the impacts of COVID-19 in developing countries was suggested. Focusing on the mitigation theme, more mitigation strategies were needed for air and seaport transport modes, as their related strategies were limited. Additionally, investigating dynamic routing and parking of mobile warehouses were suggested. Based on the recoverability theme, it was recommended to develop robust optimization models to deal with schedule disruptions and profit reduction. More detailed research gaps and future directions are represented in Figure 6.

Although the novelty of this study has been highlighted, it is, nevertheless, important to highlight some of its limitations. For instance, some scientometric analyses, such as the most prolific/active authors, were not provided to avoid making the study too long. Similarly, in the systematic review, we overlooked studies on freight transport before COVID-19. It might be interesting research to study freight transport before and during COVID-19.

Research Gaps	Impacts	Mitigation	Recoverability
	Future Directions		
Lack of studies focusing on the so-called "new norm" (July 2020)	Identify the strengths and weaknesses of each transport mode under the different "new norm" policies adopted to reopen society		
Lack of studies researching the COVID-related impacts in developing countries.	Comparing different control measures implemented by these countries and to measure the impacts of these measures on the performances of freight transport.		
Lack of studies examining the resilience of specific city-logistics initiatives	Examining the resilience of specific city logistics initiatives, e.g., smart lockers, collection points, etc., during the early and "new norm" periods of the pandemic		
Validating the prediction models proposed for the end of the year 2020	Comparing the predicted results with the actual results to develop a better understanding of the main factors that led to any deviations between both results.		
Existing studies used only traffic data in estimating the carbon emissions from freight transport during the pandemic	Developing a complete picture by calculating the reduction in CO_2 emissions concerned with the utilization of different transport facilities and infrastructure		
Most evidences of COVID impacts are based on macro perspective	Adoption of various methods based on empirical data analysis from a micro perspective		
Using limited factors while discussing the acceptance of ADVs		Delivery distance and time need to be considered	
Overlooking energy consumption and operational cost while using robots		Energy consumption and operational cost of robots are imperative considerations to improve the applicability of robots	
Ignoring traffic and weather conditions while discussing greenhouse gas emissions of ADVs with robots		Traffic and weather conditions are suggested considerations to accurately determine greenhouse gas emissions	
Ignoring many aspects while assessing the viability of using the existing drone infrastructe		More aspects need to be considered, such as legal visibility and the opinion of policymaker	
Studying drone delivery during limited conditions		Different weather conditions need to be investigated while using drone delivery	
Lack of accurate estimation of product demand delivered by mobile warehouse		Adoption of data analytic techniques to accurately estimate product demand	
Overlooking dynamic routing and packing optimzation of mobile warehouses		Investigate the dynamic routing and parking of mobile warehouses using stochastic programming approach	
Ignoring the demand fluctuations, sea weather conditions and sailing time of large ships		Develop a stochastic model considering all uncertain factors	
Limited mitigation strategies in the modes of air and sea transport modes		More mitigation strategies are needed for air and seaport transport modes	
Existing recoverability models use sole factor			A single-index multidimensional recovery model is recommended
No studies tackle the disruption due to the different COVID-19 mutations			Robust optimization models are required to deal with schedule disruptions, profit reduction, etc.
Lack of recoverability models after the lock down			Proactive actions and models should be developed to improve the recoverability and resilience of freight transport modes, not only after COVID-19, but also until the disrupting event ends

Figure 6. Research gaps and future directions matrix.

Author Contributions: Idea for the article: A.K.; Literature search and bibliometric data filtration: A.K. and I.A.S.; Scientometric analysis: I.A.S. and A.E.E.E.; Writing and drafting: A.K., A.E.E.E., E.-A.A. and I.A.S.; Critical revision of the work: A.K., A.E.E.E. and E.-A.A.; Funding acquisition: A.K. and E.-A.A. All authors have read and agreed to the published version of the manuscript.

Funding: This research received no external funding.

Institutional Review Board Statement: Not applicable.

Informed Consent Statement: Not applicable.

Data Availability Statement: The search queries used in Scopus during the study are available from the corresponding authors on reasonable requests.

Acknowledgments: This study was supported by the Danish Research Center for Freight Transport, Aalborg University.

Conflicts of Interest: The authors declare that they have no known competing financial interests or personal relationships that could have appeared to influence the work reported in this paper.

References

1. IATA. Air Cargo Capacity Crunch: Demand Plummets but Capacity Disappears Even Faster. 2020. Available online: https://www.iata.org/en/pressroom/pr/2020-06-02-01/ (accessed on 19 December 2021).
2. Maneenop, S.; Kotcharin, S. The impacts of COVID-19 on the global airline industry: An event study approach. *J. Air Transp. Manag.* **2020**, *89*, 101920. [CrossRef] [PubMed]
3. IRU. COVID-19 Impact on the Road Transport Industry. 2020. Available online: https://www.itf-oecd.org/sites/default/files/docs/covid-19_impact_on_the_road_transport_industry_-_june_2021.pdf (accessed on 20 October 2021).
4. Millefiori, L.M.; Braca, P.; Zissis, D.; Spiliopoulos, G.; Marano, S.; Willett, P.K.; Carniel, S. COVID-19 impact on global maritime mobility. *Sci. Rep.* **2021**, *11*, 18039. [CrossRef] [PubMed]
5. Bartle, J.R.; Lutte, R.K.; Leuenberger, D.Z. Sustainability and air freight transportation: Lessons from the global pandemic. *Sustainability* **2021**, *13*, 3738. [CrossRef]
6. Munawar, H.S.; Khan, S.I.; Qadir, Z.; Kouzani, A.Z.; Mahmud, M.A.P. Insight into the impact of COVID-19 on Australian transportation sector: An economic and community-based perspective. *Sustainability* **2021**, *13*, 1276. [CrossRef]
7. Michail, N.A.; Melas, K.D. Shipping markets in turmoil: An analysis of the COVID-19 outbreak and its implications. *Transp. Res. Interdiscip. Perspect.* **2020**, *7*, 100178. [CrossRef]
8. Yang, S.; Ning, L.; Jiang, T.; He, Y. Dynamic impacts of COVID-19 pandemic on the regional express logistics: Evidence from China. *Transp. Policy* **2021**, *111*, 111–124. [CrossRef]
9. Tianming, G.; Erokhin, V.; Arskiy, A.; Khudzhatov, M. Has the COVID-19 pandemic affected maritime connectivity? An estimation for China and the polar silk road countries. *Sustainability* **2021**, *13*, 3521. [CrossRef]
10. Chen, C.; Demir, E.; Huang, Y.; Qiu, R. The adoption of self-driving delivery robots in last mile logistics. *Transp. Res. Part E Logist. Transp. Rev.* **2021**, *146*, 102214. [CrossRef]
11. Srinivas, S.S.; Marathe, R.R. Moving towards "mobile warehouse": Last-mile logistics during COVID-19 and beyond. *Transp. Res. Interdiscip. Perspect.* **2021**, *10*, 100339. [CrossRef]
12. Mamani, H.; Chick, S.E.; Simchi-Levi, D. A Game-Theoretic Model of International Influenza Vaccination Coordination. *Manag. Sci.* **2013**, *59*, 1650–1670. [CrossRef]
13. Anparasan, A.; Lejeune, M. Analyzing the response to epidemics: Concept of evidence-based Haddon matrix. *J. Humanit. Logist. Supply Chain Manag.* **2017**, *7*, 266–283. [CrossRef]
14. Büyüktahtakın, İ.E.; des-Bordes, E.; Kıbış, E.Y. A new epidemics–logistics model: Insights into controlling the Ebola virus disease in West Africa. *Eur. J. Oper. Res.* **2018**, *265*, 1046–1063. [CrossRef]
15. Parvin, H.; Beygi, S.; Helm, J.E.; Larson, P.S.; van Oyen, M.P. Distribution of Medication Considering Information, Transshipment, and Clustering: Malaria in Malawi. *Prod. Oper. Manag.* **2018**, *27*, 774–797. [CrossRef]
16. Dasaklis, T.K.; Pappis, C.P.; Rachaniotis, N.P. Epidemics control and logistics operations: A review. *Int. J. Prod. Econ.* **2012**, *139*, 393–410. [CrossRef]
17. Queiroz, M.M.; Ivanov, D.; Dolgui, A.; Wamba, S.F. Impacts of epidemic outbreaks on supply chains: Mapping a research agenda amid the COVID-19 pandemic through a structured literature review. *Ann. Oper. Res.* **2020**, *291*, 504–518. [CrossRef]
18. Yuen, K.F.; Wang, X.; Ma, F.; Li, K.X. The Psychological Causes of Panic Buying Following a Health Crisis. *Int. J. Environ. Res. Public Health* **2020**, *17*, 3513. [CrossRef]
19. Chowdhury, P.; Paul, S.K.; Kaisar, S.; Moktadir, M.A. COVID-19 pandemic related supply chain studies: A systematic review. *Transp. Res. Part E Logist. Transp. Rev.* **2021**, *148*, 102271. [CrossRef]
20. Borca, B.; Putz, L.M.; Hofbauer, F. Crises and Their Effects on Freight Transport Modes: A Literature Review and Research Framework. *Sustainability* **2021**, *13*, 5740. [CrossRef]

21. Hussein, M.; Eltoukhy, A.E.E.; Karam, A.; Shaban, I.A.; Zayed, T. Modelling in off-site construction supply chain management: A review and future directions for sustainable modular integrated construction. *J. Clean. Prod.* **2021**, *310*, 127503. (In English) [CrossRef]
22. Hofmann, M.; Chisholm, A. *Text Mining and Visualization: Case Studies Using Open-Source Tools*; CRC Press: Boca Raton, FL, USA, 2016.
23. Meyer, T. Decarbonizing road freight transportation—A bibliometric and network analysis. *Transp. Res. Part D Transp. Environ.* **2020**, *89*, 102619. [CrossRef]
24. Eltoukhy, A.E.E.; Shaban, I.A.; Chan, F.T.S.; Abdel-Aal, M.A.M. Data Analytics for Predicting COVID-19 Cases in Top Affected Countries: Observations and Recommendations. *Int. J. Environ. Res. Public Health* **2020**, *17*, 7080. [CrossRef]
25. Van Eck, N.J.; Waltman, L. Software survey: VOSviewer, a computer program for bibliometric mapping. *Scientometrics* **2010**, *84*, 523–538. [CrossRef] [PubMed]
26. Smith, M.L. Regulating law enforcement's use of drones: The need for state legislation. *Harv. J. Legis.* **2015**, *52*, 423. [CrossRef]
27. Villa, R.; Monzón, A. Mobility restrictions and e-commerce: Holistic balance in madrid centre during COVID-19 lockdown. *Economies* **2021**, *9*, 57. [CrossRef]
28. Arellana, J.; Márquez, L.; Cantillo, V. COVID-19 Outbreak in Colombia: An Analysis of Its Impacts on Transport Systems. *J. Adv. Transp.* **2020**, *2020*, 8867316. [CrossRef]
29. Bartuska, L.; Masek, J. Changes in road traffic caused by the declaration of a state of emergency in the czech republic-a case study. *Transp. Res. Procedia* **2021**, *53*, 321–328. [CrossRef]
30. Cruz, C.O.; Sarmento, J.M. The impact of COVID-19 on highway traffic and management: The case study of an operator perspective. *Sustainability* **2021**, *13*, 5320. [CrossRef]
31. Cui, Q.; He, L.; Liu, Y.; Zheng, Y.; Wei, W.; Yang, B.; Zhou, M. The impacts of COVID-19 pandemic on China's transport sectors based on the CGE model coupled with a decomposition analysis approach. *Transp. Policy* **2021**, *103*, 103–115. [CrossRef]
32. Gray, R.S. Agriculture, transportation, and the COVID-19 crisis. *Can. J. Agric. Econ.* **2020**, *68*, 239–243. [CrossRef]
33. Ho, S.J.; Xing, W.; Wu, W.; Lee, C.C. The impact of COVID-19 on freight transport: Evidence from China. *MethodsX* **2021**, *8*, 101200. [CrossRef]
34. Li, T. A SWOT analysis of China's air cargo sector in the context of COVID-19 pandemic. *J. Air Transp. Manag.* **2020**, *88*, 101875. [CrossRef] [PubMed]
35. Liu, W.; Liang, Y.; Bao, X.; Qin, J.; Lim, M.K. China's logistics development trends in the post COVID-19 era. *Int. J. Logist. Res. Appl.* **2020**, *25*, 1–12. [CrossRef]
36. Meng, F.; Gong, W.; Liang, J.; Li, X.; Zeng, Y.; Yang, L. Impact of different control policies for COVID-19 outbreak on the air transportation industry: A comparison between China, the U.S. And Singapore. *PLoS ONE* **2021**, *16*, e0248361. [CrossRef] [PubMed]
37. Narasimha, P.T.; Jena, P.R.; Majhi, R. Impact of COVID-19 on the Indian seaport transportation and maritime supply chain. *Transp. Policy* **2021**, *110*, 191–203. [CrossRef]
38. Nižetić, S. Impact of coronavirus (COVID-19) pandemic on air transport mobility, energy, and environment: A case study. *Int. J. Energy Res.* **2020**, *44*, 10953–10961. [CrossRef]
39. Stanivuk, T. Impact of SARS-CoV-2 virus on Maritime Traffic in the Port of Ploce. *European Transport.* **2021**, *82*, 13. [CrossRef]
40. Statista. *COVID-19: Traffic Reduction in Selected Countries Worldwide*; Statista: Hamburg, Germany, 2020.
41. Jin, L.; Chen, J.; Chen, Z.; Sun, X.; Yu, B. Impact of COVID-19 on China's international liner shipping network based on AIS data. *Transp. Policy* **2022**, *121*, 90–99. [CrossRef]
42. Li, Q.; Bai, Q.; Hu, A.; Yu, Z.; Yan, S. How Does COVID-19 Affect Traffic on Highway Network: Evidence from Yunnan Province, China. *J. Adv. Transp.* **2022**, *2022*, 7379334. [CrossRef]
43. Fang, D.; Guo, Y. Flow of goods to the shock of COVID-19 and toll-free highway policy: Evidence from logistics data in China. *Res. Transp. Econ.* **2022**, *93*, 101185. [CrossRef]
44. Aftab, R.; Naveed, M.; Hanif, S. An analysis of COVID-19 implications for SMEs in Pakistan. *J. Chin. Econ. Foreign Trade Stud.* **2021**, *14*, 74–88. [CrossRef]
45. Hobbs, J.E. Food supply chains during the COVID-19 pandemic. *Can. J. Agric. Econ.* **2020**, *68*, 171–176. [CrossRef]
46. Loske, D. The impact of COVID-19 on transport volume and freight capacity dynamics: An empirical analysis in German food retail logistics. *Transp. Res. Interdiscip. Perspect.* **2020**, *6*, 100165. [CrossRef]
47. Shih, W. COVID-19 And Global Supply Chains: Watch Out For Bullwhip Effects. *Forbes*, 21 February 2020.
48. Xu, Z.; Elomri, A.; Kerbache, L.; el Omri, A. Impacts of COVID-19 on Global Supply Chains: Facts and Perspectives. *IEEE Eng. Manag. Rev.* **2020**, *48*, 153–166. [CrossRef]
49. Hilmola, O.P.; Lähdeaho, O.; Henttu, V.; Hilletofth, P. COVID-19 pandemic: Early implications for north european manufacturing and logistics. *Sustainability* **2020**, *12*, 8315. [CrossRef]
50. IATA. *Industry Losses to Top $84 Billion in 2020*; International Air Transport Association: Montreal, QC, Canada, 2020.
51. IATA. *Fuel Price Monitor*; International Air Transport Association: Montreal, QC, Canada, 2021.
52. Grzelakowski, A. The COVID 19 pandemic–challenges for maritime transport and global logistics supply chains. *TransNav Int. J. Mar. Navig. Saf. Sea Transp.* **2022**, *16*, 71–77. [CrossRef]
53. ATRI; OOIDA. *COVID-19 Impact on Trucking Industry*; American Transportation Research Institute: Arlington, VA, USA, 2020.

54. Koyuncu, K.; Tavacioğlu, L.; Gökmen, N.; Arican, U.Ç. Forecasting COVID-19 impact on RWI/ISL container throughput index by using SARIMA models. *Marit. Policy Manag.* **2021**, *48*, 1096–1108. [CrossRef]
55. Özden, A.T.; Celik, E. Analyzing the service quality priorities in cargo transportation before and during the COVID-19 outbreak. *Transp. Policy* **2021**, *108*, 34–46. [CrossRef]
56. Han, P.; Cai, Q.; Oda, T.; Zeng, N.; Shan, Y.; Lin, X.; Liu, D. Assessing the recent impact of COVID-19 on carbon emissions from China using domestic economic data. *Sci. Total Environ.* **2021**, *750*, 141688. [CrossRef]
57. Statista. *COVID-19 Impact Retail E-Commerce Site Traffic*; Statista: Hamburg, Germany, 2020.
58. OECD. *E-Commerce in the Time of COVID-19*; Organisation for Economic Co-operation and Development: Paris, France, 2020.
59. IATA. *Keeping Air Cargo Flying*; International Air Transport Association: Montreal, QC, Canada, 2020.
60. Ahart, M. Canada Issues Hours-of-Service Exemption for COVID-19 Relief. *Omnitracks*, 26 March 2020.
61. Statista. *Lowest Crude Oil Prices due to COVID-19 2020*; Statista: Hamburg, Germany, 2020.
62. Carrington, D. UK Road Travel Falls to 1955 Levels as COVID-19 Lockdown Takes Hold. *The Guardian*, 3 April 2020.
63. Kapser, S.; Abdelrahman, M.; Bernecker, T. Autonomous delivery vehicles to fight the spread of COVID-19—How do men and women differ in their acceptance? *Transp. Res. Part A Policy Pract.* **2021**, *148*, 183–198. [CrossRef]
64. Li, L.; He, X.; Keoleian, G.A.; Kim, H.C.; De Kleine, R.; Wallington, T.J.; Kemp, N.J. J. Life Cycle Greenhouse Gas Emissions for Last-Mile Parcel Delivery by Automated Vehicles and Robots. *Environ. Sci. Technol.* **2021**, *55*, 11360–11367. [CrossRef]
65. Liu, T.; Liao, Q.; Gan, L.; Ma, F.; Cheng, J.; Xie, X.; Liu, M. The Role of the Hercules Autonomous Vehicle During the COVID-19 Pandemic: An Autonomous Logistic Vehicle for Contactless Goods Transportation. *IEEE Robot. Autom. Mag.* **2021**, *28*, 48–58. [CrossRef]
66. Ozkan, O.; Atli, O. Transporting COVID-19 testing specimens by routing unmanned aerial vehicles with range and payload constraints: The case of Istanbul. *Transp. Lett.* **2021**, *13*, 482–491. [CrossRef]
67. Pani, A.; Mishra, S.; Golias, M.; Figliozzi, M. Evaluating public acceptance of autonomous delivery robots during COVID-19 pandemic. *Transp. Res. Part D Transp. Environ.* **2020**, *89*, 102600. [CrossRef]
68. Alsamhi, S.H.; Lee, B.; Guizani, M.; Kumar, N.; Qiao, Y.; Liu, X. Blockchain for decentralized multi-drone to combat COVID-19 and future pandemics: Framework and proposed solutions. *Trans. Emerg. Telecommun. Technol.* **2021**, *32*, e4255. [CrossRef]
69. Kunovjanek, M.; Wankmüller, C. Containing the COVID-19 pandemic with drones—Feasibility of a drone enabled back-up transport system. *Transp. Policy* **2021**, *106*, 141–152. [CrossRef]
70. Quintanilla García, I.; Vera Vélez, N.; Alcaraz Martínez, P.; Vidal Ull, J.; Fernández Gallo, B. A Quickly Deployed and UAS-Based Logistics Network for Delivery of Critical Medical Goods during Healthcare System Stress Periods: A Real Use Case in Valencia (Spain). *Drones* **2021**, *5*, 13. [CrossRef]
71. Yakushiji, K.; Fujita, H.; Murata, M.; Hiroi, N.; Hamabe, Y.; Yakushiji, F. Short-Range Transportation Using Unmanned Aerial Vehicles (UAVs) during Disasters in Japan. *Drones* **2020**, *4*, 68. [CrossRef]
72. Bathke, H.; Münch, C.; Heiko, A.; Hartmann, E. Building Resilience Through Foresight: The Case of Maritime Container Shipping Firms. *IEEE Trans. Eng. Manag.* **2022**, *69*, 1–23. [CrossRef]
73. Pasha, J.; Dulebenets, M.A.; Fathollahi-Fard, A.M.; Tian, G.; Lau, Y.Y.; Singh, P.; Liang, B. An integrated optimization method for tactical-level planning in liner shipping with heterogeneous ship fleet and environmental considerations. *Adv. Eng. Inform.* **2021**, *48*, 101299. [CrossRef]
74. Shaban, I.A.; Chan, F.T.S.; Chung, S.H. A novel model to manage air cargo disruptions caused by global catastrophes such as COVID-19. *J. Air Transp. Manag.* **2021**, *95*, 102086. [CrossRef]
75. Aloui, A.; Hamani, N.; Delahoche, L. Designing a Resilient and Sustainable Logistics Network under Epidemic Disruptions and Demand Uncertainty. *Sustainability* **2021**, *13*, 14053. [CrossRef]
76. Schofer, J.L.; Mahmassani, H.S.; Ng, M.T.M. Resilience of U.S. Rail Intermodal Freight during the COVID-19 Pandemic. *Res. Transp. Bus. Manag.* **2022**, *43*, 100791. [CrossRef]
77. Simić, V.; Lazarević, D.; Dobrodolac, M. Picture fuzzy WASPAS method for selecting last-mile delivery mode: A case study of Belgrade. *Eur. Transp. Res. Rev.* **2021**, *13*, 43. [CrossRef]
78. Shavarani, S.M.; Nejad, M.G.; Rismanchian, F.; Izbirak, G. Application of hierarchical facility location problem for optimization of a drone delivery system: A case study of Amazon prime air in the city of San Francisco. *Int. J. Adv. Manuf. Technol.* **2018**, *95*, 3141–3153. [CrossRef]
79. EUR-Lex. Available online: https://eur-lex.europa.eu/legal-content/EN/TXT/?uri=CELEX:52020XC0408(04) (accessed on 10 September 2022).
80. Gnap, J.; Senko, Š.; Kostrzewski, M.; Brídziková, M.; Cződörová, R.; Říha, Z. Research on the Relationship between Transport Infrastructure and Performance in Rail and Road Freight Transport—A Case Study of Japan and Selected European Countries. *Sustainability* **2021**, *13*, 6654. [CrossRef]
81. Tardivo, A.; Zanuy, A.C.; Martín, C.S. COVID-19 Impact on Transport: A Paper from the Railways' Systems Research Perspective. *Transp. Res. Rec.* **2021**, *2675*, 367–378. [CrossRef]
82. Van Tatenhove, J.P.M. COVID-19 and European maritime futures: Different pathways to deal with the pandemic. *Marit. Stud.* **2021**, *20*, 63–74. [CrossRef]
83. Guo, J.; Zhu, X.; Liu, C.; Ge, S. Resilience Modeling Method of Airport Network Affected by Global Public Health Events. *Math. Probl. Eng.* **2021**, *2021*, 6622031. [CrossRef]

84. Oyenuga, A. Perspectives on the impact of the COVID-19 pandemic on the global and African maritime transport sectors, and the potential implications for Africa's maritime governance. *WMU J. Marit. Aff.* **2021**, *20*, 215–245. [CrossRef]
85. Rivero Gutiérrez, L.; De Vicente Oliva, M.A.; Romero-Ania, A. Managing Sustainable Urban Public Transport Systems: An AHP Multicriteria Decision Model. *Sustainability* **2021**, *13*, 4614. [CrossRef]
86. Akyurek, E.; Bolat, P. Port state control at European Union under pandemic outbreak. *Eur. Transp. Res. Rev.* **2020**, *12*, 66. [CrossRef]
87. Notteboom, T.; Pallis, T.; Rodrigue, J.-P. Disruptions and resilience in global container shipping and ports: The COVID-19 pandemic versus the 2008–2009 financial crisis. *Marit. Econ. Logist.* **2021**, *23*, 179–210. [CrossRef]
88. Gudmundsson, S.V.; Cattaneo, M.; Redondi, R. Forecasting temporal world recovery in air transport markets in the presence of large economic shocks: The case of COVID-19. *J. Air Transp. Manag.* **2021**, *91*, 102007. [CrossRef]
89. Cheong, M.L.; Chong, U.M.; Nguyen, A.N.; Ang, S.Y.; Djojosaputro, G.P.; Adiprasetyo, G.; Gadong, K.L. *Singapore Airlines: Profit Recovery and Aircraft Allocation Models during the COVID-19 Pandemic*; Singapore Management University: Singapore, 2021.
90. Fu, X.; Qiang, Y.; Liu, X.; Jiang, Y.; Cui, Z.; Zhang, D.; Wang, J. Will multi-industry supply chains' resilience under the impact of COVID-19 pandemic be different? A perspective from China's highway freight transport. *Transp. Policy* **2022**, *118*, 165–178. [CrossRef]
91. Dwivedi, A.; Shardeo, V.; Patil, A. Analysis of recovery measures for sustainable freight transportation. *J. Asia Bus. Stud.* **2022**, *16*, 495–514. [CrossRef]
92. Nguyen, H.K. Application of Mathematical Models to Assess the Impact of the COVID-19 Pandemic on Logistics Businesses and Recovery Solutions for Sustainable Development. *Mathematics* **2021**, *9*, 1977. [CrossRef]

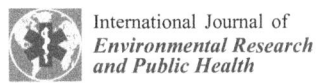

International Journal of
Environmental Research and Public Health

Article

Assessing the Nationwide COVID-19 Risk in Mexico through the Lens of Comorbidity by an XGBoost-Based Logistic Regression Model

Sonia Venancio-Guzmán [1], Alejandro Ivan Aguirre-Salado [1,*], Carlos Soubervielle-Montalvo [2] and José del Carmen Jiménez-Hernández [1]

1 Institute of Physics and Mathematics, Universidad Tecnológica de la Mixteca, Huajuapan de León C.P. 69000, Mexico
2 Faculty of Engineering, Universidad Autónoma de San Luis Potosí, San Luis Potosí C.P. 78280, Mexico
* Correspondence: aleaguirre@mixteco.utm.mx; Tel.: +55-953-532-0214

Citation: Venancio-Guzmán, S.; Aguirre-Salado, A.I.; Soubervielle-Montalvo, C.; Jiménez-Hernández, J.d.C. Assessing the Nationwide COVID-19 Risk in Mexico through the Lens of Comorbidity by an XGBoost-Based Logistic Regression Model. *Int. J. Environ. Res. Public Health* **2022**, *19*, 11992. https://doi.org/10.3390/ijerph191911992

Academic Editors: Sachiko Kodera and Essam A. Rashed

Received: 12 July 2022
Accepted: 17 September 2022
Published: 22 September 2022

Publisher's Note: MDPI stays neutral with regard to jurisdictional claims in published maps and institutional affiliations.

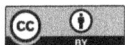

Copyright: © 2022 by the authors. Licensee MDPI, Basel, Switzerland. This article is an open access article distributed under the terms and conditions of the Creative Commons Attribution (CC BY) license (https://creativecommons.org/licenses/by/4.0/).

Abstract: The outbreak of the new COVID-19 disease is a serious health problem that has affected a large part of the world population, especially older adults and people who suffer from a previous comorbidity. In this work, we proposed a classifier model that allows for deciding whether or not a patient might suffer from the COVID-19 disease, considering spatio-temporal variables, physical characteristics of the patients and the presence of previous diseases. We used XGBoost to maximize the likelihood function of the multivariate logistic regression model. The estimated and observed values of percentage occurrence of cases were very similar, and indicated that the proposed model was suitable to predict new cases (AUC = 0.75). The main results revealed that patients without comorbidities are less likely to be COVID-19 positive, unlike people with diabetes, obesity and pneumonia. The distribution function by age group showed that, during the first and second wave of COVID-19, young people aged ≤ 20 were the least affected by the pandemic, while the most affected were people between 20 and 40 years, followed by adults older than 40 years. In the case of the third and fourth wave, there was an increased risk for young individuals (under 20 years), while older adults over 40 years decreased their chances of infection. Estimates of positive COVID cases with both the XGBoost-LR model and the multivariate logistic regression model were used to create maps to visualize the spatial distribution of positive cases across the country. Spatial analysis was carried out to determine, through the data, the main geographical areas where a greater number of positive cases occurred. The results showed that the areas most affected by COVID-19 were in the central and northern regions of Mexico.

Keywords: coronavirus; comorbidity; spatial analysis; logistic regression; ROC curve

1. Introduction

The COVID-19 pandemic has affected many countries worldwide. Among these, the United States, India, Brazil, the United Kingdom and Russia lead the list of countries with the highest number of infected [1]. The outbreak of the SARS-CoV-2 virus was declared a pandemic in March 2020, due to its rapid dissemination and its negative effects across various countries [2]. After 18 months, the United States has reported 82,613,620 confirmed cases and 999,842 deaths; India has reported 43,125,370 confirmed cases and 524,260 deaths; Brazil has reported 30,701,900 confirmed cases and 665,216 deaths, among others. In the case of Mexico (5,752,441 confirmed cases and 324,617 deaths), it is in 15th and 4th place regarding the countries with the larger number of positive cases and deaths, respectively [1].

Coronaviruses are a group of viruses that cause respiratory illnesses [3]. The most common symptoms produced by the virus include fever, dry cough, tiredness and shortness of breath, though, in more severe cases, it causes pneumonia or severe acute respiratory syndrome (SARS) that may lead to death. In other cases, some people infected by the virus do not develop any symptom, but they may still infect the rest of the population. According to the World Health Organization (WHO), the coronavirus can be transmitted from an infected person to others through droplets (also called aerosols) that are expelled when coughing, sneezing or speaking, when shaking a sick person's hand, or by touching objects or surfaces contaminated by the virus [4].

The vulnerability of a person to COVID-19 is determined by various factors; among these, the educational level, age, gender, social conditions, sociodemographic conditions, housing conditions, and even psychological and emotional factors. In their recent study, Ref. [5] analyzed the effects of living conditions on morbidity and mortality in the state of Oaxaca. In this study, it was determined that the health of the population was seriously affected by poor living conditions, and the lack of services such as electricity, gas, water, and health educational services. Therefore, several factors have contributed to the exacerbation of the coronavirus disease. Ref. [6] tested the hypothesis that social vulnerability in Mexico contributes considerably to the probability of hospitalization of people sick from COVID-19. To prove this, a cross-sectional study was carried out with public data from the General Directorate of Epidemiology of the Ministry of Health of Mexico using 5-month period data from individuals with coronavirus. The results show that patients with diabetes have 38.4% probability of being hospitalized, and for those patients whose suffer from some other comorbidity, the risk increases to 42.9% (42.2–43.7%).

Several studies have carried out for the evaluation of comorbidities associated with severe and fatal cases of COVID-19. Ref. [7] reviewed 33 systematic studies and 22 meta-analysis, concluding that, of the total cases, 40% had comorbidities, while fatal cases had about 74% had comorbidities. Hypertension, diabetes, and respiratory diseases were the most frequent comorbidities in severe and fatal cases. Ref. [8] founded that about 66.6% of the deaths caused by from COVID-19 were to men, with a mean age of 69.9 years. In addition, a high incidence of hypertension, diabetes, low platelet levels, and chronic cerebrovascular and cardiovascular diseases were observed among the deceased. Ref. [2] carried out a descriptive analysis of COVID-19 cases in Mexico with data obtained through the official website of the Ministry of Health in Mexico. The study included epidemiological, demographic, and clinical characteristics of the patients who were confirmed positive by a real-time RT-PCR test. The results determined that most of the positive cases of COVID-19 occurred in Mexico City, the average age of the patients confirmed with the disease was 46 years old, most of these cases occurred in people between 30 to 59 years, and 58% of all positive cases occurred in men. Regarding deceased patients, it was determined that they had one or more comorbidities, mainly hypertension, diabetes and obesity. Similarly, Ref. [9] determined that the most influential factor in men and women was obesity, followed by diabetes and hypertension, as well as chronic kidney failure only in the case of women. These findings indicate that these comorbidities were associated with the severity of the disease and predispose to more serious complications of COVID-19.

Multivariate logistic regression has been widely used to identify variables associated with risks of coronavirus disease. Ref. [10] adjusted a multivariable logistic regression models with 450 patients from the Massachusetts General Hospital (MGH). They found that, among patients with diabetes, 42.1% was admitted to the intensive care unit, or ICU, 37.1% required mechanical ventilation, and 15.9% died; while, among patients without diabetes, 29.8% was admitted to ICU, 23.2% required mechanical ventilation, and 7.9% died. In their results, they also found that diabetes and obesity were associated with greater odds of ICU admission and mechanical ventilation. Ref. [11] conducted a study with 220 adult patients with confirmed and suspected COVID-19 using multivariate logistic regression and found that older age was an independent risk factor for mortality. In a study with 648 COVID-19-positive patients with a median age of 34 years, using multivariate logistic regression, Ref. [12] found that independent risk factors for critical outcomes among COVID-19 cases include old age, males, cardiac patients, chronic respiratory diseases, and the presence of two or more comorbidities; all had significant p-values < 0.05. In order of predicting COVID-19 severity, Ref. [13] conducted a retrospective study with

287 patients of which 36.6% were classified as severe cases and 63.4% as non-severe cases. They used 23 covariates on blood chemistry and obtained an accuracy of 85.2% and an AUC of 0.928. Ref. [14] analyzed the survival probability of patients with COVID-19 in Mexico considering their characteristics and comorbidities. They carried out logistic regression analyses and fitted nonparametric survival curves using the Kaplan–Meier estimator. A greater risk of death was associated with diabetes, obesity, hypertension, age and gender, and at a lower degree to, obstructive pulmonary disease, kidney disease and immunosuppressive diseases. Ref. [15] implemented two logistic regression models to investigate the rate of hospitalization and mortality against other variables. In the analysis, 10,544 records published by the Epidemiological Surveillance System of Respiratory Viral Diseases of the Ministry of Health of Mexico (Ministry of Health, SSA) were used. The results showed that the majority of the positive cases were men, being 54% times more likely to be hospitalized than women. People older than 50 years and with two or more simultaneous chronic diseases were prone to a higher risk of hospitalization and death.

Currently, there is a wide variety of statistical models and machine learning techniques that allow predictions to be made given a set of characteristics. Ensemble learning uses simple models to form a more precise and efficient algorithm. Boosting is an ensemble technique where simpler algorithms are used in a sequential way to take advantage of each original model in order to improve the precision of the subsequent model (Freund and Shapire, 1996). Some assembly models that are based on the Boosting principle include the AdaBoost [16], CatBoost [17], LightGBM [18] and Extreme Gradient Boosting (XGBoost). XGBoost is an algorithm developed as a research project at the University of Washington by [19] at the SIGKDD conference. This model was built by adding simpler models based on regression trees. The optimization algorithm consisted on the gradient descent on an objective function composed of the sum of individual loss functions of each observation. These loss functions measure the distance between an observation and its prediction based on the sum of its estimate in the previous iteration plus a new function that is added sequentially in each iteration. These characteristics allow the global estimation of the model to be scalable.

The XGBoost algorithm has proven its effectiveness and scalability over other methods in recent studies. For example, Ref. [20] implemented XGBoost to predict PM2.5 concentration per hour. The method was compared to several algorithms including random forest, multiple linear regression, decision tree, and support vector machines. Their results showed that this algorithm superpassed all of these methods. Ref. [21] designed a real driving task to extract data to model driving stress dynamics. They built a driver stress management model based on driving behavior, environment and road familiarity, and performed a cluster analysis with K-means to grouping observations of psychological and driver stress data. The XGBoost was used to monitor stress within each group. Performance comparisons revealed that the XGBoost model significantly transcended support vector machines, random forest and gradient boosting decision tree.

In accordance with the current health emergency around the world, it is necessary to build models that can predict the characteristics of people at higher risk of being infected with COVID-19. Therefore, in this research work, we build an XGBoost model to predict when the patient may or may not present the disease, considering risk factors such as having previous diseases. For this, the proposed methodology to address this problem is initially described. Subsequently, the description of the data is made, as well as the main results obtained from the descriptive statistics and the results predicted by the model. Finally, a brief discussion and conclusion is made about the main results obtained, as well as the scope and limitations of the work carried out.

2. Materials and Methods

The population of Mexico is approximately 126 million people, with a proportion of 51.2% and 48.8% of women and men (Population and Housing Census 2020, [22]), with a median of 29 years old. The country has 32 states, of which the state of Mexico has the largest number of inhabitants, while the state of Colima is the least populated. The data used to carry out this study were collected for the entire country.

2.1. Available Data

The data for this study were obtained from the official website of the General Directorate of Epidemiology of the Ministry of Health of Mexico https://www.gob.mx/salud/documentos/datos-abiertos-152127 (accessed on 10 May 2022). The records obtained from the database range from February 2020 to the end of April 2022, a total of 15,119,419 registered cases, and 40 explanatory variables. The set of variables used is shown in Table 1. The only available geographic data were the name of the municipality. To obtain the geographic coordinates of the municipalities, a shapefile was used. In order to merge the data, 7,347,705 were eliminated from the database, this due to the presence of missing values on the records and the presence of variables that represented individuals with duplicate characteristics, thus leaving a total of 7,771,714 individuals to be considered for analysis; of these, 3,119,851 (40.14%) was confirmed as positive cases and the rest as negative cases.

Table 1. Explanatory variables used in the study.

	Variable	Description	Units	Input Data Source [1,2]
1	Date	–	Days	DGE
2	Gender	0: Male, 1: Female	–	DGE
3	Age	–	Years	GDE
4	Asthma	0: No, 1: Yes	–	DGE
5	Diabetes	0: No, 1: Yes	–	DGE
6	Cardiovascular disease	0: No, 1: Yes	–	DGE
7	COPD	0: No, 1: Yes	–	DGE
8	Hypertension	0: No, 1: Yes	–	DGE
9	Obesity	0: No, 1: Yes	–	DGE
10	Chronic kidney disease	0: No, 1: Yes	–	DGE
11	Smoking	0: No, 1: Yes	–	DGE
12	Pneumonia	0: No, 1: Yes	–	DGE
13	Other disease	0: No, 1: Yes	–	DGE
14	Longitude	X UTM coordinate	m	CONABIO
15	Latitude	Y UTM coordinate	m	CONABIO

[1] https://www.gob.mx/salud/documentos/datos-abiertos-152127 accessed on 10 May 2022; [2] http://www.conabio.gob.mx/informacion/gis/maps/geo/cabmun2kgw.zip accessed on 10 May 2022.

2.2. Logistic Regression

A generalized linear model is a function that relates a set of response variables with some distribution belonging to the exponential family and a set of independent variables that are obtained through a measurement or observation. This type of model allows the generalization of other existing models by varying the distribution of the response variable or the function that relates $E(Y_i) = \mu_i$ with the set of covariates [23]. This last function, commonly called the link function, is a monotonic and differentiable function, which satisfies:

$$g(\mu_i) = X^\top \beta, \qquad (1)$$

where X is an $n \times p$ matrix of explanatory covariates and $\beta \in \mathbb{R}^p$ is a $p \times 1$ vector of coefficients of the model. In the case where the response variable follow a Bernoulli distribution, the parameter $\mu_i = p_i$ represents the probability that a success will occur. The link function commonly used in this case is the *logit* function $g(\mu) = g(p) = \log\left(\frac{p}{1-p}\right)$. Consequently, the conditional probability of Y given X can be expressed as:

$$p(Y = y \mid X) = \frac{e^{X^\top \beta}}{1 + e^{X^\top \beta}} = \frac{e^{\beta_0 + \beta_1 x_1 + \beta_2 x_2 + \ldots + \beta_p x_p}}{1 + e^{\beta_0 + \beta_1 x_1 + \beta_2 x_2 + \ldots + \beta_p x_p}}, \qquad (2)$$

which satisfies (1). This model is known as the logistic regression model.

2.3. XGBoost

In this research, we used an XGBoost-based logistic regression model for the classification problem, which may be denoted XGBoost-LR, where the explanatory variables are the main risk factors described in [7,8], and the response variable is the presence or absence of COVID-19 disease.

Let be a data set: $\{(x_i, y_i) : i = 1, \ldots, n, \ x_i \in \mathbb{R}^p, \ y_i \in \mathbb{R}\}$, where x_i is the vector of characteristics, and y_i is the response variable. An assembly model based on regression trees makes use of K simpler models, to predict y_i additively:

$$\widehat{y}_i = \sum_{k=1}^{K} f_k(x_i), \quad f_k \in \mathbf{F},$$

$\widehat{y}_i$ is the prediction of y_i and $\mathbf{F}$ is the class of functions of all possible regression trees;

$$\mathbf{F} = \left\{ f(x) = w_{q(x)} \mid q : \mathbb{R}^p \to I, \ w \in \mathbb{R}^T \right\}, \quad (3)$$

T is the number of leaf, $I = \{1, 2, \ldots, T\}$, $q(x)$ represents the index $q(x)$-th in vector w, $w_{q(x)}$ represents the $q(x)$-th component of w, f_k represents an independent regression tree that corresponds to a tree structure q with leaf weights w.

Regression trees have a score on each of their leaves, w_i denotes the score on the i-th leaf of a tree. The data used in the training of the model are grouped in the leaf nodes. Thus, in the prediction of an example, the decision rules generated by these trees are considered to classify it in the corresponding leaves and calculate the final prediction adding each of the scores in the leaves given by the vector w of each tree [19].

The regularized function to minimize, and to learn each f_i is:

$$\mathcal{L} = \sum_{i=1}^{n} l(y_i, \widehat{y}_i) + \sum_{k} \Omega(f_k), \quad (4)$$

l represents the loss function between the observed value y_i and the predicted value $\widehat{y}_i$. In addition,

$$\Omega(f) = \gamma T + \frac{1}{2} \lambda \|w\|^2.$$

Ω is the regularized term that penalizes the complexity of the model to avoid overfitting of the data, γ penalizes the number of leaves or equivalently the complexity of the tree, T is the number of leaves in the tree, λ is the regularization parameter, and w is the score vector in the leaves.

The loss function is considered as the mean square error if the problem is regression, whereas in a binary classification problem, the loss function is the likelihood function obtained from Equation (2):

Let $\widehat{y}_i^{(t)} = \sum_{k=1}^{t} f_k(x_i) = \left\{ \sum_{k=1}^{t-1} f_k(x_i) \right\} + f_t(x_i)$, and Equation (4) can be written as:

$$\mathcal{L}^{(t)} = \sum_{i=1}^{n} l(y_i, \widehat{y}_i^{(t-1)} + f_t(x_i)) + \Omega(f_t). \quad (5)$$

Using the second order Taylor expansion of the loss function and denoting by $I_j = \{i \mid q(x_i) = j\}$ for some fixed structure $q(x)$ to the index set whose examples correspond to that leaf, we can rewrite (5) as:

$$\mathcal{L}^{(t)} = \sum_{j=1}^{T} \left[(\sum_{i \in I_j} g_i) w_j + \frac{1}{2} (\sum_{i \in I_j} h_i + \lambda) w_j^2 \right] + \gamma T. \quad (6)$$

The internal sums of the Equation (6) over the index set I_j of the leaf j is due to the fact that the examples present in that leaf have the same score. Subsequently, to find the optimal value of the parameters w_j in each of the leaves, fixing $q(x)$ and deriving Equation (6), it was determined that such a value is:

$$w_j^* = -\frac{\sum_{i \in I_j} g_i}{\sum_{i \in I_j} h_i + \lambda}. \tag{7}$$

Substituting (7) in (6), we found that the minimum value is reached in:

$$\mathcal{L}^{(t)}(q) = -\frac{1}{2} \sum_{j=1}^{T} \frac{(\sum_{i \in I_j} g_i)^2}{\sum_{i \in I_j} h_i + \lambda} + \gamma T.$$

In practice, the goal is to optimize one level of the tree at a time, so that branches are added iteratively to a tree. Thus, if a leaf is divided into two leaves and the index set of the examples that are on the left leaf and on the right leaf are I_I and I_D, respectively, then the reduction in loss after division is given by:

$$L_{split} = \frac{1}{2} \left[\frac{(\sum_{i \in I_I} g_i)^2}{\sum_{i \in I_I} h_i + \lambda} + \frac{(\sum_{i \in I_D} g_i)^2}{\sum_{i \in I_D} h_i + \lambda} - \frac{(\sum_{i \in I_I \cup I_D} g_i)^2}{\sum_{i \in I_I \cup I_D} h_i + \lambda} \right] - \gamma. \tag{8}$$

This last expression consists of the scores of the original leaf, the left leaf, the right leaf, and the regularization term. In addition, this formula is the gain in the loss reduction equation; therefore, it is used to evaluate the division with the candidates.

3. Results

3.1. Spatiotemporal Distribution of Daily Cases

The temporal distribution function of daily cases of COVID-19 in Mexico from February 2020 to the end of April 2022 is described in Figure 1. When analyzing the Figure 1, it can be seen that, after the arrival of the SARS-CoV-2 virus in Mexico, the daily cases of infected increased rapidly beginning in the month of May, reaching the peak of the first wave of positive cases in summer 2020 (mid-July and early August). In this first wave, the temporal distribution function considering the gender of the patient indicates that there is a greater presence of masculine cases than feminine. Subsequently, the second wave of positive cases is confirmed during the winter of 2021 (January–February). In this phase, the occurrence of positive cases was higher than in the first wave, the infection had propagated to every state in Mexico. In addition, notice from Figure 2 that the cases in women and men are quite similar, and the trend of male cases is very similar to the trend of female cases. On the other hand, the third and fourth wave of cases occurred during the months of July 2021 and January 2022. Furthermore, the last wave was the largest, with a significantly greater number of cases in men than in women. The distribution function by age group shows that, during the first and second wave, young people aged ≤ 20 were the least affected by the pandemic, while the most affected were people between 20 and 40 years, followed by adults older than 40 years. In the case of the third and fourth wave, there was an increased risk for young individuals (under 20 years), while older adults over 40 years decreased their chances of infection; see Figure 3.

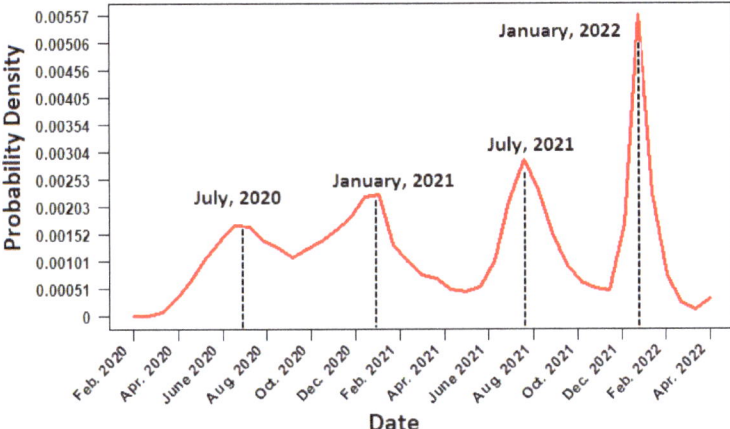

Figure 1. Temporal distribution function in terms of probability for daily COVID-19 cases from February 2022 to April 2021. The dotted line represents the date when a maximum was reached in COVID cases.

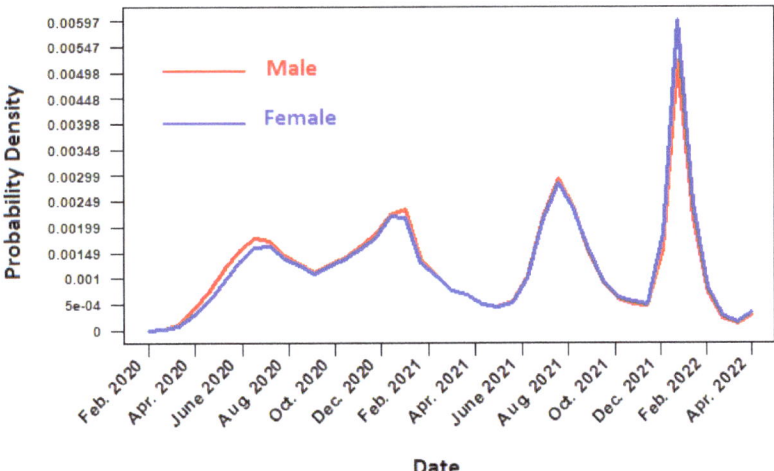

Figure 2. Temporal distribution function in terms of probability for daily COVID-19 cases by gender.

The results obtained from the statistical analysis by geographic location determined that the states with the highest occurrence of COVID-19 cases were the following: in the central zone of Mexico, the predominant states were Mexico City and the State of Mexico; in the west, Jalisco and Guanajuato; in the north of Mexico, these were Tamaulipas, Nuevo León, Sonora, and, in the south, these were Puebla, Veracruz, and Tabasco, see Figure 4. Most of the states least affected by the disease, with the exception of Chiapas, were the least populated, as is the case of Colima, Nayarit and Campeche; an exception is the state of Chiapas. On the other hand, the municipalities in Mexico with the most cases of COVID-19 were Puebla, Querétaro, León, Monterrey and Guadalajara. In the case of Mexico City, the largest number of cases occurred in the most populated municipalities, such as Iztapalapa, Gustavo A. Madero, Álvaro Obregón, Tlalpan and Benito Juarez, see Figure 5.

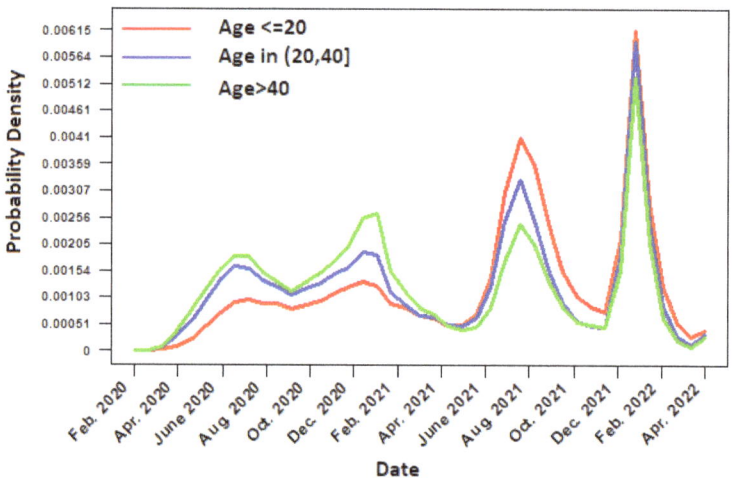

Figure 3. Temporal distribution function in terms of probability for daily COVID-19 cases by age.

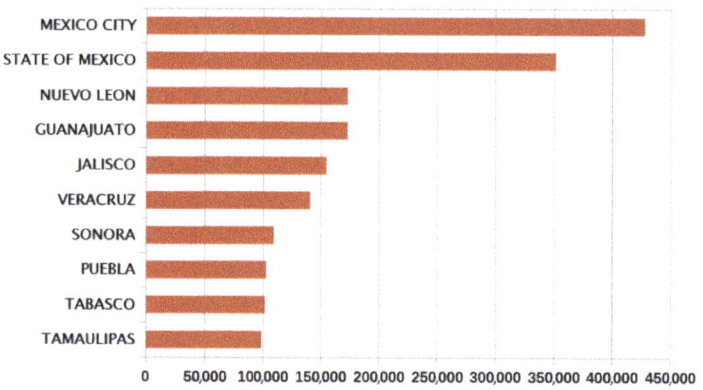

Figure 4. Mexican states with most COVID-19 cases from February 2020 to April 2022.

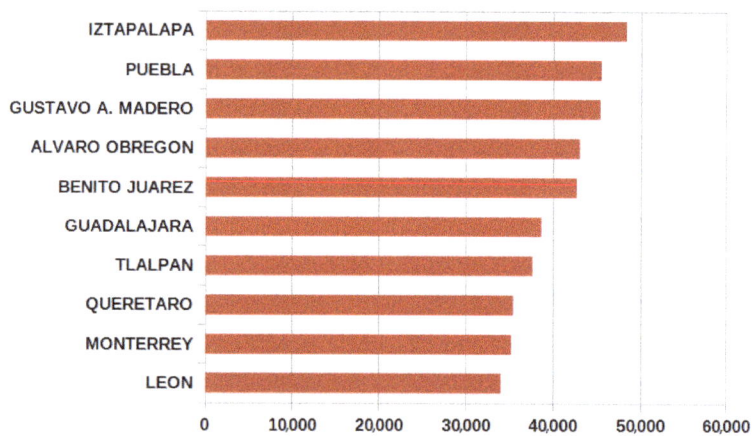

Figure 5. Municipalities with most COVID-19 cases from February 2020 to April 2022.

Additionally, the maps in Figure 6a,b show the actual frequency for each municipality of positive cases of COVID-19. Figure 6a shows that many entities in Mexico have a high number of incidents, while Figure 6b shows the center of Mexico, it can be seen that the federal district is one of the most affected entities.

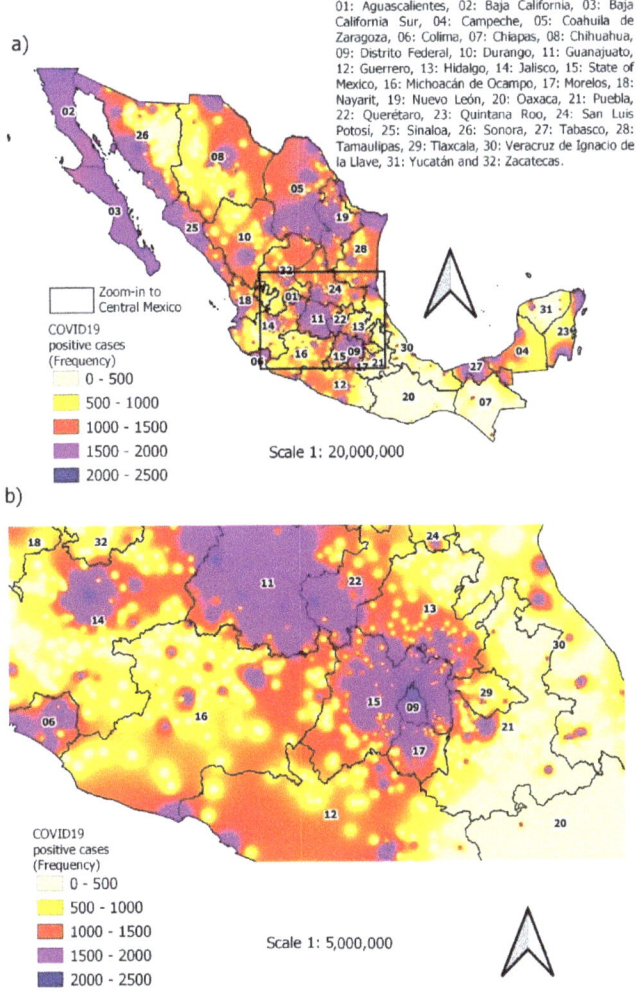

Figure 6. Spatial distribution of COVID-19 positive cases: (**a**) national context; (**b**) zoom-in to Central Mexico.

3.2. Spatiotemporal Distribution of Individuals with Comorbidities

In Mexico, a large part of the population suffers from a disease that exposes them to a higher risk of developing COVID-19 or of having serious complications once they are sick. Therefore, it is important to explore the probability of cases against the main risk factors. To do this, four groups that were diagnosed positive for COVID-19 were analyzed: (1) individuals who did not present any risk factor, (2) individuals with diabetes, (3) individuals who suffered from obesity and (4) those who presented pneumonia, Figure 7. For the group of individuals without comorbidity, it was determined that the highest number of incidences occurred in patients between the ages of 25 and 35 years, with an average of 37.75 years. In the case of individuals with diabetes, the mean was presented at

57.5 years, while, for obesity, the cases were positively skewed with a mean of 45.62 years, unlike pneumonia, where the distribution of cases was negatively skewed with a mean of 56.8 years.

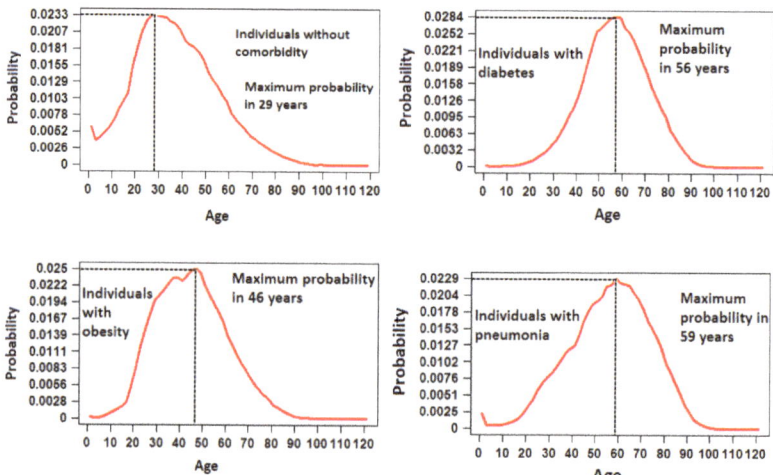

Figure 7. Probability distribution functions for positive COVID-19 cases by comorbidity against age.

The proportion of patients who presented some risk factor of the total set of records is described in Table 2. Figure 8 shows that the main risk factors present in a large part of the Mexican population are hypertension, pneumonia, obesity, diabetes and smoking. On the other hand, the spatial distribution of each of the comorbidities under study associated with the cases that tested positive for COVID-19 can be seen in Figure 8.

Table 3 shows the patients diagnosed as positive for COVID-19, who had some previous comorbidity. The main risk factors in the Mexican population included hypertension, pneumonia, obesity, and diabetes. In addition, only of the positive cases (3,119,851), 55.59% of the patients suffered at least one of the 10 diseases that were considered in the study. When analyzing the gender, it was found that 50.31% and 49.69% of the total positive cases are men and women, respectively. In the group of men, 56.16% had at least one disease, while in the case of women this was 55%.

Table 2. Percentage of patients with any comorbidity, out of a total of 7,771,714 observations.

Variable	Yes	No
Hypertension	19.00%	81.00%
Pneumonia	9.00%	91.00%
Obesity	15.50%	84.50%
Diabetes	14.17%	85.83%
Smoking	10.02%	89.98%
Asthma	3.77%	96.23%
Chronic kidney failure	1.88%	98.12%
Cardiovascular disease	1.94%	98.06%
Other disease	2.6%	97.40%
COPD	1.32%	98.68%

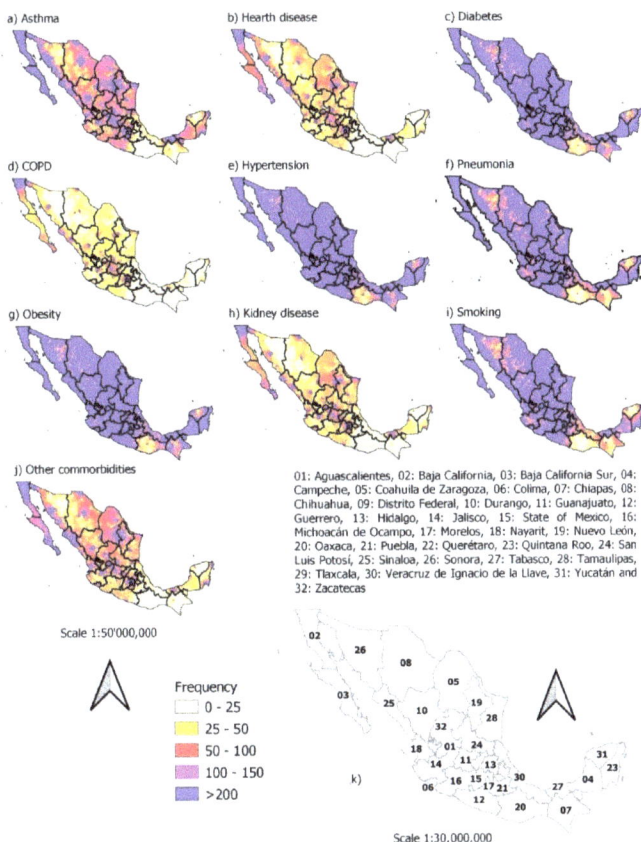

Figure 8. Spatial distribution of comorbidities associated with COVID-19 occurrence from February 2020 to April 2022: (**a**–**j**) all the comorbidities and (**k**) captions for states and countries.

Table 3. Percentage of COVID-19 patients with any comorbidity, out of a total of 3,119,851 observations.

Variable	Yes	No
Hypertension	21.62%	78.38%
Pneumonia	15.62%	84.38%
Obesity	17.67%	82.33%
Diabetes	16.53%	83.47%
Smoking	8.98%	91.02%
Asthma	3.37%	96.63%
Chronic kidney failure	1.93%	98.07%
Cardiovascular disease	1.95%	98.05%
Other disease	2.78%	97.22%
COPD	1.37%	98.63%

3.3. Classification Analysis with XGBoost-LR and Classic LR

This study is focused on determining a model capable of predicting whether or not the patient will suffer from the COVID-19 disease, considering a set of explanatory variables. Additionally, it sought to identify the importance of each of these variables in different groups of patients. The study was performed with the XBGoost-LR model described in Section 2.3 using the likelihood of a multivariate logistic regression model as a loss function. The measure of selection that determined the order of importance of variables in the context of decision trees was the gain, defined in (8). This measure allowed for deciding which attribute should go to a decision node, selecting the one whose gain is greater.

The XGBoost-LR model was built considering 70% of the data as the training set and 30% as the testing set. To measure model quality among a set of candidate models, evaluation metrics were calculated with only the test set. For the final model, we obtained a score known as sensitivity (66.11%) (i.e., recall rate or fraction of true positives), which is the proportion of positive cases that the model correctly identified. The specificity was 70.11% (true negative rate), which represented the proportion of negative cases that were correctly classified by the algorithm. The probability of how close the result of a measurement is to the true value, that is, the accuracy of the model, was 68.5%. In addition, it was determined that the most influential variables in the model (in terms of decision trees, which generate the greatest gain) for the classification were: date, pneumonia, location with latitude, longitude and age, while diseases such as asthma, hypertension, disease Chronic obstructive pulmonary disease and cardiovascular diseases were the least influential in the model classification. The importance of the variables is shown in Figure 9. This type of importance represents the average gain across all splits where feature was used. Therefore, the table shows that the variables age, latitude, longitude, pneumonia and date are the variables with the greatest importance, while that the variables associated with asthma, hypertension, COPD, cardiovascular disease, another disease, diabetes, chronic, kidney, disease, smoking obesity and gender have lower values of importance. Although the measure of importance obtained by these variables is low, this does not mean that the variables do not contribute to the adjustment; rather, it means that the number of cases in which the variable was decisive to form a new branch is lower.

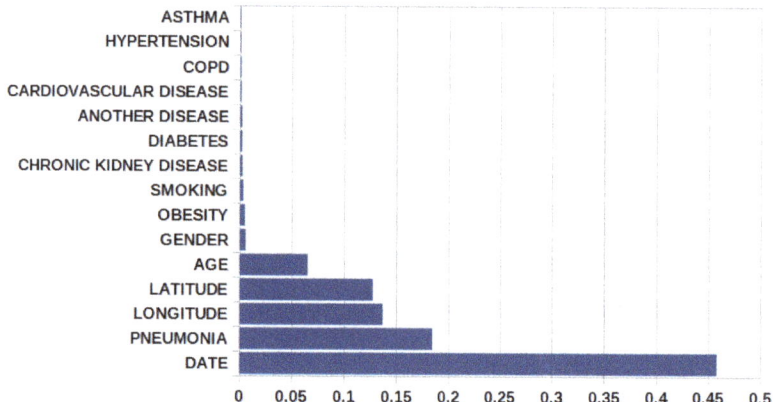

Figure 9. Importance of explanatory variables in XGBoost.

The predictive capacity of the built model was analyzed by comparing it with other classification models. To do this, it was compared with the classic multivariate logistic regression model, which allows for predicting a binary response variable [23]. For training the classical logistic regression model, the same training and testing set used with the XGBoost-LR model was employed. The results obtained for the new model were as follows: the sensitivity was 43.63%, the specificity was 70.49%, and the accuracy was 59.69%. Therefore, it can be showed that the XGBoost-LR model outperformed the classic logistic regression model in almost all the assessment metrics, except for specificity, see Table 4.

Alternatively, the predictive ability of the final model can also be viewed graphically using maps; see Figure 10a,b. The prediction of cases by municipality obtained with the XGBoost-LR model considering the entire Mexican territory can be seen in Figure 10a, while the zoom-in to Central Mexico is found in Figure 10b. Figure 10a shows the level of risk present in each of the municipalities, even more so the areas with the highest probability of risk include the north, coast and center of the country. Note that the map is quite similar to the map in Figure 6, so it can be assumed that the model has good predictive capacity on the data. We also elaborate a map with the predictions using the multivariate logistic regression model to contrast the results of the proposed model. The results are shown in Figure 11, in which we observe a significant difference with respect to the map of the observed values shown in Figure 6.

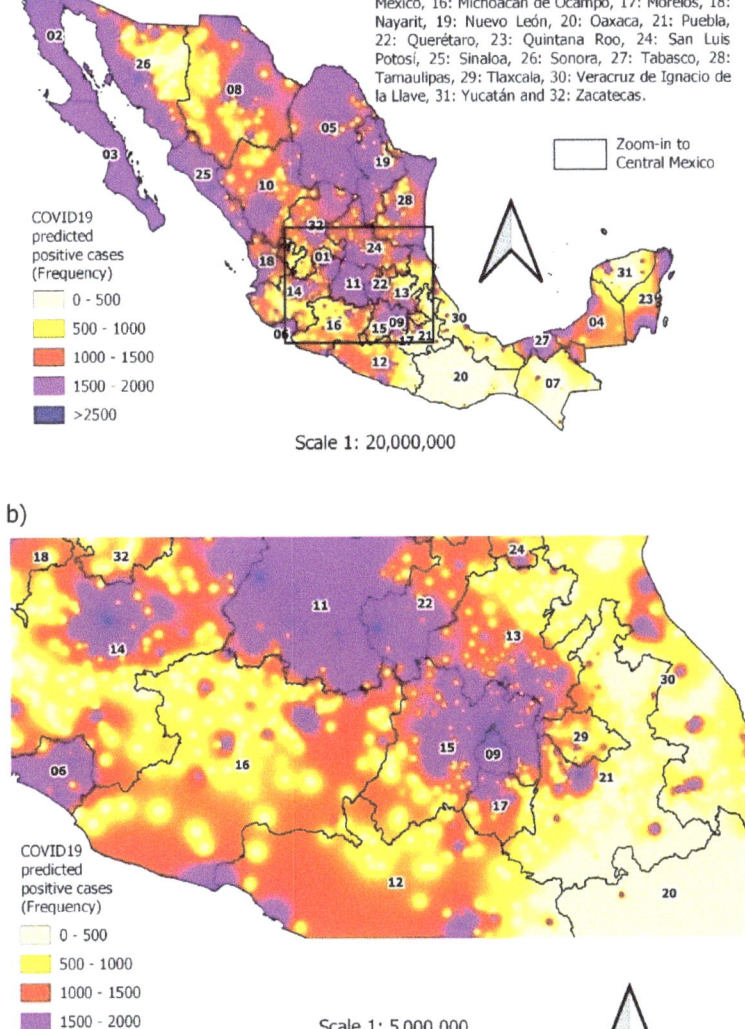

Figure 10. Predicted spatial distribution of COVID-19 occurrence from February 2020 to April 2022: (**a**) average actual occurrence with XGBoost-based logistic regression; (**b**) zoom-in to Central México.

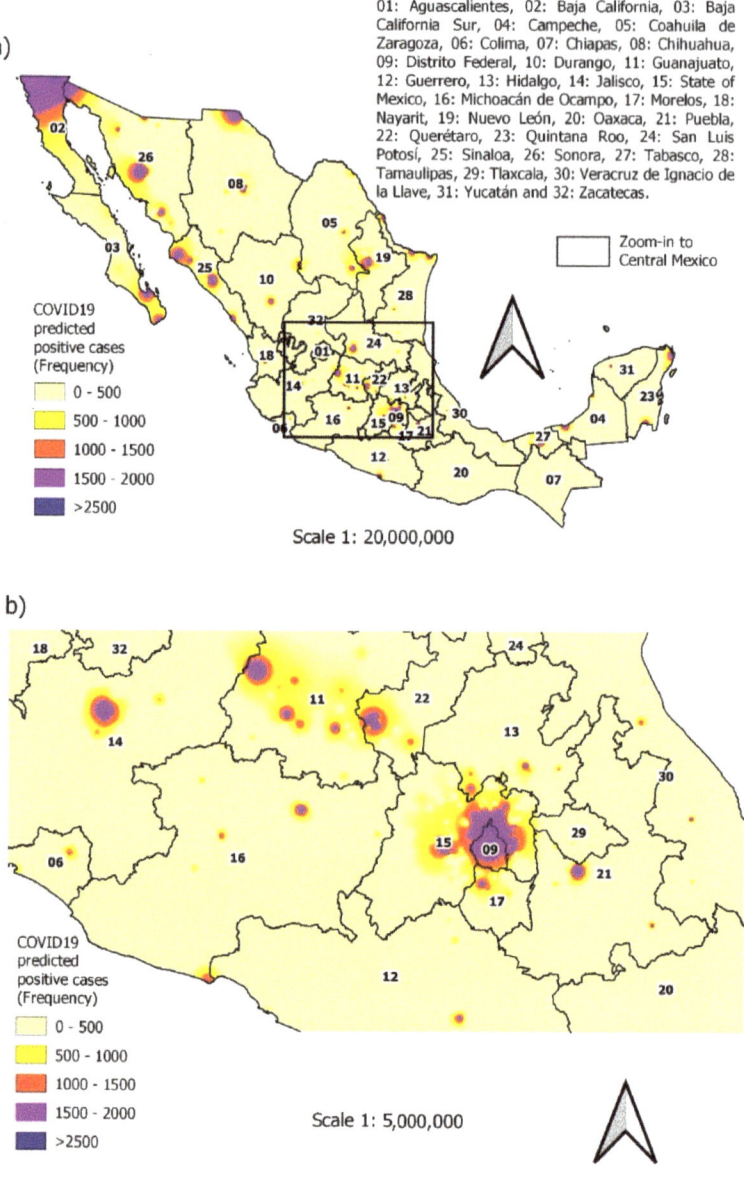

Figure 11. Predicted spatial distribution of COVID-19 occurrence from February 2020 to April 2022: (a) average actual occurrence with multivariate logistic regression; (b) zoom-in to Central México.

The XGBoost-LR model was analytically evaluated by calculating the area under the ROC curve called AUC. The AUC value obtained was 0.75, which indicates that, if an individual is randomly selected, then there is a probability of 0.75 that the diagnosis made by the model is correct. Thus, the constructed model is considered appropriate to predict the risk of acquiring the COVID-19 disease. Figure 12a, shows the ROC curve with the performance of the XGBoost model. Specificity evaluates the proportion of real negatives that are correctly identified, while sensitivity describes the proportion of real positives that were correctly identified. In this way, the ROC curve also provides a perspective on the behavior of the predictive potential of the proposed model. In addition, the optimal cut-off point was also determined, which maximizes the difference between sensitivity and 1-specificity (Figure 12b). Figure 12c shows the ROC curve and AUC obtained for the multivariate logistic regression model. The value of the AUC obtained for this model shows that the proposed model is better than the multivariate logistic regression model. In this model, the cut-off was 0.37, which is slightly lower than the cut-off obtained by the XGBoost model.

Table 4. Evaluation metrics of the XGBoost-LR and classic multivariate logistic regression models.

Model	Sensitivity	Specificity	Accuracy
XGBoost	66.11%	70.11%	68.50%
Multivariate logistic regression	43.63%	70.49%	59.69%

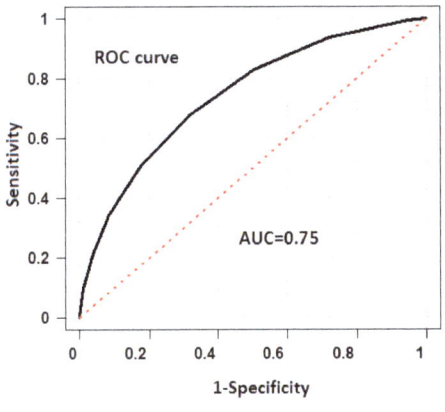

(a) ROC curve and AUC of the XGBoost-LR model.

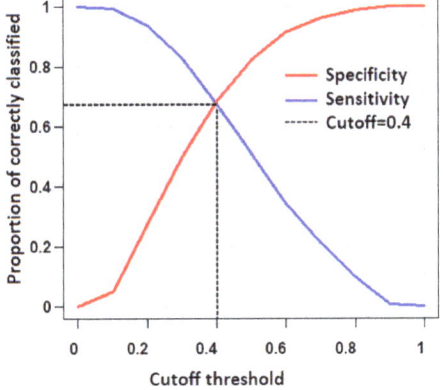

(b) Global optimal cut-off in 0.4 of the of the XGBoost-LR model.

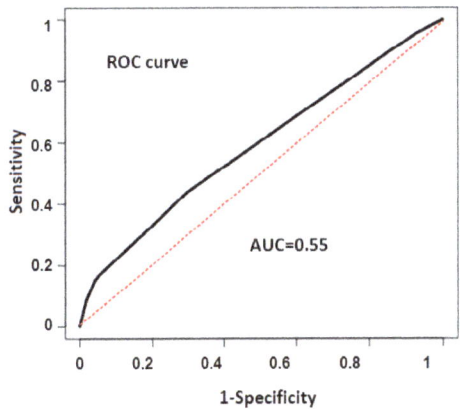

(c) ROC curve and AUC of the logistic regression model.

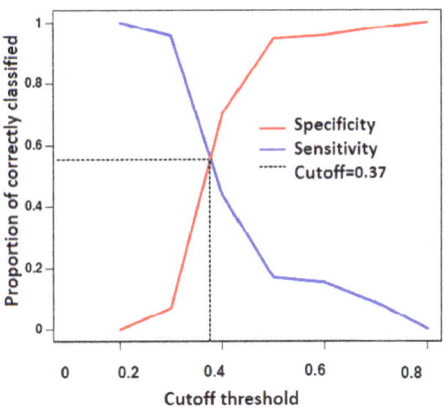

(d) Global optimal cut-off in 0.37 of the logistic regression model.

Figure 12. ROC curve (**a**,**c**), area under the AUC curve (**b**,**d**) and optimal cut-off value of the models: XGBoost-LR and logistic regression, respectively, to estimate the risk of suffering from COVID-19.

3.4. Predicting New Cases

Figure 9 shows that pneumonia is the most important variable of the variables associated with previous comorbidities. In addition, the rest of the variables associated with previous comorbidities also contribute to the construction of the model. The reason is because the decision tree considers spatial and temporal variables, and consequently, in certain geographical places, these variables play an important role for prediction. However, because these places are less numerous within the study region, the importance assigned to the variable is considerably lower. In the case of patients with no history, it was observed that the estimated probability of risk is low, so the aforementioned probability does not exceed the optimal threshold of 0.4, for which the model classifies these observations as negative cases for COVID-19. In the case of patients suffering from obesity and diabetes, it was determined that the probability of risk increases slightly compared to individuals who do not present comorbidity; however, this probability is also below the optimal threshold; thus, they are considered as cases negative for the disease. Finally, in the case of pneumonia, the probability of risk increases beyond the optimal threshold after 10 years.

4. Discussion

Our findings based on descriptive statistics determined that the most prevalent comorbidities in the studied population were obesity, diabetes, hypertension and pneumonia. When analyzed variables of location, the data reflected a notable spatial differentiation in the number of incidents of positive and non-positive COVID-19 cases. That is, urban areas in the central, northern and coastal region of the country, presented a high risk of infection compared to less populated places, such as Chiapas, Campeche and Colima, as can be seen in the maps.

Another result of the descriptive analysis was the ability to determine the time periods with a high rate of contagion in Mexico, which occurred shortly after the holiday seasons of each year. This is reasonable given the enormous mobility on those dates. Additionally, when analyzing the distribution function of positive cases of COVID-19 grouped by comorbidity, it was observed that older adults were more likely at least one of the comorbidities considered in the study. Depending on gender, there was almost the same proportion of positive cases in men and women, which suggests that the risk is independent of gender. On the other hand, after using the XGBoost-LR model, we were able to confirm that, indeed, a large part of the Mexican population was affected by the COVID-19 disease.

Our results also revealed that some vulnerable groups have a greater risk, which may be characterized by their health status and geographic location. This fact is of vital importance not only for the study of the new coronavirus disease, but to show the health status of a large part of the Mexican population. In fact, the Mexican Ministry of Health indicated that, after the United States, Mexico ranks second in terms of obesity rate, a disease that is highly related to diabetes, being one of the main causes of death in the country. On the other hand, the analysis of the geographical locations makes it possible to analyze the existing risk in densely populated places, and encourages the relevant authorities to take better measures, for example, to strengthen security protocols, in touristic areas of the country.

Treviño [24] found the presence of the same comorbidities, finding that men suffer from COVID-19 disease more often than women. In addition, he indicated that admission to the Intensive Care Unit was related to the gender patients, as verified by the Chi-square test. Our result probably differs in that, during the first year of the pandemic, there were more positive cases in men than in women; however, during the second year, this could change. On the other hand Ref. [15] performed a logistic regression analysis and determined that men were 1.54 times more likely to be hospitalized than women. Furthermore, both [25] and [9] found that, in addition to diabetes and obesity, high blood pressure and chronic kidney damage can increase mortality in COVID-19 patients. Regarding the analysis by geographic location of each state of Mexico, Refs. [2,26] analyzed the cases of COVID-19 in Mexico. In both studies, the results agreed with our analysis, since the same spatial pattern was detected throughout the country: State of Mexico, Nuevo León, among others, were the most affected by the pandemic.

Having a predictive model that allows for identifying individuals with particular characteristics is important for taking preventive measures to avoid further deaths. On the other hand, the constant appearance of new variants of the virus worries stakeholders around the world and makes it difficult to pinpoint an end date for the pandemic. Therefore, the authorities must strengthen surveillance and adopt systematic approaches to provide health indications to the entire population, based on each local context.

5. Conclusions

In the present study, positive and non-positive cases of COVID-19 in Mexico were analyzed at the municipal level using data from the Mexican Ministry of Health. A descriptive analysis was performed to explore the spatial and temporal distribution of positive cases, and subsequently an XGBoost-LR model was trained to estimate the risk of infection using the main comorbidities in patients as covariates. According to the results, we confirm that pneumonia, obesity and diabetes were variables of utmost importance to predict new cases. The estimated and observed values of percentage occurrence of cases were very similar, and indicated that the proposed model was suitable to predict new cases (AUC = 0.75). The optimal global cutoff to identify when a case is positive for COVID-19 was 0.41. Our results revealed that patients without comorbidities are less likely to be COVID-19 positive, unlike people with diabetes, obesity and pneumonia with ages close to 56, 46 and 59 years old, respectively. The current worldwide situation regarding COVID-19 is still serious, especially with the emergence of new SARS-CoV-2 virus variants. Therefore, we recommend reviewing and adapting government policies concerning the establishment of preventative measures to avoid the spread of virus and mitigate the pandemic effects.

Author Contributions: Conceptualization, S.V.-G., A.I.A.-S., C.S.-M. and J.d.C.J.-H.; Data curation, S.V.-G., A.I.A.-S., C.S.-M. and J.d.C.J.-H.; Formal analysis, S.V.-G., A.I.A.-S., C.S.-M. and J.d.C.J.-H.; Funding acquisition, S.V.-G., A.I.A.-S., C.S.-M. and J.d.C.J.-H.; Investigation, S.V.-G., A.I.A.-S., C.S.-M. and J.d.C.J.-H.; Methodology, S.V.-G., A.I.A.-S., C.S.-M. and J.d.C.J.-H.; Project administration, S.V.-G., A.I.A.-S., C.S.-M. and J.d.C.J.-H.; Resources, S.V.-G., A.I.A.-S., C.S.-M. and J.d.C.J.-H.; Software, S.V.-G., A.I.A.-S., C.S.-M. and J.d.C.J.-H.; Supervision, S.V.-G., A.I.A.-S., C.S.-M. and J.d.C.J.-H.; Validation, S.V.-G. and A.I.A.-S.; Visualization, S.V.-G. and A.I.A.-S.; Writing—original draft, S.V.-G. and A.I.A.-S.; Writing—review & editing, S.V.-G. and A.I.A.-S. All authors have read and agreed to the published version of the manuscript.

Funding: This work was supported by a CONACYT Grant scholarship: 2021–2023, for the doctoral studies of the first author. This research was funded by CONACYT through the grant "Convocatoria de Ciencia Básica y/o Ciencia de Frontera 2022", project ID 320036.

Institutional Review Board Statement: Not applicable.

Informed Consent Statement: Informed consent was obtained from all subjects involved in the study.

Data Availability Statement: The analyzed data sets can be consulted at the following links: https://www.gob.mx/salud/documentos/datos-abiertos-152127 accessed on 10 May 2022; http://www.conabio.gob.mx/informacion/gis/maps/geo/cabmun2kgw.zip accessed on 10 May 2022.

Acknowledgments: The authors thank the Secretary of Health of Mexico (https://www.gob.mx/salud/documentos/datos-abiertos-152127, accessed on 10 May 2022) for providing the data used in this research. Special thanks are also given to two anonymous reviewers who shared insightful observations that deeply improved our work.

Conflicts of Interest: The authors declare no conflict of interest.

Abbreviations

The following abbreviations are used in this manuscript:

COVID-19	'CO' stands for corona, 'VI' for virus, 'D' for disease, and '19' for 2019
CONABIO	National Commission for the Knowledge and Use of Biodiversity
COPD	Chronic obstructive pulmonary disease
DGE	Directorate General for Epidemiology
ROC	Receiver Operating Characteristic
SARS-CoV-2	Severe acute respiratory syndrome coronavirus 2
WHO	World Health Organization

References

1. Johns Hopkins University. Center for Systems Science and Engineering (CSSE). COVID-19 Dashboard. Available online: https://coronavirus.jhu.edu/map.html (accessed on 10 March 2021).
2. Suárez, V.; Quezada, M.S.; Ruiz, S.O.; De Jesús, E.R. Epidemiología de COVID-19 en México: Del 27 de febrero al 30 de abril de 2020. *Rev. Clínica Española* **2020**, *220*, 463–471. [CrossRef] [PubMed]
3. Ena, J.; Wenzel, R. Un nuevo coronavirus emerge. *Rev. Clínica Española* **2020**, *220*, 115–116. [CrossRef] [PubMed]
4. World Health Organization. Modes of Transmission of Virus Causing COVID-19: Implications for Ipc Precaution Recommendations. Available online: https://www.who.int/news-room/commentaries/detail/modes-of-transmission-of-virus-causing-COVID-19-implications-for-ipc-precaution-recommendations (accessed on 1 December 2021).
5. González-Villoria, A.M.; Zuñiga, R.A.A. Social vulnerability and its possible relation to the principal causes of morbidity and mortality in the Mexican state of Oaxaca. *Int. J. Equity Health* **2018**, *17*. [CrossRef] [PubMed]
6. Sosa-Rubí, S.G.; Seiglie, J.A.; Chivardi, C.; Manne-Goehler, J.; Meigs, J.B.; Wexler, D.J.; Wirtz, V.J.; Gómez-Dantés, O.; Serván-Mori, E. Incremental Risk of Developing Severe COVID-19 Among Mexican Patients with Diabetes Attributed to Social and Health Care Access Disadvantages. *Diabetes Care* **2020**, *44*, 373–380. [CrossRef] [PubMed]
7. Gold, M.S.; Sehayek, D.; Gabrielli, S.; Zhang, X.; McCusker, C.; Ben-Shoshan, M. COVID-19 and comorbidities: A systematic review and meta-analysis. *Postgrad. Med.* **2020**, *132*, 749–755. [CrossRef] [PubMed]
8. Qiu, P.; Zhou, Y.; Wang, F.; Wang, H.; Zhang, M.; Pan, X.; Zhao, Q.; Liu, J. Clinical characteristics, laboratory outcome characteristics, comorbidities, and complications of related COVID-19 deceased: A systematic review and meta-analysis. *Aging Clin. Exp. Res.* **2020**, *32*, 1869–1878. [CrossRef] [PubMed]
9. Hernández-Garduño, E. Obesity is the comorbidity more strongly associated for Covid-19 in Mexico. A case-control study. *Obes. Res. Clin. Pract.* **2020**, *14*, 375–379. [CrossRef] [PubMed]
10. Seiglie, J.; Platt, J.; Cromer, S.J.; Bunda, B.; Foulkes, A.S.; Bassett, I.V.; Hsu, J.; Meigs, J.B.; Leong, A.; Putman, M.S.; et al. Diabetes as a Risk Factor for Poor Early Outcomes in Patients Hospitalized With COVID-19. *Diabetes Care* **2020**, *43*, 2938–2944. [CrossRef] [PubMed]
11. Zhou, S.; Mi, S.; Luo, S.; Wang, Y.; Ren, B.; Cai, L.; Wu, M. Risk Factors for Mortality in 220 Patients with COVID-19 in Wuhan, China: A Single-Center, Retrospective Study. *Ear Nose Throat J.* **2020**, *100*, 140S–147S. [CrossRef] [PubMed]
12. Khan, A.; Althunayyan, S.; Alsofayan, Y.; Alotaibi, R.; Mubarak, A.; Arafat, M.; Assiri, A.; Jokhdar, H. Risk factors associated with worse outcomes in COVID-19: A retrospective study in Saudi Arabia. *East. Mediterr. Health J.* **2020**, *26*, 1371–1380. [CrossRef] [PubMed]
13. Xiong, Y.; Ma, Y.; Ruan, L.; Li, D.; Lu, C.; Huang, L. Comparing different machine learning techniques for predicting COVID-19 severity. *Infect. Dis. Poverty* **2022**, *11*, 1–9. [CrossRef] [PubMed]
14. Parra-Bracamonte, G.M.; Lopez-Villalobos, N.; Parra-Bracamonte, F.E. Clinical characteristics and risk factors for mortality of patients with COVID-19 in a large data set from Mexico. *Ann. Epidemiol.* **2020**, *52*, 93–98.e2. [CrossRef] [PubMed]
15. Carrillo-Vega, M.F.; Salinas-Escudero, G.; García-Peña, C.; Gutiérrez-Robledo, L.M.; Parra-Rodríguez, L. Early estimation of the risk factors for hospitalization and mortality by COVID-19 in Mexico. *PLoS ONE* **2020**, *15*, e0238905. [CrossRef] [PubMed]
16. Freund, Y.; Schapire, R.E. A Decision-Theoretic Generalization of On-Line Learning and an Application to Boosting. *J. Comput. Syst. Sci.* **1997**, *55*, 119–139. [CrossRef]
17. Prokhorenkova, L.; Gusev, G.; Vorobev, A.; Dorogush, A.V.; Gulin, A. CatBoost: Unbiased boosting with categorical features. In Proceedings of the Advances in Neural Information Processing Systems, Montreal, QC, Canada, 3–8 December 2018. [CrossRef]
18. Ke, G.; Meng, Q.; Finley, T.; Wang, T.; Chen, W.; Ma, W.; Ye, Q.; Liu, T.Y. LightGBM: A Highly Efficient Gradient Boosting Decision Tree. In Proceedings of the 31st International Conference on Neural Information Processing Systems, Long Beach, CA, USA, 4–9 Dcember 2017; Curran Associates Inc.: Red Hook, NY, USA, 2017; pp. 3149–3157.
19. Chen, T.; Guestrin, C. XGBoost: A Scalable Tree Boosting System. In Proceedings of the 22nd ACM SIGKDD International Conference on Knowledge Discovery and Data Mining, San Francisco, CA, USA, 13–17 August 2016.
20. Ma, J.; Yu, Z.; Qu, Y.; Xu, J.; Cao, Y. Application of the XGBoost Machine Learning Method in PM2.5 Prediction: A Case Study of Shanghai. *Aerosol Air Qual. Res.* **2020**, *20*, 128–138. [CrossRef]
21. Lu, Y.; Fu, X.; Guo, E.; Tang, F. XGBoost Algorithm-Based Monitoring Model for Urban Driving Stress: Combining Driving Behaviour, Driving Environment, and Route Familiarity. *IEEE Access* **2021**, *9*, 21921–21938. [CrossRef]

22. Instituto Nacional de Estadística, Geografía e Informática. Población 2020. Available online: http://cuentame.inegi.org.mx/poblacion/habitantes.aspx?tema=p (accessed on 20 March 2021).
23. Dobson, A.J.; Barnett, A.G. *An Introduction to Generalized Linear Models*, 4th ed.; Chapman and Hall/CRC: Boca Raton, FL, USA, 2018. [CrossRef]
24. Treviño, J.A. Demografía, comorbilidad y condiciones médicas de los pacientes hospitalizados por COVID-19 en México. *Middle Atl. Rev. Lat. Am. Stud.* **2020**, *4*, 49. [CrossRef]
25. Salinas-Aguirre, J.; Sánchez-García, C.; Rodríguez-Sanchez, R.; Rodríguez-Muñoz, L.; Díaz-Castaño, A.; Bernal-Gómez, R. Características clínicas y comorbilidades asociadas a mortalidad en pacientes con COVID-19 en Coahuila (México). *Rev. Clínica Española* **2022**, *222*, 288–292. [CrossRef] [PubMed]
26. Juárez, M.V.S. COVID-19 en México: Análisis de su comportamiento espacio—Temporal a partir de los Condicionantes Socio espaciales de la Salud. *Pers. Soc.* **2021**, *35*, 15. [CrossRef]

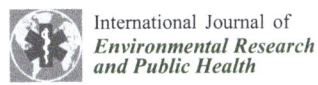

Review

The Atmospheric Environment Effects of the COVID-19 Pandemic: A Metrological Study

Zhong Chen [1] and Dongping Shi [1,2,*]

1. College of Environment and Resources, Xiangtan University, Xiangtan 411105, China
2. Key Laboratory of Large Structure Health Monitoring and Control, Shijiazhuang 050043, China
* Correspondence: shidongping@xtu.edu.cn

Abstract: Since the COVID-19 outbreak, the scientific community has been trying to clarify various problems, such as the mechanism of virus transmission, environmental impact, and socio-economic impact. The spread of COVID-19 in the atmospheric environment is variable and uncertain, potentially resulting in differences in air pollution. Many scholars are striving to explore the relationship between air quality, meteorological indicators, and COVID-19 to understand the interaction between COVID-19 and the atmospheric environment. In this study, we try to summarize COVID-19 studies related to the atmospheric environment by reviewing publications since January 2020. We used metrological methods to analyze many publications in Web of Science Core Collection. To clarify the current situation, hotspots, and development trends in the field. According to the study, COVID-19 research based on the atmospheric environment has attracted global attention. COVID-19 and air quality, meteorological factors affecting the spread of COVID-19, air pollution, and human health are the main topics. Environmental variables have a certain impact on the spread of SARS-CoV-2, and the prevalence of COVID-19 has improved the atmospheric environment to some extent. The findings of this study will aid scholars to understand the current situation in this field and provide guidance for future research.

Keywords: COVID-19; metrology; data analysis; atmospheric environment; pollution

1. Introduction

The COVID-19 pandemic caused by SARS-CoV-2 has been recognized as a global public health emergency by The World Health Organization [1]. The outbreak and continued prevalence of COVID-19 has had a severe impact on all aspects of human life worldwide. In response to the strong infectivity and spread of COVID-19, many countries have adopted policies of lockdown and restriction of activities to strictly control the occurrence of the infection. Lockdown is the most direct way to stop COVID-19, but it cannot be sustained in the context of a global pandemic. Research into specific drugs to prevent or treat COVID-19 have yet to yield results [2]. Vaccination is the most effective and cost-effective intervention to control the spread of COVID-19, but the continuous emergence of new variants of SARS-CoV-2 undoubtedly poses another great challenge to vaccine development [3].

Under the current circumstances, COVID-19 is likely to coexist with humans for a long time. Its normalization will lead to a significant decrease in the mobility of the population, making a big change in the way people live and travel, and having a great impact on the functioning of society and the policies of the state. Both natural and human behavioral changes resulting from COVID-19 have direct or indirect effects on the atmospheric environment. These influences are multifaceted, with many positive and negative influences. Also, the atmospheric environment has an important relationship to the spread of COVID-19. Understanding the interrelationship between air quality, meteorological indicators, and COVID-19 is significant for saving human lives.

We need to comprehensively understand the relationship between COVID-19 and the atmospheric environment, which has attracted the attention of many authors. But there is no metrological analysis type of review study in this field. Metrological analysis overcomes the subjective factors in the traditional literature review, completely covers all literature in the selected period, avoids the loss of key literature, and can quantitatively explore the knowledge structure, research hotspots, and the latest insights in some scientific fields [4]. The metrological study of COVID-19 and the atmospheric environment simultaneously, aiming to present the overall picture of this field by analyzing and exploring the current situation and research hotspots in this field [5].

2. Research Methodology

This section details the process of research design (Section 2.1), data collection (Section 2.2), and data processing (Section 2.3) used in this research.

2.1. Research Design

The bibliometric approach is good at uncovering the underlying knowledge structure in literature and integrating the visualization results for further analysis [4]. In this paper, we use bibliometric analysis methods and data visualization analysis tools to synthesize and comb the literature related to COVID-19 and the atmospheric environment, quantitatively analyze the data, and generate visualization and content analysis results. Drawing with AutoCAD as shown in Figure 1. To understand the complex relationship between COVID-19 and the atmospheric environment as well as the degree and trend of its impact on the atmospheric environment.

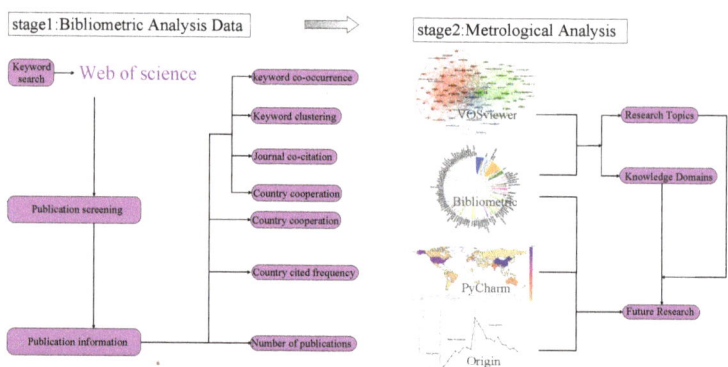

Figure 1. Workflow of the systematic.

2.2. Data Collection

The data in this paper are all from Web of Science Core Collection, which was selected because it covers a wide range of outstanding publications in the entire academic field and is one of the largest databases from 1900 to the present. The database contains authors, citations, journals, and much more bibliographic information that can be used for analysis [5,6]. The World Health Organization named the new coronavirus infection pneumonia as COVID-19, and the International Committee on Classification of Viruses named the new coronavirus SARS-CoV-2. Therefore, the search strategy was set to (COVID-19) OR (SARS-CoV-2) AND (atmosphere OR air). The search record includes title, author, abstract, keywords, and references [7]. In the Web of Science Core Collection database, the Boolean operators "OR" and "AND" are used to merge the individual components of a search query.

An initial search using these keywords from the Web of Science Core Collection database for the period 1 January 2020–31 December 2021. After filtering by publication type and research direction, a total of 1781 relevant publications were obtained by removing duplicates, including 1684 papers and 144 reviews. Research interests include environmental sciences, public environmental and occupational health, meteorology and atmospheric sciences, multidisciplinary sciences, and green and sustainable technologies, which are related to the environmental field.

2.3. Data Processing

We analyzed and evaluated the collected data, including country, source, title, author, publication year, affiliation, document type, field of interest, keywords, citation, etc. We consider the number of published publications as a quantitative indicator of the research productivity of authors, countries, institutions, sources, etc. The bibliometric analysis in this study was conducted mainly on VOSviewer, and the co-occurrence network visualization map was constructed based on the information extracted from 1781 publications to present the publication data. VOSviewer can combine network visualization and spectral clustering to analyze the underlying knowledge structure contained in many publications [8]. In addition, the software can perform network analysis on different aspects of the data collected, and quickly process text data downloaded directly from the Web of Science site [5]. This study also utilizes the integrated development environment PyCharm, the scientific drawing software Origin, and the spreadsheet software Excel to further assist in the analysis and processing of the data.

3. Results of the Metrological Analysis

This section conducts a qualitative and in-depth metrological analysis of publication data from selected studies. It includes the trend of publication volume in the last two years (Section 3.1), research content of high-influence authors (Section 3.2), national cooperation relationship (Section 3.3), analysis of the number of national citations (Section 3.4), and analysis of publication sources (Section 3.5). In addition, high co-occurrence keywords are analyzed (Section 3.6) and keyword co-occurrence cluster analysis is elaborated (Section 3.7).

3.1. The Number of Publications in the Past Two Years

The variation in a research field's publication output can be used to assess its development status, knowledge accumulation, and maturity [9]. As can be seen in Figure 2, the number of publications in this research area has grown rapidly over time and is divided into three phases. There were 474 publications in 2020 and 1307 publications in 2021.

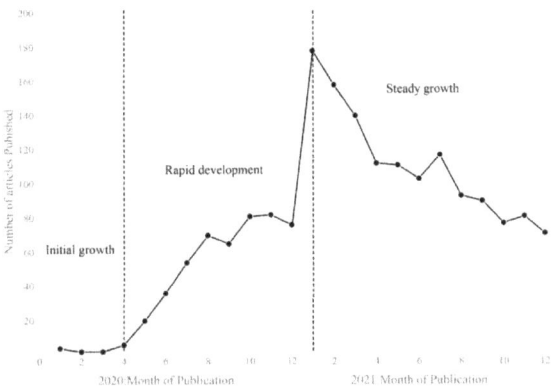

Figure 2. The number of publications in the past two years.

The first phase is from January to March 2020, this phase is the initial growth phase. At the beginning of the COVID-19 epidemic, many countries began to focus on and study the correlation between COVID-19 and the atmospheric environment, especially the influence of the atmospheric environment on COVID-19 transmission and mortality. The first publication was published in January 2020 and focused on the extent of air and surface contamination in a COVID-19 non-intensive care unit [10]. The second publication was published in January 2020 and the study focused on the driving role of travel numbers on the spread of COVID-19 [11]. Both publications were published in Bioscience.

The second phase is from April 2020 to January 2021, and this phase is the rapid development phase. At this time, the COVID-19 outbreak has been going on for some time, research in the field expanded and the number of publications exploded. With a buffer of time and sufficient data to support it, studies on the effects of COVID-19 on air quality began to emerge and develop rapidly. The impact of COVID-19 on the atmosphere is clear and immediate. A study on NO_x reduction and recovery during COVID-19 in East China was published in Atmosphere in April 2020 [12]. The paper shows that NO_x emissions in most parts of eastern China have decreased significantly due to the lockdown after the outbreak of COVID-19. After the lockdown period, NO_x emissions began to rise to various degrees. Among them, January 2021 saw the maximum number of papers published, far higher than other months. The main reason may be that papers published at the beginning of the year have a longer time to accumulate citations than papers published at the end of the year, which helps to improve the impact factor.

The third phase is from February 2021 to December 2021, and this phase is the stable growth phase. The number of publications in this period began to fall from the peak, but still maintained a certain number of publications. The research focuses more on changes in air quality and emissions of atmospheric pollutants caused by COVID-19. This will be a research direction of lasting interest.

3.2. Influential Authors and Their Research Interests

Authors with many highly cited papers often accompany the research hotspots and methodological trends in this field and play an important role in the development of this field. In this study, the top five authors were determined by a comprehensive evaluation of the number of authors' publications and citation times, as shown in Table 1.

Table 1. Top 5 most productive authors on COVID-19 and air environment research.

Rank	Author	Institution	TP	TC	AC	Main Research Interests
1	Zhang, Hongliang	Fudan University	7	852	121.7	The impact of lockdown measures on air quality in China and India
2	Coccia, Mario	CNR Natl Res Council Italy	6	558	93	The impact of air pollution on the spread of outbreaks
3	Bashir, Muhammad Farhan	Cent South University	6	539	89.8	Environmental quality, climate indicators and the COVID-19 pandemic
4	Querol, Xavier	Spanish Res Council CSIC	5	423	84.6	Changes in air quality caused by COVID-19 lockdown and its implications
5	Wang, Peng	Hong Kong Polytech University	7	358	51.1	Changes and causes of air pollutant concentration under epidemic lockdown

Notes: TP = Total publications; TC = Total citations; AC = Average number of citations per paper.

Zhang, Hongliang of Fudan University published 7 papers and was cited 852 times, with an average of 121.7 times [13–19]. His papers were cited the most frequently and had the highest average number of citations per paper, indicating that his research received high attention from other authors. In general, the research content of these five authors has attracted much attention, and the research direction tends to be about the impact of COVID-19 lockdowns on air quality and the impact of meteorological indicators on the spread of the epidemic.

3.3. Cluster Analysis of National Cooperation

The number of publications is an important indicator to measure the development trend of a certain field. To some extent, the number of publications in this field can reflect the research strength of a country in this field [7]. As shown in Figure 3a, through the online bibliometric analysis website bibliometric.com (accessed on 30 April 2022), we can directly obtain the inter-country partnership map, where the area occupied by countries represents the number of national publications and the total linkage intensity represents the degree of inter-country partnership.

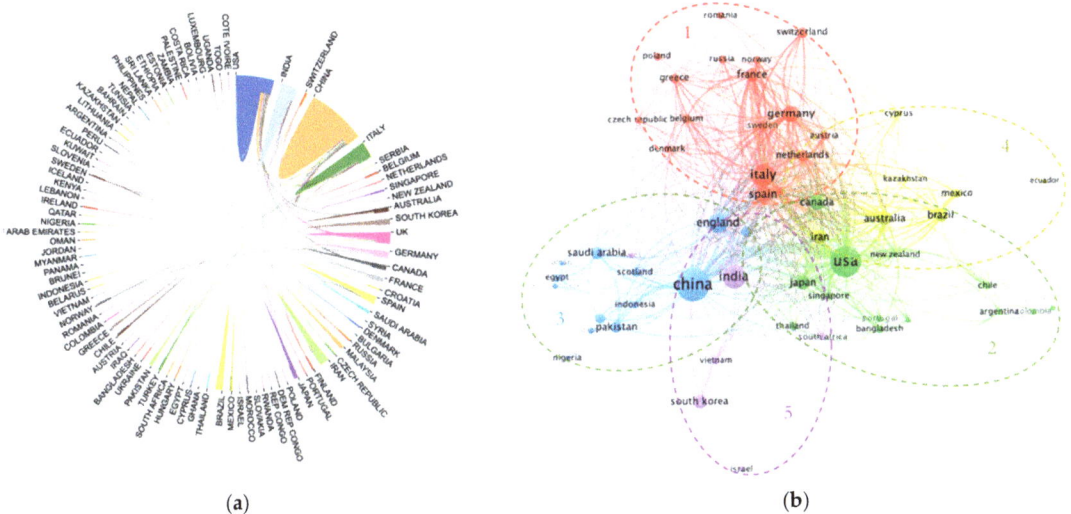

Figure 3. (a) Country partnership chart; (b) Country partnership clustering chart.

Figure 3b shows the graph of VOSviewer to generate the clustering analysis of country cooperation relations. In this paper, the analysis process of clustering algorithm is divided into three steps.

1. Construct an association matrix for the analysis object. The co-occurrence matrix based on the quantitative relationship between objects is a data-based square matrix. It is assumed that there are n variables in the research matrix, x_{ij} is the co-occurrence observed value of the i-th variable and the j-th variable, and the co-occurrence observed values of all variables form a $n \times n$ square matrix [20]. The formula is as follows.

$$M = \begin{bmatrix} x_{11} & \cdots & x_{1n} \\ \vdots & \ddots & \vdots \\ x_{n1} & \cdots & x_{nn} \end{bmatrix} \quad (1)$$

2. Calculate the similarity relation value or dissimilarity relation value (distance) between any two data objects in the matrix.
3. A certain clustering algorithm is used to divide or merge data objects to form a certain clustering result.

VOSviewer clustering algorithm can be regarded as a weighted variant based on modular clustering. The modular Q value calculation formula of VOSviewer is as follows, and the optimal clustering result is obtained when the modular Q value is the largest [20,21].

$$Q = \frac{1}{2m} \Sigma_{i<j} \delta(x_i, x_j) w_{ij} \left(c_{ij} - \gamma \frac{c_i c_j}{2m} \right) \quad (2)$$

In the above formula, m represents the total number of connections in the network; c_{ij} represents the number of connections between nodes i and j ($c_{ij} = c_{ji} \geq 0$); c_i represents all connections of node i; x_i represents the cluster to which the node belongs, the δ function is

1 for $x_i = x_j$ and 0 otherwise; w_{ij} represents the weight value $w_{ij} = 2m/c_i c_j$, and γ represents the clustering parameter.

The essence of VOSviewer co-occurrence clustering is that two related items appear simultaneously and aggregate together. Different types of clustering groups can be obtained based on the measure of index clustering of the strength and direction of item correlation. VOSviewer adopts the algorithm of limiting parameter variables. By adjusting the value of limiting parameter variables, it can control small clusters, and the generated clusters have strong consistency and high stability. Using VOSviewer, the minimum number of publications is set to 7, and the minimum citation frequency is set to 10. Finally, a total of 56 countries were obtained, divided into 5 clusters. The color of the spheres represents different regions, the size of the spheres represents the number of national publications, and the total link strength indicates the intensity of cooperation between the two countries.

The first cluster (red) is dominated by Italy, which mainly cooperates closely with European countries; the second cluster (green) is dominated by the United States, which has frequent cooperation with the Americas, Oceania, Asia, Europe, and Africa; the third cluster (blue) is dominated by China, which cooperates more with European, Asian, and African countries; the fourth cluster (yellow) is dominated by Australia, which cooperates more closely with American countries; the fifth cluster (purple) is dominated by India, which cooperates more with Asian and European countries. We can find Italy, the United States, China, Australia, and India as regional leading countries, as the close cooperation between countries has played a substantial role.

The papers on COVID-19 and the atmospheric environment field are mainly concentrated in China (469), the United States (399), India (209), Italy (173), the United Kingdom (137), and other countries such as Germany (94) and Spain (89), which also have more prominent research capacity in this field. Among them, the United States is the country with the most cooperation with several countries in the world, and it frequently cooperates with China, the United Kingdom, Italy, and Canada. Globally, the international cooperation links in research in the field of the atmospheric environment under COVID-19 are strong, and many countries pay attention to research and cooperation in this field.

3.4. Country Cited Frequency Analysis

The number of citations is an important indicator of the influence of papers in a certain field. The total number of citations and the average number of citations of a country in the field can reflect the international influence and research strength of the country in the field to a certain extent. The average number of citations can also show the quality of a country's papers, thus reflecting the country's scientific research capacity and level. This paper uses a simple average method. The average citation frequency is the total citation frequency divided by the total number of publications. In Figure 4a,b, the darker the color, the higher the total or the average number of citations for a country. The total number of citations in China was 13,568, with an average citation rate of 28.93. Meanwhile, the total number of citations in the United States was 11,263, with an average citation rate of 28.23. These two countries have the highest total citations, which are much higher than other countries, and the average citations are relatively good, indicating that both countries have strong research strength and influence in the field. The total number of citations in India is 4135 and the average number of citations is 19.78, which indicates that India has some research strength and influence in the field. The total citations of Australia and the United Kingdom are relatively high, with 2805 and 5781 respectively; the average citations are high, with 48.36 and 42.20, respectively, indicating the profound academic influence and first-class research level of these two countries in the field. The total number of citations in Ecuador, Norway, and Denmark is low, only 577, 1194 and 938 respectively, but the average number of citations is high, 82.43, 59.70 and 58.65, respectively, which indicates that these countries have great potential for research in this field. In contrast, it can be found that the average citation frequency data of most European countries and Australia are more prominent. This shows that the overall quality of these countries' papers may be higher, and subject to more attention and recognition by scholars.

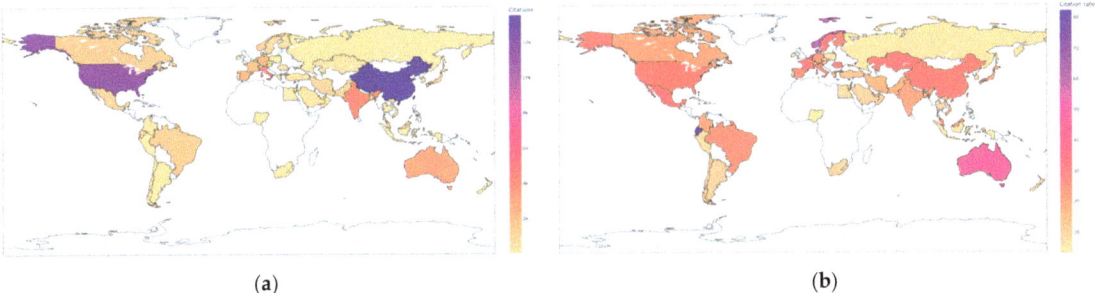

Figure 4. (**a**) The total number of citations by country; (**b**) The average citation rate by country.

3.5. Analysis of Journal Publications and Co-Citation

A total of 137 journals have published relevant research between 2020 and 2021. Table 2 shows the information on the 10 most productive journals in this research area. In terms of the number of publications, Science of The Total Environment (203, 11.39%) is the most active journal, followed by International Journal of Environmental Research and Public Health (140, 7.86%), Environmental Research (134, 7.52%), and Aerosol and Air Quality Research (125, 7.02%). Among them, Science of The Total Environment has an impact factor of 10.753 and a citation frequency of 12,176, which is quite influential. Environmental Pollution has an impact factor of 9.988 and a citation frequency of 1644. Environmental Research has an impact factor of 8.431 and a citation frequency of 2323. They are among the most influential journals in the field of the atmospheric environment. Next, Air Quality, Atmosphere & Health has an impact factor of 5.804 and a citation frequency of 1115. Environmental Science and Pollution Research has an impact factor of 5.190 and a citation frequency of 565. These two journals are also influential in the field of the atmospheric environment.

Table 2. The top 10 most active journals in terms of publication.

Rank	Journal Title	TP	TP (%)	TC	IF (2021)	Subject Category of the Journal
1	Science of The Total Environment	203	11.39%	12,176	10.753	Environmental Sciences
2	International Journal of Environmental Research and Public Health	140	7.86%	1368	4.614	Public Environmental & Occupational Health
3	Environmental Research	134	7.52%	2323	8.431	Environmental Sciences
4	Aerosol and Air Quality Research	125	7.02%	1384	4.53	Environmental Sciences
5	Sustainability	109	6.12%	542	3.889	Green & Sustainable Science & technology
6	Environmental Science and Pollution Research	89	5.00%	565	5.190	Environmental Sciences
7	Atmosphere	81	4.55%	466	3.110	Meteorology & Atmospheric Sciences
8	Scientific Reports	75	4.21%	832	4.996	Multidisciplinary Sciences
9	Environmental Pollution	60	3.37%	1644	9.988	Environmental Sciences
10	Air Quality Atmosphere and Health	55	3.09%	1115	5.804	Environmental Sciences

Notes: TP = Total publications, TP (%) = Total publications (%), IF (2021) = Impact factor in 2021, TC = Total citations.

Journal co-citation is determined based on the number of times they are cited together. Journal co-citation analysis can be used to classify journals on different topics and identify the core journals in each category. This is very helpful for authors to understand the most relevant and influential journals for a particular research topic [22]. In this paper, we use VOSviewer to perform a co-citation analysis of the collected data according to different sources, setting the minimum number of citations for a source to 200. The minimum threshold can be adjusted according to the number of publications rendered and clustering groupings. The color of the sphere represents different journal topics, and the size of the sphere indicates the number of citations. The total link strength then indicates the closeness between journals.

The journals shown in Figure 5 have a significant impact on authors studying COVID-19 and the atmospheric environment. Science of the Total Environment is the most-cited journal, followed by Atmospheric Environment, Atmospheric Chemistry and Physics, Environment Pollution and Environmental research. These journals are grouped into three main groups: Environmental Science and Ecology (blue) includes science of the Total Environment, Aerosol and Air Quality Research, Environment Pollution. Environmental public health and Medicine (red) includes Environmental research, Lancet, International Journal of Environmental Research and Public Health, Science. Meteorology and Atmospheric Sciences (green) includes atmospheric Environment, Atmospheric Chemistry and Physics, Environment Science & Technology, Journal of Geophysical Research: Atmospheres. The medical journal The Lancet (202.731) and the comprehensive journal Science (63.714) have higher impact factors. The more influential journal in the environmental field is Environment Science & Technology (11.357).

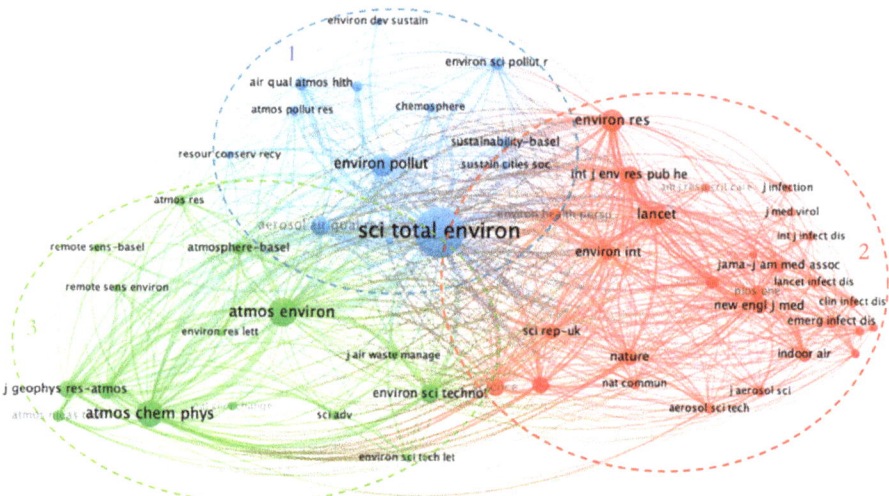

Figure 5. Journal co-occurrence chart.

3.6. Research Keywords

Keywords are highly generalized and concise to the subject of a paper. High-frequency keywords also reflect the research direction to some extent. The keyword density visualization can be used to quickly observe the knowledge and research density of a certain field. VOSviewer sets the minimum keyword frequency to 20 and gets a co-occurrence graph of 86 keywords after removing nonsense words. Each keyword in the figure will fill the color according to the density of its surrounding keywords. The greater the density, the closer it is to red; conversely, the smaller the density, the closer to blue. The density depends on the number and importance of keywords in the surrounding area.

It can be seen from Figure 6 that in addition to air pollution and air quality, keywords related to COVID-19 mortality and environmental factors, SARS-CoV-2 and meteorological conditions also appear frequently.

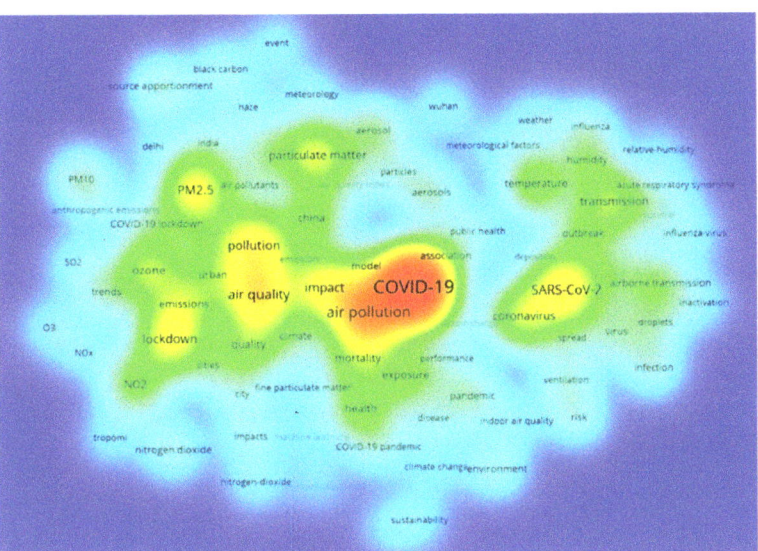

Figure 6. Keyword density visualization.

3.7. Keyword Co-Occurrence Cluster Analysis

VOSviewer takes a distance-based approach to visualizing bibliometric networks. After the construction of the normalized network is completed, the keywords are positioned to make the position of the strongly related keywords closer and the position of the weak related keywords further away [23]. The keyword co-occurrence networks analyze the link strength between co-occurrence keywords by studying their co-occurrence relationship in many publications. Its purpose is to describe the internal composition relationship and structure in a certain academic domain as well as to provide insights into the main research themes of the domain [24,25]. The clusters group keywords that are frequently combined in a set of keywords [26]. Different color spheres indicate different clusters, and the same sphere color represents clusters that are consistent with the research topic. The size of the spheres is proportional to the frequency of keywords. The lines between the keywords reflect the strength of their relevance [27]. A total of 5630 keywords were obtained from publications by setting the minimum keyword frequency to 20, and 86 keywords were obtained after removing meaningless words. They were divided into three major clusters, as in Figure 7.

(1) Air quality indicators (red) contain keywords "pollution", "air quality", "$PM_{2.5}$", "ozone", "lockdown", "NO_2", "particulate matter", etc. Cluster 1 focuses on changes in the atmospheric environment and air quality in the context of COVID-19 and describes how lockdowns due to COVID-19 affect air quality.

(2) Meteorological factors affecting the spread of the outbreak (green) contain keywords "COVID-19", "SARS-CoV-2", "temperature", "transmission", "humidity", "weather", etc. Cluster 2 focuses on meteorological factors influencing the spread of COVID-19 and the special relationship between COVID-19 and environmental variables.

(3) Air pollution and human health (blue) contain keywords "air pollution", "exposure", "mortality", "health", "pandemic", etc. Cluster 3 focuses on the effects of air pollution on human health and mortality.

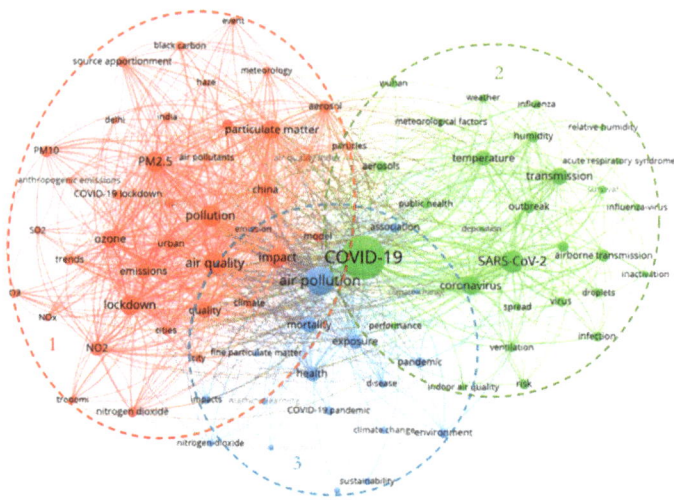

Figure 7. Keyword co-occurrence clustering.

3.7.1. COVID-19 and Air Quality

The COVID-19 outbreak has had a significant impact on almost every aspect of people's lives around the globe, resulting in a variety of direct and indirect impacts on the atmospheric environment. Shutdowns or closures of factories have reduced the amount of pollution, with an estimated 50 percent reduction in N_2O and CO due to the closure of heavy industry during China's lockdown [28]. Restrictions on travel, reduced mobility of people, and reduced transport and related activities have significantly reduced mobile pollution sources and pollutant emissions. $PM_{2.5}$, PM_{10}, CO_2, and NO_2 concentrations have all declined to various degrees during the lockdown period compared to those before the lockdown [13,29,30]. Volatile organic compounds (VOCs), including benzene, are mainly produced by vehicular traffic and other incomplete combustion processes that lockdown has increasingly limited [31]. NO_2, one of the main indicators of world economic activity, shows signs of decline in many countries, including the United States, Canada, China, India, Italy, and Brazil [1,28,32]. At the same time, reduced activities following the lockdown have led to a broad reduction in greenhouse gas emissions. One estimate suggests that global daily CO_2 emissions during the lockdown were 17 percent lower than the 2019 average [33]. It can be seen that the environmental conditions of various countries have changed greatly during the COVID-19 pandemic, indicating that policy intervention has played a great role.

Different studies have shown that urban lockdowns have led to considerable improvements in air quality. The positive impact of urban lockdowns on air quality is greater in cities with larger economies, more industrial activities, and higher traffic volumes [33]. According to data from the Meteorological bulletin of the atmospheric environment, the national average number of haze days in 2020 and 2021 will decrease by 1.5 and 4.4 days, respectively, compared with 2019. In 2020, the meteorological data of Shanghai during the lockdown period and before and after the lockdown were consistent. The comparison of 14 trace elements in $PM_{2.5}$ found that the concentration of trace elements in most fine particles showed a "V" shape trend, indicating that the lockdown measures had a significant impact [34]. Comparing the air quality index (AQI) results before and after the impact of COVID-19 across India shows that most pollutant concentrations (PM_{10}, $PM_{2.5}$, CO, SO_2, NO_x) show different patterns of gradual to rapid decreases [35,36]. A wavelet analysis of COVID-19 confirmed data and weather data in California from 1 March to 24 May 2020 found that AQI and COVID-19 showed negative correlation circles during the observation period, suggesting that COVID-19 leads to better AQI and less environmental pollution [37].

However, with the end of the lockdown and the resumption of normal activities, pollutant emissions rebounded somewhat, and air pollution gradually returned to near pre-COVID-19 levels. NO, NO_2, and NO_x all exhibit abrupt decreases at the time the United Kingdom locked down. But the return of vehicles to the road during early lockdown has already offset much of the air quality improvement seen when locked down [38]. Most of the lockdown's impact on the atmosphere is short-term, but changes in human activities caused by the ongoing COVID-19 pandemic can also have lasting effects on the atmosphere.

COVID-19 has also had some adverse effects on the atmospheric environment, with changes in O_3 due to changes in NO_x and VOC_s emissions. The significant reduction of NO_x during the lockdown was the main reason for the significant increase in O_3. Compared with the same period of the previous year, O_3 in most parts of the world showed various degrees of increase during the epidemic lockdown period [39–41]. AQI results in some parts of India comparing the 2020 lockdown period with 2019 show a sharp decrease in NO_2 and an increase in O_3 [13,35]. During the nationwide implementation of restrictions in China in 2020, NO_x generated during transportation decreased significantly (>50%), O_3 concentration in the air increased significantly, and the atmospheric oxidation capacity (AOC) in the Yangtze River Delta region increased significantly (up to 25%), which was also a major reason for the increase of O_3 level during city lockdown [14].

3.7.2. Meteorological Factors Affecting the Spread of COVID-19

Meteorological factors are unstable and diverse, and the impact of meteorological indicators on the spread of COVID-19 is comprehensive and complex. Analysis of Canadian meteorological data and COVID-19 confirmed cases for 2020 revealed a direct negative correlation between air quality, temperature, humidity, and COVID-19 infection [42]. A study of meteorological data and COVID-19 data in Istanbul and other regions also came to the same conclusion that air quality and temperature significantly affect the number of COVID-19 deaths in Istanbul [43]. In the same analysis of Wuhan, there was also a significant agreement between AQI, humidity, and mortality rates. Humidity was negatively correlated with related COVID-19 deaths [44]. Temperature is the only significant meteorological indicator that has a significant correlation with the spread of COVID-19 [45]. Although only in the short term, daily temperatures in Madrid, Spain, and California, the United States show a negative correlation between COVID-19 outbreaks and death rates [37,46]. This means that temperature plays an important role in limiting COVID-19, suggesting that temperature may help contain COVID-19. Overall, empirical results suggest that rising temperatures may reduce transmission of the SARS-CoV-2.

Statistical analysis of confirmed COVID-19 data and local meteorological variables in Manaus revealed that low solar radiation cycles may lead to increased COVID-19 deaths due to reduced solar radiation. Dry spells may impair nasal functions that prevent viruses and bacteria from entering the body, leading to increased mortality from COVID-19 [47]. A study in Italy found that cities with high wind speeds had fewer COVID-19 infections, and inland cities with low wind speeds and high air pollution had higher COVID-19 infections [48]. Low wind speeds and high concentrations of air pollutants may contribute to the persistence of virus particles in urban air and thus to the indirect transmission of SARS-CoV-2.

3.7.3. Air Pollution and Human Health

Air pollution is one of the biggest environmental threats to human health. It is harmful to the human body in many ways, mainly in the form of respiratory diseases and physiological disorders. It is of great practical significance to study the impact of air pollution on aggravating COVID-19 infection in the population. People living in areas with high levels of pollutants are more likely to develop chronic respiratory diseases and infections with pathogens [49].

An analysis of the link between air pollution and COVID-19 in Indian cities found an asymmetric relationship between $PM_{2.5}$ and COVID-19 cases, where the positive impact of $PM_{2.5}$ concentration intensifies the spread of COVID-19. Environmental pollutants CO, O_3, and NO_2 are also positively correlated with confirmed cases and deaths of COVID-19 [50]. Atmospheric particulate matter, upon exceeding the satisfactory level, serves as an important cofactor in increasing the risk of SARS-CoV-2 transmission and related mortality [51].

Data from Tehran also shows a significant link between COVID-19 mortality and exposure to environmental pollution, with increased $PM_{2.5}$ levels in the air likely to increase SARS-CoV-2 mortality [52]. A similar study conducted in Germany showed that $PM_{2.5}$, O_3, and NO_2 were significantly correlated with COVID-19 outbreaks [45]. In many Italian provinces, long-term air quality data are significantly associated with COVID-19 cases, further demonstrating that long-term exposure to air pollution may be an enabling environment for virus transmission [53]. Data from Wuhan also points to an increase in deaths due to poor air quality [44]. Environmental pollution is an important factor affecting the incidence and death of COVID-19. Areas with higher levels of environmental pollution are prone to respiratory syndrome, which reduces the immunity of residents and affects their susceptibility to COVID-19 [54]. The mortality rate decreases more significantly in countries with high levels of greenery than in countries with low levels of greenery. A good air environment and a green environment are conducive to human survival and development [55].

4. Conclusions

At the beginning of COVID-19, many authors began to study the meteorological factors affecting the spread of COVID-19 and the impact of air pollution on human health and mortality, which is also a continuing hot research direction. Studies have shown that good air quality, high temperature, and humidity are relatively adverse to COVID-19 infection. Dry air may impair nasal functions that prevent viruses and bacteria from entering the body, leading to increased mortality from COVID-19. Low solar radiation cycles may lead to higher COVID-19 mortality due to reduced solar radiation [47]. Rising temperatures could help curb the spread of COVID-19. Low wind speed and high concentration of air pollutants may promote the persistence of virus particles in urban air, thus facilitating the indirect transmission of SARS-CoV-2 [48]. People living in areas with high levels of pollutants are more likely to suffer from chronic respiratory diseases and to be infected with pathogens [49]. The higher the level of environmental pollution, the more likely it is to affect the susceptibility to COVID-19 [54]. Understanding SARS-CoV-2 transmission under environmental variables can help provide supporting evidence to healthcare policymakers for formulating strategies to combat COVID-19.

Subsequently, there have been more and more papers on the impact of COVID-19 on the atmospheric environment and air quality, which has become the hottest topic in the field of the atmospheric environment under the impact of COVID-19. Obtaining sufficient atmospheric environment data requires a time buffer, so papers on this topic appeared relatively late. Air pollution is already a serious environmental problem. The COVID-19 pandemic has had a great impact on the atmospheric environment and improved the atmospheric environment to a certain extent. During the COVID-19 pandemic, lockdowns, travel restrictions, and reductions in industry, transportation, and related activities have significantly reduced mobile sources of pollution and emissions of pollutants. The lockdown has also led to widespread reductions in air pollutants and greenhouse gas emissions, and considerable improvements in air quality. In general, the concentrations of the environmental pollutants $PM_{2.5}$, PM_{10}, CO_2, CO, SO_2, and NO_2 all declined to various degrees, while the concentration of O_3 showed an increasing trend. Studying the special and complex relationship between COVID-19 and the atmospheric environment can provide new insights for environmental managers to control good air quality and manage air pollution under the impact of COVID-19.

Author Contributions: Conceptualization, Z.C. and D.S.; methodology, Z.C. and D.S.; software, Z.C.; formal analysis, Z.C.; resources, Z.C. and D.S.; data curation, Z.C.; writing—original draft preparation, Z.C. and D.S.; writing—review and editing, Z.C.; visualization, Z.C.; supervision, D.S.; project administration, D.S.; funding acquisition, D.S. All authors have read and agreed to the published version of the manuscript.

Funding: This research was funded by National Natural Science Foundation of Hunan Provincial (2021JJ40538), Scientific research project of Hunan Provincial Department of Education (21B0133), Foundation of Key Laboratory of Large Structure Health Monitoring and Control in Hebei Province (KLLSHMC2104).

Institutional Review Board Statement: Not applicable.

Informed Consent Statement: Not applicable.

Data Availability Statement: Not applicable.

Conflicts of Interest: The authors declare no conflict of interest.

References

1. Biswal, A.; Singh, T.; Singh, V.; Ravindra, K.; Mor, S. COVID-19 lockdown and its impact on tropospheric NO_2 concentrations over India using satellite-based data. *Heliyon* **2020**, *6*, e04764. [CrossRef]
2. Fang, E.Y.; Liu, X.H.; Li, M.; Zhang, Z.L.; Song, L.F.; Zhu, B.Y.; Wu, X.H.; Liu, J.J.; Zhao, D.H.; Li, Y.H. Advances in COVID-19 mRNA vaccine development. *Signal Transduct. Tar.* **2022**, *7*, 94.
3. Fernandes, Q.; Inchakalody, V.P.; Merhi, M.; Mestiri, S.; Taib, N.; El-Ella, D.M.A.; Bedhiafi, T.; Raza, A.; Al-Zaidan, L.; Mohsen, M.O.; et al. Emerging COVID-19 variants and their impact on SARS-CoV-2 diagnosis, therapeutics and vaccines. *Ann. Med.* **2022**, *54*, 524–540. [CrossRef]
4. Zhang, J.D.; Jiang, L.P.; Liu, Z.H.; Li, Y.A.; Liu, K.L.; Fang, R.Y.; Li, H.H.; Qu, Z.G.; Liu, C.Y.; Li, F. A bibliometric and visual analysis of indoor occupation environmental health risks: Development, hotspots and trend directions. *J. Clean. Prod.* **2021**, *300*, 126824.
5. Ye, N.; Kueh, T.B.; Hou, L.S.; Liu, Y.X.; Yu, H. A bibliometric analysis of corporate social responsibility in sustainable development. *J. Clean. Prod.* **2020**, *272*, 122679. [CrossRef]
6. Gou, X.; Liu, H.; Qiang, Y.; Lang, Z.; Wang, H.; Ye, D.; Wang, Z.; Wang, H. In-depth analysis on safety and security research based on system dynamics: A bibliometric mapping approach-based study. *Saf. Sci.* **2021**, *147*, 105617. [CrossRef]
7. Wang, Z.H.; Zhao, Y.D.; Wang, B. A bibliometric analysis of climate change adaptation based on massive research literature data. *J. Clean. Prod.* **2018**, *199*, 1072–1082. [CrossRef]
8. van Eck, N.J.; Waltman, L. Software survey: VOSviewer, a computer program for bibliometric mapping. *Scientometrics* **2010**, *84*, 523–538. [CrossRef]
9. Liu, H.; Hong, R.; Xiang, C.L.; Lv, C.; Li, H.H. Visualization and analysis of mapping knowledge domains for spontaneous combustion studies. *Fuel* **2020**, *262*, 13. [CrossRef]
10. Declementi, M.; Godono, A.; Mansour, I.; Milanesio, N.; Garzaro, G.; Clari, M.; Fedele, L.; Passini, V.; Bongiorno, C.; Pira, E. Assessment of air and surfaces contamination in a COVID-19 non-Intensive Care Unit. *Med. Lav.* **2020**, *111*, 372–378.
11. Ribeiro, S.P.; Silva, A.C.E.; Dattilo, W.; Reis, A.B.; Goes-Neto, A.; Alcantara, L.C.J.; Giovanetti, M.; Coura-Vital, W.; Fernandes, G.W.; Azevedo, V.A.C. Severe airport sanitarian control could slow down the spreading of COVID-19 pandemics in Brazil. *Peerj* **2020**, *8*, e9446. [CrossRef] [PubMed]
12. Zhang, R.X.; Zhang, Y.Z.; Lin, H.P.; Feng, X.; Fu, T.M.; Wang, Y.H. NOx Emission Reduction and Recovery during COVID-19 in East China. *Atmosphere* **2020**, *11*, 433. [CrossRef]
13. Sharma, S.; Zhang, M.Y.; Anshika; Gao, J.S.; Zhang, H.L.; Kota, S.H. Effect of restricted emissions during COVID-19 on air quality in India. *Sci. Total Environ.* **2020**, *728*, 8. [CrossRef]
14. Wang, Y.; Zhu, S.Q.; Ma, J.L.; Shen, J.Y.; Wang, P.F.; Wang, P.; Zhang, H.L. Enhanced atmospheric oxidation capacity and associated ozone increases during COVID-19 lockdown in the Yangtze River Delta. *Sci. Total Environ.* **2021**, *768*, 8. [CrossRef]
15. Zhang, M.Y.; Katiyar, A.; Zhu, S.Q.; Shen, J.Y.; Xia, M.; Ma, J.L.; Kota, S.H.; Wang, P.; Zhang, H.L. Impact of reduced anthropogenic emissions during COVID-19 on air quality in India. *Atmos. Chem. Phys.* **2021**, *21*, 4025–4037. [CrossRef]
16. Ma, J.L.; Shen, J.Y.; Wang, P.; Zhu, S.Q.; Wang, Y.; Wang, P.F.; Wang, G.H.; Chen, J.M.; Zhang, H.L. Modeled changes in source contributions of particulate matter during the COVID-19 pandemic in the Yangtze River Delta, China. *Atmos. Chem. Phys.* **2021**, *21*, 7343–7355. [CrossRef]
17. Kang, M.J.; Zhang, J.; Zhang, H.L.; Ying, Q. On the Relevancy of Observed Ozone Increase during COVID-19 Lockdown to Summertime Ozone and $PM_{2.5}$ Control Policies in China. *Environ. Sci. Technol. Lett.* **2021**, *8*, 289–294. [CrossRef]
18. Wang, S.Y.; Zhang, Y.L.; Ma, J.L.; Zhu, S.Q.; Shen, J.Y.; Wang, P.; Zhang, H.L. Responses of decline in air pollution and recovery associated with COVID-19 lockdown in the Pearl River Delta. *Sci. Total Environ.* **2021**, *756*, 143868. [CrossRef]
19. Wang, P.F.; Chen, K.Y.; Zhu, S.Q.; Wang, P.; Zhang, H.L. Severe air pollution events not avoided by reduced anthropogenic activities during COVID-19 outbreak. *Resour. Conserv. Recycl.* **2020**, *158*, 9. [CrossRef]
20. Huang, F.; Hou, H.; Liang, G.; Wang, Y.; Hu, Z. Analysis of Clustering Algorithm in Software of Scientometrics. *Sci. Technol. Manag. Res.* **2018**, *38*, 232–238.
21. Waltman, L.; van Eck, N.J.; Noyons, E.C.M. A unified approach to mapping and clustering of bibliometric networks. *J. Informetr.* **2010**, *4*, 629–635. [CrossRef]
22. Yang, Y.F.; Chen, G.H.; Reniers, G.; Goerlandt, F. A bibliometric analysis of process safety research in China: Understanding safety research progress as a basis for making China's chemical industry more sustainable. *J. Clean. Prod.* **2020**, *263*, 121433.

23. van Eck, N.J.; Waltman, L. Visualizing Bibliometric Networks. In *Measuring Scholarly Impact*; Springer: Berlin, Germany, 2014; pp. 285–320.
24. Bamel, U.K.; Pandey, R.; Gupta, A. Safety climate: Systematic literature network analysis of 38 years (1980–2018) of research. *Accid. Anal. Prev.* **2020**, *135*, 105387. [CrossRef]
25. Zou, X.; Yue, W.L.; Vu, H.L. Visualization and analysis of mapping knowledge domain of road safety studies. *Accid. Anal. Prev.* **2018**, *118*, 131–145. [CrossRef] [PubMed]
26. Ho, L.; Alonso, A.; Forio, M.A.E.; Vanclooster, M.; Goethals, P.L.M. Water research in support of the Sustainable Development Goal 6: A case study in Belgium. *J. Clean. Prod.* **2020**, *277*, 124082. [CrossRef]
27. Tao, J.; Qiu, D.Y.; Yang, F.Q.; Duan, Z.P. A bibliometric analysis of human reliability research. *J. Clean. Prod.* **2020**, *260*, 11. [CrossRef]
28. Rume, T.; Didar-Ul Islam, S.M. Environmental effects of COVID-19 pandemic and potential strategies of sustainability. *Heliyon* **2020**, *6*, e04965.
29. Li, L.; Li, Q.; Huang, L.; Wang, Q.; Zhu, A.S.; Xu, J.; Liu, Z.Y.; Li, H.L.; Shi, L.S.; Li, R.; et al. Air quality changes during the COVID-19 lockdown over the Yangtze River Delta Region: An insight into the impact of human activity pattern changes on air pollution variation. *Sci. Total Environ.* **2020**, *732*, 11. [CrossRef]
30. Fasso, A.; Maranzano, P.; Otto, P. Spatiotemporal variable selection and air quality impact assessment of COVID-19 lockdown. *Spat. Stat.* **2022**, *49*, 100549. [CrossRef]
31. Collivignarelli, M.C.; Abba, A.; Bertanza, G.; Pedrazzani, R.; Ricciardi, P.; Miino, M.C. Lockdown for COVID-2019 in Milan: What are the effects on air quality? *Sci. Total Environ.* **2020**, *732*, 9. [CrossRef]
32. Saadat, S.; Rawtani, D.; Hussain, C.M. Environmental perspective of COVID-19. *Sci. Total Environ.* **2020**, *728*, 138870. [CrossRef]
33. He, C.; Hong, S.; Zhang, L.; Mu, H.; Xin, A.X.; Zhou, Y.Q.; Liu, J.K.; Liu, N.J.; Su, Y.M.; Tian, Y.; et al. Global, continental, and national variation in $PM_{2.5}$, O_3, and NO_2 concentrations during the early 2020 COVID-19 lockdown. *Atmos. Pollut. Res.* **2021**, *12*, 136–145. [CrossRef] [PubMed]
34. Cheng, K.; Chang, Y.H.; Kuang, Y.Q.; Khan, R.; Zou, Z. Elucidating the responses of highly time-resolved $PM_{2.5}$ related elements to extreme emission reductions. *Environ. Res.* **2022**, *206*, 7. [CrossRef]
35. Nigam, R.; Pandya, K.; Luis, A.J.; Sengupta, R.; Kotha, M. Positive effects of COVID-19 lockdown on air quality of industrial cities (Ankleshwar and Vapi) of Western India. *Sci. Rep.* **2021**, *11*, 12. [CrossRef]
36. Tibrewal, K.; Venkataraman, C. COVID-19 lockdown closures of emissions sources in India: Lessons for air quality and climate policy. *J. Environ. Manage.* **2022**, *302*, 114079. [CrossRef]
37. Fareed, Z.; Bashir, M.F.; Bilal; Salem, S. Investigating the Co-movement Nexus Between Air Quality, Temperature, and COVID-19 in California: Implications for Public Health. *Front. Public Health* **2021**, *9*, 8. [CrossRef]
38. Ropkins, K.; Tate, J.E. Early observations on the impact of the COVID-19 lockdown on air quality trends across the UK. *Sci. Total Environ.* **2021**, *754*, 8. [CrossRef]
39. Souri, A.H.; Chance, K.; Bak, J.; Nowlan, C.R.; Abad, G.G.; Jung, Y.; Wong, D.C.; Mao, J.Q.; Liu, X. Unraveling pathways of elevated ozone induced by the 2020 lockdown in Europe by an observationally constrained regional model using TROPOMI. *Atmos. Chem. Phys.* **2021**, *21*, 18227–18245. [CrossRef]
40. Torkmahalleh, M.A.; Akhmetvaliyeva, Z.; Omran, A.D.; Omran, F.F.D.; Kazemitabar, M.; Naseri, M.; Naseri, M.; Sharifi, H.; Malekipirbazari, M.; Adotey, E.K.; et al. Global Air Quality and COVID-19 Pandemic: Do We Breathe Cleaner Air? *Aerosol Air Qual. Res.* **2021**, *21*, 200567. [CrossRef]
41. Ching, J.; Kajino, M. Rethinking Air Quality and Climate Change after COVID-19. *Int. J. Environ. Res. Public Health* **2020**, *17*, 5167. [CrossRef]
42. Sarwar, S.; Shahzad, K.; Fareed, Z.; Shahzad, U. A study on the effects of meteorological and climatic factors on the COVID-19 spread in Canada during 2020. *J. Environ. Health Sci. Eng.* **2021**, *19*, 1513–1521. [CrossRef] [PubMed]
43. Shahzad, K.; Farooq, T.H.; Dogan, B.; Hu, L.Z.; Shahzad, U. Does environmental quality and weather induce COVID-19: Case study of Istanbul, Turkey. *Environ. Forensics* **2021**. [CrossRef]
44. Fareed, Z.; Iqbal, N.; Shahzad, F.; Shah, S.G.M.; Zulfiqar, B.; Shahzad, K.; Hashmi, S.H.; Shahzad, U. Co-variance nexus between COVID-19 mortality, humidity, and air quality index in Wuhan, China: New insights from partial and multiple wavelet coherence. *Air Qual. Atmos. Health* **2020**, *13*, 673–682. [CrossRef] [PubMed]
45. Bashir, M.F.; Benghoul, M.; Numan, U.; Shakoor, A.; Komal, B.; Bashir, M.A.; Bashir, M.; Tan, D.J. Environmental pollution and COVID-19 outbreak: Insights from Germany. *Air Qual. Atmos. Health* **2020**, *13*, 1385–1394. [CrossRef]
46. Linares, C.; Belda, F.; Lopez-Bueno, J.A.; Luna, M.Y.; Sanchez-Martinez, G.; Hervella, B.; Culqui, D.; Diaz, J. Short-term associations of air pollution and meteorological variables on the incidence and severity of COVID-19 in Madrid (Spain): A time series study. *Environ. Sci. Eur.* **2021**, *33*, 1–13. [CrossRef]
47. Barcellos, D.D.; Fernandes, G.M.K.; de Souza, F.T. Data based model for predicting COVID-19 morbidity and mortality in metropolis. *Sci. Rep.* **2021**, *11*, 24491. [CrossRef]
48. Coccia, M. How do low wind speeds and high levels of air pollution support the spread of COVID-19? *Atmos. Pollut. Res.* **2021**, *12*, 437–445. [CrossRef]
49. Conticini, E.; Frediani, B.; Caro, D. Can atmospheric pollution be considered a co-factor in extremely high level of SARS-CoV-2 lethality in Northern Italy? *Environ. Pollut.* **2020**, *261*, 3. [CrossRef]

50. Meo, S.A.; Alqahtani, S.A.; Binmeather, F.S.; AlRasheed, R.A.; Aljedaie, G.M.; Albarrak, R.M. Effect of environmental pollutants PM$_{2.5}$, CO, O$_3$ and NO$_2$, on the incidence and mortality of SARS-CoV-2 in largest metropolitan cities, Delhi, Mumbai and Kolkata, India. *J. King Saud Univ. Sci.* **2022**, *34*, 101687. [CrossRef]
51. Aggarwal, S.; Balaji, S.; Singh, T.; Menon, G.R.; Mandal, S.; Madhumathi, J.; Mahajan, N.; Kohli, S.; Kaur, J.; Singh, H.; et al. Association between ambient air pollutants and meteorological factors with SARS-CoV-2 transmission and mortality in India: An exploratory study. *Environ. Health* **2021**, *20*, 120. [CrossRef]
52. Faridi, S.; Yousefian, F.; Niazi, S.; Ghalhari, M.R.; Hassanvand, M.S.; Naddafi, K. Impact of SARS-CoV-2 on Ambient Air Particulate Matter in Tehran. *Aerosol Air Qual. Res.* **2020**, *20*, 1805–1811. [CrossRef]
53. Fattorini, D.; Regoli, F. Role of the chronic air pollution levels in the COVID-19 outbreak risk in Italy. *Environ. Pollut.* **2020**, *264*, 5. [CrossRef]
54. Wen, C.; Akram, R.; Irfan, M.; Iqbal, W.; Dagar, V.; Acevedo-Duqued, A.; Saydaliev, H.B. The asymmetric nexus between air pollution and COVID-19: Evidence from a non-linear panel autoregressive distributed lag model. *Environ. Res.* **2022**, *209*, 112848. [CrossRef] [PubMed]
55. Meo, S.A.; Almutairi, F.J.; Abukhalaf, A.A.; Usmani, A.M. Effect of Green Space Environment on Air Pollutants PM$_{2.5}$, PM$_{10}$, CO, O$_3$, and Incidence and Mortality of SARS-CoV-2 in Highly Green and Less-Green Countries. *Int. J. Environ. Res. Public Health* **2021**, *18*, 13151. [CrossRef]

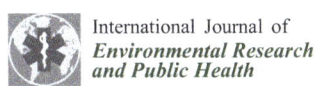

Article

Coronavirus Disease Pandemic Effect on Medical-Seeking Behaviors Even in One Resource-Competent Community: A Case Controlled Study

Fang Wang [1,†], Jin-Ming Wu [2,3,†], Yi-Chieh Lin [4], Te-Wei Ho [2], Hui-Lin Lin [1], Hsi-Yu Yu [2,*] and I-Rue Lai [2,*]

1. Department of Nursing, National Taiwan University Hospital, Taipei 100, Taiwan
2. Department of Surgery, National Taiwan University Hospital and National Taiwan University College of Medicine, Taipei 100, Taiwan
3. Department of Surgery, National Taiwan University Hospital Hsin-Chu Branch, Hsinchu 300, Taiwan
4. Department of Public Health, College of Health Sciences, Kaohsiung Medical University, Kaohsiung City 807, Taiwan
* Correspondence: hyyvpn@ntu.edu.tw (H.-Y.Y.); iruelai@gmail.com (I.-R.L.); Tel.: +886-2-23123456 (ext. 65107) (I.-R.L.)
† These authors contributed equally to this work.

Citation: Wang, F.; Wu, J.-M.; Lin, Y.-C.; Ho, T.-W.; Lin, H.-L.; Yu, H.-Y.; Lai, I.-R. Coronavirus Disease Pandemic Effect on Medical-Seeking Behaviors Even in One Resource-Competent Community: A Case Controlled Study. *Int. J. Environ. Res. Public Health* **2022**, *19*, 10822. https://doi.org/10.3390/ijerph191710822

Academic Editors: Sachiko Kodera and Essam A. Rashed

Received: 18 July 2022
Accepted: 24 August 2022
Published: 30 August 2022

Publisher's Note: MDPI stays neutral with regard to jurisdictional claims in published maps and institutional affiliations.

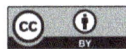

Copyright: © 2022 by the authors. Licensee MDPI, Basel, Switzerland. This article is an open access article distributed under the terms and conditions of the Creative Commons Attribution (CC BY) license (https://creativecommons.org/licenses/by/4.0/).

Abstract: (1) Background: The coronavirus disease 2019 (COVID-19) pandemic had overwhelming impacts on medical services. During its initial surge, Taiwan was unique in maintaining its medical services without imposing travel restrictions, which provided an ideal environment in which to test if the fear of becoming infected with COVID-19 interfered with health-seeking behavior (HSB). We tested this hypothesis among adults with acute complicated appendicitis (ACA). (2) Methods: Adults with acute appendicitis were enrolled between 1 January and 30 June 2020 (COVID-19 period). The first two quarters of the preceding 3 years were defined as a historical control group. Outcome measures included the rate of ACA and the number of hospital stays. (3) Results: The COVID-19 era included 145 patients with acute appendicitis. Compared to the historical control (320 patients), the COVID-19 era was significantly associated with a higher length of symptom duration until presentation to the emergency room within >48 h (17.2% vs. 9.1%, $p = 0.011$), a higher incidence of ACA (29.7% vs. 19.4%, $p = 0.014$), and a longer length of hospital stays (5.0 days vs. 4.0 days, $p = 0.043$). The adjusted models showed that the COVID-19 period had a significant relationship with a higher rate of ACA (odds ratio (OR) = 1.87; 95% confidence interval (CI): 1.23–2.52; $p = 0.008$) and longer length of hospital stays (OR= 2.10; 95% CI: 0.92 to 3.31; $p < 0.001$). (4) Conclusions: The fear of COVID-19 may prohibit patients from seeking medical help, worsening their clinical outcomes. The surgical community should take action to provide scientific information to relive mental stress.

Keywords: health-seeking behavior; COVID-19; appendicitis; surgical care

1. Introduction

Health-seeking behavior is described as "steps taken by a patient who perceives a need for help when he or she tries to solve a medical disease" [1]. In other words, health-seeking behavior is the behavioral element of healthcare utilization and is conceptually associated with clinicodemographics, socioeconomic status, access to healthcare institutes, and the views and experiences of both the patient and medical provider [2,3]. Andersen developed a serial behavioral model to elucidate the mechanisms associated with healthcare utilization [2,4], defined as the quantity of people using healthcare services and estimated by costs and medical visits [5].

The new variant of severe acute respiratory syndrome coronavirus disease 2 (SARS-CoV-2), also known as coronavirus disease 2019 (COVID-19), first broke out in China in December 2019 and rapidly spread worldwide [6]. As of 30 September 2020, 33.83 million confirmed cases and >1.01 million deaths have been cumulatively recorded worldwide since the start of the pandemic according to the World Health Organization statistics [7]. The highly contagious potential of COVID-19 deepened the strain on healthcare institutes and resulted in reduced healthcare utilization worldwide under a limited supply of medical resources. Furthermore, patients with severe illnesses might be unwilling to visit a highly contagious hospital due to their fear of being infected by the virus [8].

Acute appendicitis is not only one of the most common causes of acute abdominal diseases in adults [9], but also one of the most common reasons for general emergency surgery worldwide [10]. With the advancement of minimally invasive surgery, most patients can recover early after a timely appendectomy [11]. However, the COVID-19 pandemic became a barrier to timely surgical treatment, which increased the ACA rate in countries with compromised medical supplies [12,13].

Taiwan is very close to the coast of China and was predicted to be likely to experience a high number of cases in 2020 due to the many flights that occur between the countries. However, Taiwan surprisingly controlled its sporadic outbreaks of COVID-19 well by implementing several public health responses [14] and did not suffer a shortage of medical resources. As a result, it provides a unique environment in which to validate if health-seeking behavior may have interfered with clinical outcomes even in a resource-unlimited setting. In this study, we hypothesized that the mental panic caused by the COVID-19 pandemic may have worsened the clinical outcomes of patients. Thus, we aimed to analyze the rates of uncomplicated/complicated appendicitis during the COVID-19 pandemic and compare them with those of previous years.

The rest of this paper is organized as follows. Section 2 is the Materials and Methods, Section 3 is the Results, Section 4 is the Discussion, and Section 5 is the Research Conclusions.

2. Materials and Methods

A retrospective study was conducted to review the records of adult patients with acute appendicitis ($\geq$20 years) in one academic center during the COVID-19 epidemic period from January to June 2020. Next, patients with acute appendicitis from the same months, January to June, in 2017, 2018, and 2019 were considered as the control group. The same interval every year was analyzed because a previous study demonstrated that the incidence of acute appendicitis was associated with seasonal variation [15]. The exclusion criteria were being pregnant or pathological findings of appendiceal tumors.

The data analyzed included clinical demographics such as age, gender, body mass index (BMI), residence in Taipei/New Taipei City, body temperature measured at the emergency room (ER), white blood-cell count (WBC), and the time interval from symptom onset to ER arrival. The weighted Charlson comorbidity index (CCI) score was used to account for the comorbidity burden [16,17]. Further, daily confirmed COVID-19 cases were recorded to represent the severity of the pandemic. The primary outcome measures were the occurrence of ACA defined as abscess observed in computed tomography, presence of appendiceal perforation determined by surgical documentation, or a description of gangrenous appendicitis assessed by pathological reports [10]. The secondary outcome measure was inpatient length of stay.

Furthermore, the trend of the total number of surgeries (elective and emergent operations) during the study periods was analyzed to reflect the overall impact of COVID-19 on surgical patients seeking medical services.

Statistical analyses were performed using the Statistical Package for the Social Sciences (SPSS) version 26.0 software (IBM SPSS 26.0, Armonk, NY, USA). Continuous variables (age, body mass index, time from ER visit to surgery, white blood count, and length of hospital stays) were presented as medians with interquartile ranges (IQRs), and categorical variables (gender, category of Charlson comorbidity index score, residence in Taipei/New Taipei City, category of duration of symptoms until presentation to ER, body temperature > 38 degrees Celsius, and appendectomy performed) were expressed as numbers (percentages). Categorical variables were compared using the Chi-square test or Fisher's exact test (the numbers were <5). Continuous variables between groups were compared using the Mann–Whitney U test. The binary logistic regression model was used on associated variables to determine the odds of ACA occurrence. Furthermore, a linear regression model was created to predict the length of hospital stays. Statistical significance was assumed at $p < 0.05$.

3. Results

During the 26-week COVID-19 study period, 145 patients with acute appendicitis were treated in our institute (Table 1). No patient was diagnosed with COVID-19. Among them, 43 (29.7%) patients had ACA. The rates of appendectomy in the ACA and non-ACA groups were 83.7% and 98.0%, respectively. Patients with ACA had a significantly higher rate of body temperature > 38 °C (46.5% vs. 26.5%, $p = 0.019$) and a significantly higher rate of symptom duration until presentation to the ER within >48 h (20.9% vs. 8.8%, $p = 0.001$) in comparison with the non-ACA group. No differences were observed in the median age, gender, BMI, or CCI score category between adults with ACA and non-ACA.

Table 1. Clinical variables among 145 adult patients with acute appendicitis during the COVID-19 outbreak.

	Non-Complicated Appendicitis (N = 102)	Complicated Appendicitis (N = 43)	p Value
Age, year, median (IQR)	55.5 (36.8, 65.1)	53.3 (36.4, 65.5)	0.710
Gender			0.360
Female	46 (45.1%)	23 (53.5%)	
Male	56 (54.9%)	20 (46.5%)	
Body mass index, median (IQR)	23.0 (21.3, 25.2)	23.5 (21.0, 25.1)	0.970
Charlson comorbidity index score			0.140
≤2	97 (95.1%)	38 (88.4%)	
>2	5 (4.9%)	5 (11.6%)	
Residence in Taipei/New Taipei City	93 (91.2%)	38 (88.4%)	0.690
Duration of symptoms until presentation to ER, n (%)			0.001
≤48 h	93 (91.2%)	33 (79.1%)	
>48 h	9 (8.8%)	9 (20.9%)	
Time from ER visit to surgery (hours), median (IQR)	11.0 (10.0, 14.0)	13.0 (11.0, 15.0)	0.190
Body temperature > 38 degrees Celsius	27 (26.5%)	20 (46.5%)	0.019
White blood count, 10^9/L, median (IQR)	11.0 (9.0, 14.8)	10.2 (7.9, 11.7)	0.170
Appendectomy performed	100 (98.0%)	36 (83.7%)	0.001
Length of hospital stays (day), median (IQR)	4.0 (3.0, 7.0)	5.0 (3.0, 11.0)	0.080

ER: emergency room.

To determine the impact of the COVID-19 pandemic on the severity of appendicitis, Figure 1 shows the association between the number of confirmed COVID-19 cases in Taiwan and the distribution of patients with acute appendicitis. The majority of COVID-19 cases were diagnosed from week 6 to 16. The ACA ratio during the same period was also increased.

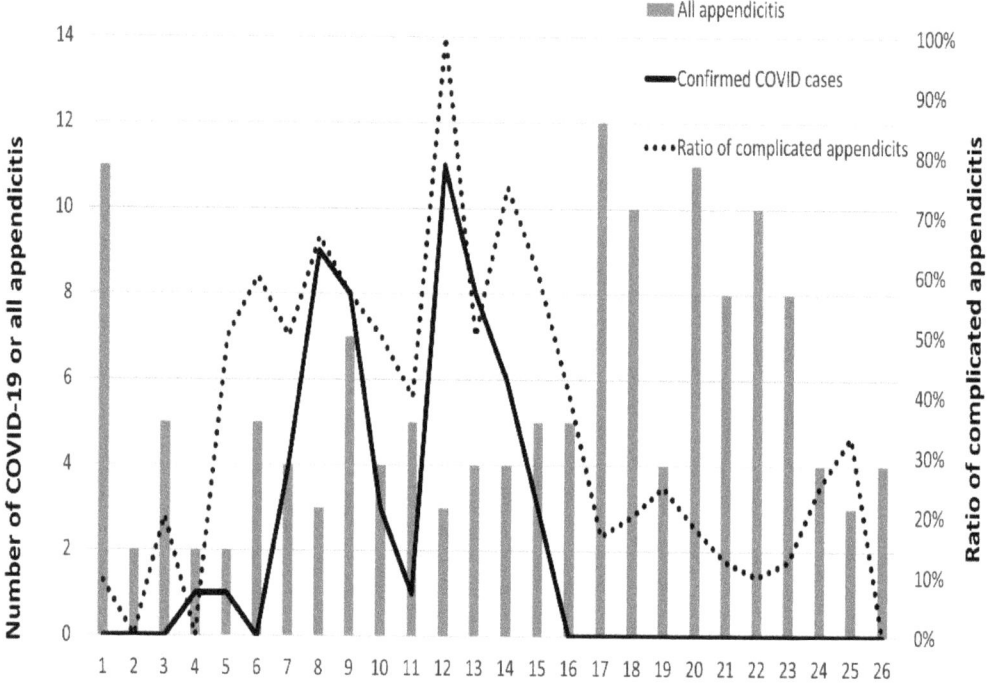

Figure 1. Weekly statistics for the number of adult patients with acute appendicitis (dotted vertical bar), the number of cases of complicated appendicitis (solid vertical bar), and the number of confirmed COVID-19 cases in Taiwan (dashed line).

For comparisons during the COVID-19 period, a control cohort comprising 320 patients was identified over 18 months between 2017 and 2019 (Table 2). No differences were observed between the two groups in terms of median age, gender, median BMI, category of CCI score, and residence in Taipei/New Taipei City. The median WBC count (10.8 vs. 9.4×10^9/L, $p = 0.010$) and rate of symptom duration until presentation to the ER within >48 h (17.2% vs. 9.1%, $p = 0.011$) were significantly higher during the COVID-19 period compared to the control period. Overall, a higher incidence of ACA (29.7% vs. 19.4%, $p = 0.014$) and a longer median length of hospital stays (5.0 days vs. 4.0 days, $p = 0.043$) were observed during the COVID-19 period.

To validate the association between the COVID-19 period and ACA onset, one binary multivariate model was developed to predict ACA occurrence (Table 3), showing that both the COVID-19 period (odds ratio (OR) = 1.87; 95% confidence interval (CI): 1.23–2.52; $p = 0.008$) and symptom duration until presentation to the ER within >48 h (OR = 1.70; 95% CI: 1.06–2.36; $p = 0.044$) were significantly associated with ACA development. Further, the adjusted linear regression model was used to predict the length of hospital stays (Table 4), demonstrating that both CCI scores of >2 (coefficient = 2.51; 95% CI: 1.25 to 3.16; $p < 0.001$) and the COVID-19 period (coefficient = 2.10; 95% CI: 0.92 to 3.31; $p < 0.001$) were significantly associated with a longer length of hospital stays.

Table 2. Comparison of clinical characteristics between adult patients with acute appendicitis during the COVID-19 epidemic period and the preceding 3-year control period.

	Control Period (N = 320)	COVID-19 Period (N = 145)	p Value
Age, year, median (IQR)	47.9 (33.4, 63.4)	55.2 (36.8, 65.4)	0.088
Gender			0.220
Female	172 (53.8%)	69 (47.6%)	
Male	148 (46.3%)	76 (52.4%)	
Body mass index, median (IQR)	23.0 (21.0, 24.7)	23.1 (21.3, 25.1)	0.210
Charlson comorbidity index score			0.690
≤2	301 (94.1%)	135 (93.1%)	
>2	19 (5.9%)	10 (6.9%)	
Residence in Taipei/New Taipei City	290 (90.6%)	131 (90.3%)	0.920
Duration of symptoms until presentation to ER, n (%)			0.011
≤48 h	291 (90.9%)	120 (82.8%)	
>48 h	29 (9.1%)	25 (17.2%)	
Time from ER visit to surgery (hours), median (IQR)	10.0 (9.0, 13.0)	11.0 (10.0, 14.0)	0.340
Body temperature > 38 degrees Celsius	129 (40.3%)	47 (32.4%)	0.100
White blood count, 10^9/L, median (IQR)	9.4 (7.6, 11.6)	10.8 (8.9, 13.2)	0.010
Complicated appendicitis	62 (19.4%)	43 (29.7%)	0.014
Length of hospital stays (day), median (IQR)	4.0 (3.0, 6.0)	5.0 (3.0, 8.0)	0.043

ER: emergency room.

Table 3. Adjusted multivariate analysis used to predict complicated appendicitis.

Variables	Odds Ratio	95% CI	p Value
Age (every one-year increment)	1.01	0.99–1.02	0.245
Male gender (ref: female)	0.93	0.58–1.50	0.793
Body mass index	0.93	0.86–1.01	0.132
Charlson comorbidity index score > 2 (ref: ≤2)	1.38	0.58–3.28	0.459
Residence in Taipei/New Taipei City	0.76	0.40–1.42	0.395
Duration of symptoms until presentation >48 h (ref: ≤48 h)	1.70	1.06–2.36	0.044
Body temperature > 38 degrees Celsius	0.74	0.35–1.57	0.446
White blood counts	1.01	0.76–2.97	0.985
COVID-19 period (ref: control period: 2017–2019)	1.87	1.23–2.52	0.008

Table 4. Adjusted multivariate analysis to predict inpatient length of stay.

Variables	Coefficients	95% Confident Interval		p Value
		Lower Limit	Upper Limit	
Age (every one-year increment)	0.16	−0.02	0.13	0.524
Male gender (ref: female)	0.64	−1.93	3.21	0.627
Body mass index	−0.15	−0.60	0.31	0.530
Charlson comorbidity index score>2 (ref: ≤2)	2.51	1.25	3.16	<0.001
Residence in Taipei/New Taipei City	−3.05	−7.4	1.29	0.168
Complicated appendicitis	2.10	0.92	3.31	<0.001

On the other hand, the trend of the total number of surgeries during the study periods is shown in Figure 2. The mean numbers of elective operations in the control period and the COVID-19 period were 23,288 and 21,526 ($p = 0.180$), respectively, whereas the mean numbers of emergent operations in the control period and the COVID-19 period were 4576 and 4601 ($p = 0.650$), respectively. Although both were not statistically significant, the COVID-19 pandemic caused a more significantly decreased number of elective operations compared to emergent operations. This implies that the COVID-19 pandemic not only changed the behavior-seeking surgical services of patients without emergent needs but also worsened the surgical outcomes of patients with emergent needs.

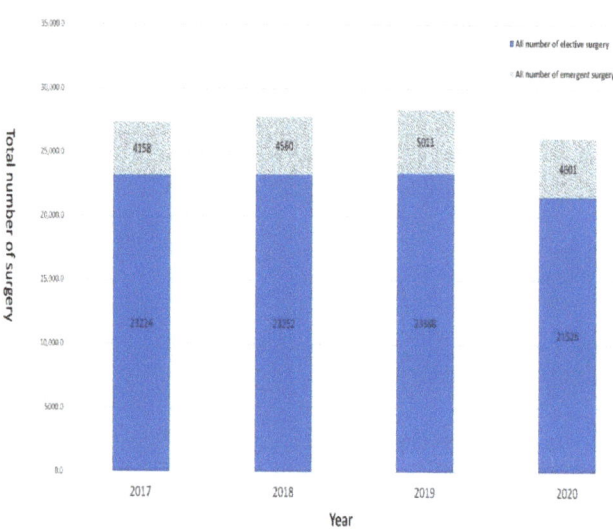

Figure 2. The trend of total number of surgeries (elective and emergent operations) during the study periods.

4. Discussion

The COVID-19 pandemic was the most concerning health problem in 2020 because it caused not only health disorders but also extensive restrictions on people's daily lives worldwide. During our study period, Taiwan avoided the worst effects of the pandemic due to its implementation of a broad public health infrastructure and domains of effective screening, isolation/quarantine, and facial mask use [18]. Although Taiwan's government did not implement travel restrictions and its medical services were sufficient, this study demonstrated that there were fewer elective operations compared to emergent operations due to the pandemic. Further, a higher rate of ACA and a longer length of hospital stays in patients with acute appendicitis during the COVID-19 period in comparison to the control period were noticed. Notably, the number of confirmed COVID-19 cases was positively correlated with the ACA rate. Therefore, patients' fear of being contaminated by COVID-19 influenced their health-seeking behavior and worsened their clinical outcomes.

In our study, symptom duration from ER presentation to >48 h after was found to be significantly associated with ACA, which was similar to the results of a previous report [19]. Prolonged appendicitis without prompt treatment might lead to more severe inflammation of the appendiceal wall and result in perforation or abscess formation [20]. Furthermore, a more significant association was observed between patients with acute appendicitis during the COVID-19 period and ACA as compared with that in the last 3 years. Our findings coincided with those of published reports on children [12,21] and adults [22].

In addition to the impact of clinical and socioeconomic determinants on outcomes, poor health-seeking behavior has been proven to increase morbidity and mortality [23]. Patients' behaviors should be understood at this level in order to improve their clinical outcomes [24]. Based on our findings, one epidemic communicable disease could interfere with the need to seek out medical services even in a resource-competent community. We hypothesize that fake news or misinformation on social media may have caused people to feel excessive fear, diminishing their willingness to travel and seek medical services [25]. Conversely, scientific information and medical knowledge can help to improve health-seeking behavior, which in turn leads to a healthy condition [23]. While social media can rapidly disseminate information, the spreading of false information can confuse and distract people. Therefore, reliable evidence is a cornerstone for promoting health awareness and implementing health policies, especially during the COVID-19 pandemic. Moreover, as educated scientists and physicians should be the leaders in delivering heath-related information to the public [25,26], governments should implement anti-misinformation actions to minimize possible adverse effects.

Although healthcare systems, disparities of medical supplies, and socioeconomic status are the main barriers to medical services [27,28], the extensive health crisis that took place during the COVID-19 pandemic may become an additional obstacle in providing timely surgical intervention, a key aspect of any healthcare system with both elective and emergency procedures. To overcome the shortage of medical supplies, healthcare systems should aim to rapidly prioritize available resources and adopt new policies to deliver clinical services [29,30]. Although surgical management varies widely according to the regional culture and healthcare system, each institution has customized plans to maintain appropriate surgical services to are sufficiently protect surgical staff.

Based on our experiences, surgical need declined during the COVID-19 pandemic even if the outbreak was not severe in Taiwan. We allocated the members of surgical teams to other departments in order to prevent infection and enable better care for patients with COVID-19. During the study period, more than 24,000 man-hours of labor were provided by our surgical teams. With this help, the workload of the departments in charge of care relating to COVID-19 was partially relieved.

This study had some limitations. The study design was retrospective and it was conducted in one universal healthcare system, which alleviated part of the barrier of access to healthcare services. Second, the period from 1 January to 30 June 2020 was selected because the spread of COVID-19 was more severe during this period. The use of different study periods might lead to different results. Third, the referral policy was associated with delayed medical visits but was consistent during the study period in Taiwan. Some studies addressed the fact that general practitioners preferred to offer medical treatment for patients with acute appendicitis without referring them to the ER [31]. Based on our findings, the number of patients with acute appendicitis (145) was higher than the average number during the control period (around 107). Therefore, we considered that the number of patients who were not referred for or who received no medical treatment to be rather low.

5. Conclusions

Based on our findings, the COVID-19 era had a significant relationship with a delayed presentation to the ER and led to an increased rate of acute complicated appendicitis in a community with normally functioning medical services and no travel restrictions. Medical professionals play a key role in delivering accurate information and knowledge, helping to eliminate panic, and encouraging patients to pursue medical attention promptly. With the recommendations made in this study, the collateral impact of this communicable disease may be partially alleviated. However, if the COVID-19 outbreak continues, medical services will be further negatively affected. Under these circumstances, healthcare systems should adopt other policies and rationally allocate medical resources in order to effectively maintain medical services.

Author Contributions: Conceptualization, F.W., J.-M.W., Y.-C.L., T.-W.H., H.-L.L., H.-Y.Y. and I.-R.L.; methodology, F.W., J.-M.W., T.-W.H., H.-Y.Y. and I.-R.L.; software, J.-M.W. and T.-W.H.; validation, J.-M.W., T.-W.H., H.-Y.Y. and I.-R.L.; formal analysis, F.W., J.-M.W., Y.-C.L., T.-W.H., H.-L.L., H.-Y.Y. and I.-R.L.; investigation, J.-M.W., T.-W.H., H.-Y.Y. and I.-R.L.; resources, J.-M.W. and T.-W.H.; data curation, F.W., J.-M.W., T.-W.H., H.-Y.Y. and I.-R.L.; writing—original draft preparation, J.-M.W., T.-W.H., H.-Y.Y. and I.-R.L.; writing—review and editing, F.W., J.-M.W., Y.-C.L., T.-W.H., H.-L.L., H.-Y.Y. and I.-R.L.; visualization, J.-M.W., T.-W.H., H.-Y.Y. and I.-R.L.; supervision, H.-Y.Y. and I.-R.L.; project administration, H.-Y.Y. and I.-R.L.; funding acquisition, H.-Y.Y. and I.-R.L. All authors have read and agreed to the published version of the manuscript.

Funding: This study was supported by a grant from NTUH (109-P22) and grants from the Ministry of Science and Technology (Numbers 110-2634-F-002-032 and 110-2811-E-002-528-MY3), Taiwan, which had no role in the study design, data collection and analysis, decision to publish, or preparation of the manuscript.

Institutional Review Board Statement: This study was reviewed and approved by the research ethics committee of the National Taiwan University Hospital (202008052RINC).

Informed Consent Statement: Patient consent was waived due to retrospective analysis from de-identification data.

Data Availability Statement: The data are available upon requested from the authors.

Acknowledgments: We thank the staff of the Department of Medical Research, National Taiwan University Hospital, for the Integrated Medical Database (NTUH-iMD).

Conflicts of Interest: The authors declare no conflict of interest.

References

1. Chrisman, N.J. The health seeking process: An approach to the natural history of illness. *Cult. Med. Psychiatry* **1977**, *1*, 351–377. [CrossRef] [PubMed]
2. Andersen, R.M. Revisiting the behavioral model and access to medical care: Does it matter? *J. Health Soc. Behav.* **1995**, *36*, 1–10. [CrossRef] [PubMed]
3. Clewley, D.; Rhon, D.; Flynn, T.; Koppenhaver, S.; Cook, C. Health seeking behavior as a predictor of healthcare utilization in a population of patients with spinal pain. *PLoS ONE* **2018**, *13*, e0201348. [CrossRef] [PubMed]
4. Andersen, R.M. National health surveys and the behavioral model of health services use. *Med. Care* **2008**, *46*, 647–653. [CrossRef] [PubMed]
5. Blackwell, D.L.; Martinez, M.E.; Gentleman, J.F.; Sanmartin, C.; Berthelot, J.M. Socioeconomic status and utilization of health care services in Canada and the United States: Findings from a binational health survey. *Med. Care* **2009**, *47*, 1136–1146. [CrossRef]
6. Zhu, N.; Zhang, D.; Wang, W.; Li, X.; Yang, B.; Song, J.; Zhao, X.; Huang, B.; Shi, W.; Lu, R.; et al. A Novel Coronavirus from Patients with Pneumonia in China, 2019. *N. Engl. J. Med.* **2020**, *382*, 727–733. [CrossRef]
7. Listings of WHO's Response to COVID-19. Available online: https://www.who.int/news-room/detail/29-06-2020-covidtimeline (accessed on 18 July 2022).
8. Boserup, B.; McKenney, M.; Elkbuli, A. The impact of the COVID-19 pandemic on emergency department visits and patient safety in the United States. *Am. J. Emerg. Med.* **2020**, *38*, 1732–1736. [CrossRef]
9. Addiss, D.G.; Shaffer, N.; Fowler, B.S.; Tauxe, R.V. The epidemiology of appendicitis and appendectomy in the United States. *Am. J. Epidemiol.* **1990**, *132*, 910–925. [CrossRef]
10. Bhangu, A.; Soreide, K.; Di Saverio, S.; Assarsson, J.H.; Drake, F.T. Acute appendicitis: Modern understanding of pathogenesis, diagnosis, and management. *Lancet* **2015**, *386*, 1278–1287. [CrossRef]
11. Sartelli, M.; Baiocchi, G.L.; Di Saverio, S.; Ferrara, F.; Labricciosa, F.M.; Ansaloni, L.; Coccolini, F.; Vijayan, D.; Abbas, A.; Abongwa, H.K.; et al. Prospective Observational Study on acute Appendicitis Worldwide (POSAW). *World J. Emerg. Surg.* **2018**, *13*, 19. [CrossRef]
12. Fisher, J.C.; Tomita, S.S.; Ginsburg, H.B.; Gordon, A.; Walker, D.; Kuenzler, K.A. Increase in Pediatric Perforated Appendicitis in the New York City Metropolitan Region at the Epicenter of the COVID-19 Outbreak. *Ann. Surg.* **2021**, *273*, 410–415. [CrossRef] [PubMed]
13. Burgard, M.; Cherbanyk, F.; Nassiopoulos, K.; Malekzadeh, S.; Pugin, F.; Egger, B. An effect of the COVID-19 pandemic: Significantly more complicated appendicitis due to delayed presentation of patients! *PLoS ONE* **2021**, *16*, e0249171. [CrossRef]
14. Wang, C.J.; Ng, C.Y.; Brook, R.H. Response to COVID-19 in Taiwan: Big Data Analytics, New Technology, and Proactive Testing. *JAMA* **2020**, *323*, 1341–1342. [CrossRef] [PubMed]
15. Zangbar, B.; Rhee, P.; Pandit, V.; Hsu, C.H.; Khalil, M.; Okeefe, T.; Neumayer, L.; Joseph, B. Seasonal Variation in Emergency General Surgery. *Ann. Surg.* **2016**, *263*, 76–81. [CrossRef]
16. Quan, H.; Li, B.; Couris, C.M.; Fushimi, K.; Graham, P.; Hider, P.; Januel, J.M.; Sundararajan, V. Updating and validating the Charlson comorbidity index and score for risk adjustment in hospital discharge abstracts using data from 6 countries. *Am. J. Epidemiol.* **2011**, *173*, 676–682. [CrossRef] [PubMed]
17. Wu, J.M.; Ho, T.W.; Yen, H.H.; Wu, C.H.; Kuo, T.C.; Yang, C.Y.; Tien, Y.W. Endoscopic Retrograde Biliary Drainage Causes Intra-Abdominal Abscess in Pancreaticoduodenectomy Patients: An Important But Neglected Risk Factor. *Ann. Surg. Oncol.* **2019**, *26*, 1086–1092. [CrossRef] [PubMed]
18. Summers, J.; Cheng, H.Y.; Lin, H.H.; Barnard, L.T.; Kvalsvig, A.; Wilson, N.; Baker, M.G. Potential lessons from the Taiwan and New Zealand health responses to the COVID-19 pandemic. *Lancet Reg. Health West Pac.* **2020**, *4*, 100044. [CrossRef] [PubMed]
19. Tsioplis, C.; Brockschmidt, C.; Sander, S.; Henne-Bruns, D.; Kornmann, M. Factors influencing the course of acute appendicitis in adults and children. *Langenbecks Arch. Surg.* **2013**, *398*, 857–867. [CrossRef]

20. Perez, K.S.; Allen, S.R. Complicated appendicitis and considerations for interval appendectomy. *JAAPA* **2018**, *31*, 35–41. [CrossRef]
21. Schafer, F.M.; Meyer, J.; Kellnar, S.; Warmbrunn, J.; Schuster, T.; Simon, S.; Meyer, T.; Platzer, J.; Hubertus, J.; Seitz, S.T.; et al. Increased Incidence of Perforated Appendicitis in Children During COVID-19 Pandemic in a Bavarian Multi-Center Study. *Front. Pediatr.* **2021**, *9*, 683607. [CrossRef]
22. Orthopoulos, G.; Santone, E.; Izzo, F.; Tirabassi, M.; Perez-Caraballo, A.M.; Corriveau, N.; Jabbour, N. Increasing incidence of complicated appendicitis during COVID-19 pandemic. *Am. J. Surg.* **2021**, *221*, 1056–1060. [CrossRef] [PubMed]
23. Saah, F.I.; Amu, H.; Seidu, A.A.; Bain, L.E. Health knowledge and care seeking behaviour in resource-limited settings amidst the COVID-19 pandemic: A qualitative study in Ghana. *PLoS ONE* **2021**, *16*, e0250940. [CrossRef] [PubMed]
24. Boslaugh, S. *Encyclopedia of Epidemiology*; Sage Publications: Thousand Oaks, CA, USA, 2007.
25. Venegas-Vera, A.V.; Colbert, G.B.; Lerma, E.V. Positive and negative impact of social media in the COVID-19 era. *Rev. Cardiovasc. Med.* **2020**, *21*, 561–564. [CrossRef] [PubMed]
26. Mheidly, N.; Fares, J. Leveraging media and health communication strategies to overcome the COVID-19 infodemic. *J. Public Health Policy* **2020**, *41*, 410–420. [CrossRef]
27. Kishore, S.P.; Kolappa, K.; Jarvis, J.D.; Park, P.H.; Belt, R.; Balasubramaniam, T.; Kiddell-Monroe, R. Overcoming Obstacles To Enable Access To Medicines For Noncommunicable Diseases In Poor Countries. *Health Aff.* **2015**, *34*, 1569–1577. [CrossRef]
28. Wu, J.M.; Ho, T.W.; Tien, Y.W. Correlation Between the Increased Hospital Volume and Decreased Overall Perioperative Mortality in One Universal Health Care System. *World J. Surg.* **2019**, *43*, 2194–2202. [CrossRef]
29. Berlin, N.L.; Dimick, J.B.; Kerr, E.A.; Skolarus, T.A.; Dossett, L.A. Demand for Surgical Procedures Following COVID-19: The Need for Operational Strategies That Optimize Resource Utilization and Value. *Ann. Surg.* **2020**, *272*, e272–e274. [CrossRef]
30. Al-Jabir, A.; Kerwan, A.; Nicola, M.; Alsafi, Z.; Khan, M.; Sohrabi, C.; O'Neill, N.; Iosifidis, C.; Griffin, M.; Mathew, G.; et al. Impact of the Coronavirus (COVID-19) pandemic on surgical practice—Part 1. *Int. J. Surg.* **2020**, *79*, 168–179. [CrossRef]
31. Tankel, J.; Keinan, A.; Blich, O.; Koussa, M.; Helou, B.; Shay, S.; Zugayar, D.; Pikarsky, A.; Mazeh, H.; Spira, R.; et al. The Decreasing Incidence of Acute Appendicitis During COVID-19: A Retrospective Multi-centre Study. *World J. Surg.* **2020**, *44*, 2458–2463. [CrossRef]

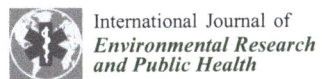

Article

The Lived Experiences of Women without COVID-19 in Breastfeeding Their Infants during the Pandemic: A Descriptive Phenomenological Study

Ka-Huen Yip *, Yuk-Chiu Yip and Wai-King Tsui

Caritas Institute of Higher Education, School of Health Sciences, 2 Chui Ling Lane, Tseung Kwan O, New Territories, Hong Kong SAR, China; jeffreyycyip@gmail.com (Y.-C.Y.); ztsui@cihe.edu.hk (W.-K.T.)
* Correspondence: khyip@cihe.edu.hk

Abstract: The coronavirus disease 2019 (COVID-19) outbreak in 2020 has led to several changes and disturbances in the daily lives of the general public. Particularly for new (first-time) mothers, there has been a significant impact on the practices of raising and feeding their babies. Social distancing measures everywhere have made mothers hesitant to breastfeed their babies anywhere else but at home. Combined with the fear of being infected with COVID-19, the present situation has created unprecedented barriers for breastfeeding mothers to accessing various types of support: emotional, instrumental, informational, and appraisal. There has been no research on the influence of the pandemic on social support regarding breastfeeding in Hong Kong. This study aimed to explore the social support and impact of COVID-19 on mothers breastfeeding their babies. Semi-structured interviews were conducted with 20 currently breastfeeding women in Hong Kong. Colaizzi's seven-step method was used for data analysis. Two key themes emerged from the interview data: (1) positive influences on breastfeeding support during COVID-19 and (2) negative influences on breastfeeding support during COVID-19. Our findings may help mothers prepare to breastfeed their babies in places other than their homes.

Keywords: burnout; COVID-19 pandemic; postnatal care; psychological distress; psychosocial support

Citation: Yip, K.-H.; Yip, Y.-C.; Tsui, W.-K. The Lived Experiences of Women without COVID-19 in Breastfeeding Their Infants during the Pandemic: A Descriptive Phenomenological Study. *Int. J. Environ. Res. Public Health* **2022**, *19*, 9511. https://doi.org/10.3390/ijerph19159511

Academic Editors: Sachiko Kodera and Essam A. Rashed

Received: 7 June 2022
Accepted: 1 August 2022
Published: 2 August 2022

Publisher's Note: MDPI stays neutral with regard to jurisdictional claims in published maps and institutional affiliations.

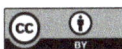

Copyright: © 2022 by the authors. Licensee MDPI, Basel, Switzerland. This article is an open access article distributed under the terms and conditions of the Creative Commons Attribution (CC BY) license (https://creativecommons.org/licenses/by/4.0/).

1. Introduction

The coronavirus [SARS-CoV-2] disease or COVID-19 rapidly spread, infecting over five hundred million people worldwide and causing over six million deaths [1]. People with COVID-19, as an acute respiratory, disease may have varied symptom severity [2,3]. The World Health Organization declared COVID-19 a public health emergency of international concern in January 2020 [4,5]. According to studies, the low mortality rates of people under 65 years, and those with no underlying health conditions, highlight that the death rates are higher among individuals with clinical vulnerabilities [6–8]. There is a higher predisposition to contract COVID-19 during the third trimester of pregnancy, and among early postpartum women [9–11]. All of these women are advised to seek urgent medical advice and care and stay at home to protect themselves and their babies, to prevent preterm birth and pregnancy loss during the COVID-19 pandemic [12,13]. However, this vulnerable group of women suffer a greater impact of COVID-19 during pregnancy compared to other groups, especially during the final trimester [9,14–16]. The main impact concerns the awareness of social support and the impact of COVID-19 on mothers breastfeeding their babies, and the need to seek more understanding about how to provide better resources and emotional support for those breastfeeding women, thus decreasing their stress and improving relationships.

COVID-19, Social Distancing Restrictions, and Postnatal Vulnerabilities

Although breastfeeding initiation rates are high in Hong Kong, where over 87% of mothers initiate breastfeeding, only half of these mothers exclusively breastfeed their babies [17]. Moreover, this 2019 survey reported that Hong Kong demonstrates a big drop in the number of mothers who practice exclusive breastfeeding in the first two months following birth, while the proportion of infants who are exclusively breastfed in the first 4–6 months is low [17]. In 2020, the Hong Kong Government increasing statutory maternity leave to 14 weeks, and forbidding discrimination on the ground of breastfeeding, was a new contribution to breastfeeding progress [18] and increased the number of Baby-Friendly Hospitals to deliver the continuum of care that supports mothers to feed their babies optimally [19]. Breastfeeding in public is still considered taboo; 40% of breastfeeding mothers who fed their babies in public have encountered uncomfortable conditions [20]. However, breastfeeding in Hong Kong is hard; most of the women who discontinue breastfeeding do not terminate voluntarily but due to breastfeeding issues, including the lack of preparation for breastfeeding, in-hospital support services, post-natal support, and public areas for breastfeeding [21,22].

With the higher transmissibility and risk of infection of the omicron strain, on 3 March 2022 [23] the Hong Kong Government strongly urged its citizens to abide by social distancing measures, to avoid going out, and to abstain from participating in unnecessary or crowded activities and gatherings, such as religious or family activities. A similar stay-at-home order was implemented by the United Kingdom Government [24]. This would prevent the spread of COVID-19 and limit COVID-19 deaths in the community.

Studies have reported that pregnant women can easily be infected during epidemics [25–27]. During the severe acute respiratory syndrome (SARS) outbreak in Hong Kong [28], women described their psychological distress, such as frustration, anxiety, sleeping disturbance, and interference in their daily lives. The postnatal period is an important transition period for women and can alter many aspects of life, including the role and identification of the infant's mother, motherhood [29], lifestyle [30], mother-infant bonding, confidence, and satisfaction [31]. Postnatal mothers may, in part, face an increased risk of experiencing mental distress during the COVID-19 pandemic [32]. Hence, transitioning into motherhood during COVID-19 presents unique stressors, which may worsen an already vulnerable period in a woman's life [33]. The findings of a qualitative study that explored the perinatal experiences of mothers during COVID-19, highlighted that virtual consultations from healthcare professionals were viewed as impersonal and caused women to feel too embarrassed to talk about their mental health concerns [34].

A web-based survey investigated the psychological experiences of women during COVID-19 [35]. A rapid literature review on the impact of COVID-19 on maternal mental health and perinatal mental health services, between October 2019 and September 2020, indicated depression and anxiety levels among mothers before October 2019 as approximately 11% and 18%, respectively [32]. A percentage of anxious mothers attained above the relevant cut-off for September 2020 indicated levels of depression (43%) and anxiety (61%) in clinical settings. A large percentage of mothers felt worry and panic because they may not have adequate support to fulfill their needs. There are only a few qualitative studies that have assessed women's psychological experiences during the COVID-19 pandemic [36,37]. Most literature has focused exclusively on the higher transmissibility and risk of infection of the omicron strain in Hong Kong [35–37]. Using qualitative research methods can provide a richer and more in-depth insight into which elements of social distancing restrictions have generated an impact on mothers' emotional health. The experiences of women breastfeeding their babies, while not being infected with COVID-19, have not been investigated. Therefore, this study aimed to explore the in-depth experiences of this vulnerable group of women during the COVID-19 pandemic in Hong Kong, with regards to their psychological state, perspectives, feeding methods, personal life, the experience of home quarantine, and the impact of COVID-19 on their mental health.

2. Materials and Methods

2.1. Ethical Review

The participants were informed of the details of the study and informed consent was obtained from all of them. Information about the study was provided to the participants before conducting interviews, including its background, purpose, and procedure. Participation was voluntary, and all participants were informed that they could withdraw from the study without any consequences. The confidentiality and anonymity of the participants were strictly ensured through encryption. Only the researchers had access to the study data. Ethical approval was obtained from the Caritas Institute of Higher Education, Research and Ethics Committee (HRE210136).

2.2. Design

A qualitative research design was used and data were collected through individual, semi-structured interviews, on the women's psychological experiences with breastfeeding their babies during COVID-19. The data were analyzed based on the phenomenological methodology suggested by Colaizzi [38]. With this method, the researchers attempted to understand the participants' subjective feelings and experiences by having them mentally return to the situation itself.

2.3. Participants

The participants in this study were 20 women breastfeeding their babies in Hong Kong. Purposive sampling was used, and to recruit participants our research team approached peer support groups from online media platforms such as Facebook, and groups related to mothers in Hong Kong, such as "Hong Kong Moms," "Little Steps," and "Mother Kingdom." The interviews were conducted by telephone or video calls (e.g., Zoom). The research team members then individually followed up with the participants who showed interest in participating in this study, who obtained our contact information (e-mail and/or phone) through these online platforms.

All participants met the following inclusion criteria: (1) women having experiences in providing their child with breast milk in any form (such as direct breastfeeding or using a bottle to feed their babies with their own milk) at least once during the COVID-19 pandemic, (2) women having lived in Hong Kong during the 12-month period as aforementioned, and (3) women whose babies were within an age range of 0 to 12 months.

Individual interviews continued until data saturation was reached at the 17th interview, after which no new information arose in the next three individual interviews. Table 1 shows the participants' characteristics. We enrolled 20 women between the ages of 22 and 46, with an average age of 32 years, who breastfed their babies during the COVID-19 pandemic. Among the participants, two women completed secondary education, nine possessed a bachelor's degree, three possessed a master's degree, and six graduated with a higher diploma. Regarding the breastfeeding period, 12 participants were first-time mothers using different feeding methods, seven participants had two children, and one participant had three children.

Table 1. Participant demographic characteristics.

Characteristic	All n = 20	
	n	%
Age		
≤21	0	0
22–26	3	15
27–31	6	30
32–36	8	40
37–41	2	10

Table 1. *Cont.*

Characteristic	All n = 20	
	n	%
42–46	1	5
≥47	0	0
Education level		
Secondary	2	10
Higher diploma	6	30
Bachelor's degree	9	45
Master degree	3	15
Number of children		
1	12	60
2	7	35
3	1	5

2.4. Data Collection

From December 2021 to February 2022, all interviews were conducted in Chinese by the researcher (W.K.) at the participant's preferred time schedule in a private password-protected Zoom (Nasdaq, San Jose, CA, USA) meeting room. Each interview took about 60–130 min, and the same interview guide was always used to reduce variation in the data collection process. In addition, field notes were taken during the interviews to facilitate the collection of contextual information for data analysis. The interview guide questions are presented in Table 2. An academic qualitative scholar and a psychological consulting specialist were employed to form an expert panel to review and affirm the validity of the interview questions. All participants' interviews were audio-recorded, with their written consent. If the participant exhibited emotional distress during the interview, adequate psychological support was provided to prevent further psychological harm.

Table 2. Interview guide.

No.	Probing Questions
1.	How did you feel when you were breastfeeding your baby during the COVID-19 pandemic?
2.	How long have you been breastfeeding your baby? Other than breastfeeding, what other feeding methods have you been practicing for your baby?
3.	Have your feelings changed over time when you were feeding your baby day and night during the COVID-19 pandemic?
4.	Can you tell me how you coped with your own psychological needs concerning breastfeeding?
5.	In what ways do you think your coping strategies have helped you on a psychological level upon breastfeeding experience?
6.	Do you think you are ready to stop breastfeeding, and what makes you think you should stop breastfeeding?
7.	Recalling on your months of breastfeeding, what are your negative and positive feelings towards breastfeeding in your experience during the COVID-19 pandemic?

2.5. Data Analysis and Trustworthiness

In addition, data analysis was conducted immediately after data collection using NVivo Version 12, QSR International [39]. Two research team members (K.H.Y. and Y.C.Y.) transcribed the interview tapes verbatim and, subsequently, translated all transcripts into English. Back translation was undertaken by another team member (W.K.T.) and a professional translator to ensure semantic equivalence. The data and field notes of all interviews were organized systematically according to Colaizzi's phenomenological analysis method [38]. This method follows a seven-step approach to expose emergent themes, namely (i) to familiarize the researchers with the collected data, (ii) to identify the significant statements, (iii) to formulate the meanings and the use of reflection by the researchers,

(iv) to cluster and define themes, (v) to formulate an exhaustive description, (vi) to create a fundamental composition of the phenomenon, and (vii) to verify the exhaustive description and fundamental composition [38].

In particular, all recorded interview data were transcribed verbatim and analyzed throughout the data analysis process [38]. All the interview data included meaningful statements and gave rise to different themes, which were independently reviewed by two research team members (K.H.Y. and Y.C.Y.). They looked at all the analyzed data and compared the subthemes, identifying the differences and similarities between them. The authors of this study (K.H.Y., Y.C.Y., and W.K.T.) discussed the results of their analyses to reach a consensus. The study referenced the stringent criteria established by Lincoln and Guba to ensure a high level of rigor in this study [40–42]. It demonstrates how each criterion regarding credibility, dependability, confirmability, and transferability was achieved through member checking.

Given credibility in creating confidence that the results are accurate, true, credible, reliable, and believable in: (1) prolonging and diversifying engagement with each composition, (2) having interviews with comprehensive process and techniques, (3) building investigators' authority, (4) gathering all referential adequacy materials, and (5) having peer debriefing sessions regularly.

Engagement through participant observation in the field was infeasible at the time of this research. There was a strict "multi-household gatherings at private premises" policy (as imposed by the Government of Hong Kong Special Administrative Region) that prohibited more than two households and groups gathering in the community. This policy was to prevent the spread of the virus to the community. However, several participants from different living and working venues were approached through peer support groups that had regular communications about the research with the authors' affiliated institution. After being granted ethical approval of this study, the interview guide was assessed at two induction meetings. Two pilot interviews via Zoom were performed, and these two interviews' data were also integrated in the final data analysis. All research team members had the required data management skills, knowledge, and practical experience and involvement of more than 4 years in qualitative research to conduct their roles.

Furthermore, field notes were applied as a tool to analyze the transcripts and utilized to aid the documentation of the contextual information mentioned by the participants for accurate data analysis. Moreover, the research team members were scheduled for debriefing sessions held regularly at 2-week intervals with the Fellows from the Hong Kong Academy of Nursing, to guarantee that there were no taken-for-granted biases, attitudes, perspectives, or assumptions on the part of researchers.

Enhancing dependability to guarantee the results of this qualitative inquiry would be duplicable if the inquiry existed within the same cohort: (1) to apply rich description of study methods, (2) to set up an audit trail, (3) to progress in a series of distinct stages in the replication of data.

The research team tried to present the study methods in detail and clearly in the research papers; they set up a detailed track-record of the data-collection process by all research team members. Additionally, to ensure the validity of the accounts from the participants, member-checking was conducted to enhance the clarity of the meanings derived from the participants. Research team members read the transcripts to the participants via telephone to clarify the interpretative meanings. It provided participants the opportunity to recognize and accept their narrative contributions, once they have been put into the research report in rough and final draft forms. All research team members appraised coding accuracy and inter-coder reliability throughout the data-analysis process.

Confirmability was maintained by empowering confidence that the results would be confirmed/corroborated by other researchers; it had self-reflection and reflexivity. This approach evaluates reflexive journals and weekly investigator meetings were applied.

Moreover, transferability was enhanced by developing the degree to which the results can be summarized/transferred to further contexts/settings; it was achieved through data saturation and possessing thick description. This approach comprised two main issues: (1) data saturation was satisfied when no new themes appeared from the participants; all research team members gained a consensus on the attainment of data saturation; (2) lengthy description was presented in the quotes of the participants, such that the meanings of the narrative statements from the participants could be translated and interpreted in context.

3. Results

Using phenomenological methods, we explored the psychological experiences of women breastfeeding their babies during the COVID-19 pandemic. Two themes were identified from our observations (summarized in Table 3).

Table 3. Themes and subthemes of the study.

Themes	Subthemes
Positive influences on breastfeeding support during COVID-19	Mothers' Desire for Support COVID is Not All bad for Mothers
Negative influences on breastfeeding support during COVID-19	Absence of Close and Personal Professional Coaching Mothers Being Forced to Focus on Breastfeeding Mothers Going Back to 'Normal' Life

3.1. Theme 1. Positive Influences on Breastfeeding Support during COVID-19

Participants were asked a series of questions about their daily activities and how they cared for their child while breastfeeding during the COVID pandemic, including how various personal protective measures and restricted movement to curb the spread of the virus had affected their breastfeeding and motherhood experience.

3.1.1. Mothers' Desire for Support

Participants described both positive and negative breastfeeding experiences due to the COVID-19 pandemic. They did not generally tend to need support for steps toward a good breastfeeding latch. However, regarding empathic and understanding support, they had established friendships and peer support groups to share their questions or concerns related to breastfeeding and caring for the baby, which, in turn, aided their ability to be open and frank. Some participants tried to search for more information, including special Chinese traditions recommended for postpartum dietary practices during this period.

"As a breastfeeding mother, I recognize that I need a lot of support in the early stages of feeding. Thank goodness my son has grown up and I do not need any support during COVID-19."

"In that time, I felt alone. She (breastfeeding mothers from peer support groups via online platform) felt like someone who is close to me and gives me all experience that I need. It was almost like we were friends. I did not even know her face-to-face. However, I really valued what she said; I would call it a friendship, I would think."

"If I had a young child and was without any support, I would think hard to decide if I should continue breastfeeding. I am lucky to have joined the 'Hong Kong Moms,' which is an online social platform group for breastfeeding mothers. I came across other breastfeeding mothers in this baby group in this online social platform during COVID-19. I mean it is different because I know I am talking to someone whom I only know by their nickname, someone who has experienced it on some level, which I think is very important, and is helpful with different kinds of advice and neutral opinions, such as how to deal with their own disasters. Besides, being anonymous, I think, was also important. It was nice to have that support . . . I have searched some interesting new ways of ginger vinegar soup and pig's trotter (delivering service), online or by phone, which I shall continue to establish and use in the future. I do not need to worry about it all, and take my time for rest."

"In the mothers' group, we would chat mostly about breastfeeding, although we also chatted about other topics. They would inquire how my baby was sleeping and provided help that way; they were reliable. The other mothers in my mothers' group were coping with their own catastrophes. It was wonderful to have that support."

During the analysis of other interviewees' responses, the findings relating to many subthemes expanded. It was interesting to note how a similar issue that took place for various interviewees could often be interpreted as either positive or negative, depending on the individual and their perception of the circumstances.

Some participants described that they had more privilege in their living environments without financial burdens. They enjoyed the breastfeeding journey with a better living environment and family support, which impacted the health outcomes of breastfeeding and baby care. With a shift in the mindset of men toward family care, some participants reported that their partners were willing to stay at home longer to take care of their newborn babies. Some fathers were granted paternity leave and spent extra time to support their spouses in breastfeeding and maternal recovery, both physically and emotionally. Some participants' partners were working from home and could spend more time being present than if they were out at work all day. This shared and collaborative care increased the bonds between partners and their babies, and strengthened the relationship between the parent and infant:

"My husband is working from home because of COVID-19 and has taken 10 days off. He enjoys so many special moments with us every day. He can help with diaper changes and baths, take care of our baby, and let me sleep when I need it ... Our family lives in a house of two floors. My husband slept in the other bedroom. He is afraid of affecting my rest and lets me have enough space to rest and exercise. Maya (Filipino domestic helper) also helped to cook lot of ginger, eggs, and chicken to increase the nutritional content in my diet. Basically, my husband and I share every little bit of happiness that is happening in our lives. The two of us have been here with each other for the baby, which means I have more time to focus on breastfeeding our baby."

3.1.2. COVID-19 Is Not All Bad for Mothers

Some participants stated that during the social distancing period, they could only allow a few visits from their friends and relatives to greet their newborn babies. They could therefore relax at home and spend more time attending to their babies, and rest instead of entertaining many friends and relatives eager to see their babies. Besides, with fewer visitors, there was less unsolicited advice, and the mothers could focus on their own way of breastfeeding their babies:

"Oh! I recall being overwhelmed by my family and friends visiting me and my son during the first to fourth weeks after giving birth to my first son. They felt that I did not know how to breastfeed my son because my son often burst into tears. When they wanted to help comfort my son, I was often unable to react at that time. As such, my son could easily become irritated most of the time, which was not good for his mental growth. At that time, I especially felt a lot of pressure from my grandma and I needed to supplement my breastfeeding with formula milk. Now that I am breastfeeding my second son during COVID-19, I do not have that stress, and this time I can really feel the enormous difference in feeding him and my mental health."

Several participants expressed that during the period of social distancing, they could experience a slow pace of life. There was no place to go and hence, they would have all the time to focus on how and when to breastfeed their children. Some participants, especially those who were struggling with the pain of bleeding nipples, breast engorgement, stress, and anxiety, welcomed this peace of mind. They believed that before social distancing, they would be busy going out and meeting friends and family to introduce them to their babies. As they would still be experiencing the pain and pressure of visiting friends and family, they would rather stop breastfeeding.

> "I find it very difficult for me as a breastfeeding mother because I have breastfeeding problems, such as bleeding nipples, tearing, and a lot of pain. Having been home for maternity leave because of COVID-19, I was able to spend time to focus on breastfeeding; my daughter is the only reason I persist in continuing breastfeeding. I am having a lot of visits from family, mom, or other friends and I need to put up with the stress that they cause to me. If it were not for the COVID-19 pandemic to reduce social gatherings, I am not sure I would be successful in breastfeeding my little daughter. I now have had six weeks of feeding!"

Coupled with the aforementioned factors, most participants were also concerned about maintaining their own privacy during breastfeeding. All participants were Chinese, and the common reason they had for stopping breastfeeding sooner than planned was the discomfort and embarrassment of feeding in front of somebody else.

Participants expressed that they felt at ease at home. On the contrary, they were embarrassed and uncomfortable breastfeeding their baby this way outside, in front of visitors, or in public. Several participants were accustomed to feeding their baby on a comfortable chair, shirtless, and through a lot of skin-to-skin contact with the baby. This allowed them to gain breastfeeding confidence to position and support their baby for a good latch, the most natural and beneficial activity for the mother and baby.

> "Not having family and friends visiting me after giving birth to my baby has allowed me time to practice how to breastfeed my daughter without having to worry about people coming, and not being able to go out during the COVID-19 pandemic has given and enhanced my confidence in breastfeeding. Having said that, I am scared and do not have faith to take my daughter to shopping malls and parks and feed her in public. I think there should be suitable and appropriate facilities for privacy for breastfeeding in the malls and parks before I breastfeed my daughter in those areas."

During the COVID-19 pandemic, participants felt that they had extra time without any pressure regarding breastfeeding. They could perform more natural feeding in responding to hunger cues and satiety from their baby, rather than following a mother-led routine. Some participants also appreciated the additional help from healthcare professionals via online communicating support systems, granted without social isolation during the COVID-19 pandemic. Participants stated that they breastfed their babies more often due to no planning in their daily activities; for instance, they did not need to plan things like going out to work on time or getting home quickly. This positively affected perceptions of milk supply by mothers and increased the early weight gain of their baby.

> "I am working from home during COVID-19, so I have more time to focus on feeding my little princess as and when she wants to be fed, and not feeling rushed because I do not need to go anywhere ... It was nice to have somebody who could maybe talk through text-based communication on mobile applications. I really valued that this support was able to listen and understand what I said. They can absolutely direct me to correct information without any confusion. Moreover, through interactions, I had no feelings of social isolation, and it also helped me relax."

Some participants stated that their return to work after maternity leave collided with the worsening of the COVID-19 pandemic. Some companies allowed employees to work from home. This relieved the mothers' worries about sending their babies to a nursery, or asking family members to take up babysitting while they were away for work. The mother could have more intimate contact with her baby and more breastfeeding; hence, the baby could have more breast milk rather than formula milk. The participants also felt relaxed under such work arrangements.

> "I am going back to work next Monday after maternity leave, and I do not actually know what uncontrollable circumstances this will bring. Despite the public panic of the COVID-19 pandemic, it is unlikely I will not be at work. This means relief from anxiety, and I can continue my breastfeeding because after maternity leave, the company allowed me to work from home, so I am still at home. I do not need to ask my mother to come over to my house to take care of my daughter. At the same time, I do not need to worry about pumping breast milk as reserve for feeding my daughter."

3.2. Theme 2. Negative Influences on Breastfeeding Support during COVID-19

Various participants explained the pessimistic impact on their own breastfeeding experience during the COVID-19 pandemic.

3.2.1. Absence of Close and Personal Professional Coaching

During the stay-at-home requirement during the COVID-19 pandemic, most mothers with first babies came across a common problem of having less counseling support in breastfeeding. Instead of healthcare providers standing close by during breastfeeding, the participants could only describe their difficulties through phone calls and online messaging. They could not come near, observe, and note the incorrect breastfeeding steps or practices of the new mothers. This is considered a significant barrier for first time mothers to start breastfeeding. The new mothers were concerned about the lack of personal support and only having support through phone calls.

Most participants really missed having someone who could look at what was happening and help them make small changes to improve their breastfeeding. This feeling meant that the participants lacked close and professional coaching during breastfeeding. They expressed a sense of sadness, anxiety, and unhappiness at losing the idea of breastfeeding they hoped to have.

> "The breastfeeding class was cancelled due to the COVID-19 pandemic. He is my first child; I have no experience at all. I feel I am not breastfeeding properly. I do not know what to do, I am depressed and retarded, and I am scared that my baby needs to lose weight. I do not stop using my mobile phone to search for a lot of information via the Internet. I do not know if it is right or wrong, and I am afraid that my baby will be infected with COVID-19. I am experiencing great levels of anxiety, stress, and uncertainty . . . I cannot have a get diagnosis due to the current situation. I am also experiencing a lot of pressure from the stress that my baby might have to be hospitalized because of his excessive weight. This has been a very difficult process, and I have been in great pain and confusion. Three days since we have returned home, we have received no further support. I was crying on the phone when asking for help from the medical support. I prefer face-to-face coaching and guidance. Hands-on demonstrations could also help me to learn the position for holding my baby properly for breastfeeding. It is more effective than a Zoom video call on a mobile device . . . My fear is that I will look back with unhappiness on what I have endured during this time. I think the trauma will be ongoing and far-reaching."

A typical housing phenomenon in Hong Kong involves many underprivileged people living in tiny "coffin homes" (accommodation in a living unit subdivided into smaller units, each of not more than 150 square feet). Poor living environment, lower educational level, and economic burden impact the emotional stress of participants' continuation of breastfeeding and affect baby care. Maintaining social distancing among the residents of these "coffin homes" is impossible, and mothers with newborn babies were concerned about becoming infected with COVID-19 easily. Further, due to social distancing restrictions, some participants felt that medical support was becoming remote and only available through online messaging or phone calls.

"My husband is a hawker with leg amputation, and I have a huge financial burden of the family. Contrarily to other families, I have only obtained secondary education level without any professional qualification. Everything made me afraid and anxious, and I do not know how to express. After the completion of my maternity leave, I must return to work as soon as possible. I do not think I would have continued breastfeeding; it was a really big impact for me . . . I was so stressed because I could not convey and do not know how to convey. Having been seriously disturbed by COVID-19 now, I need to stay in my tiny coffin home with my baby, which is making me worried and anxious, fearing that my baby and I will be infected. I also avoid going to the Maternal and Child Health Center for routine health checks. So, I have not been seeing nurses and receiving their coaching on breastfeeding for a while. I did not realize there was any support elsewhere . . . My failures in breastfeeding made me feel very frustrated; tears always streamed down my face at night."

Many participants mentioned that during social distancing restrictions, they could not get together and have physical meetings with other breastfeeding mothers' support groups. They stated that they wished to connect with others by sharing their experience and seeking support for their breastfeeding. Some participants felt they were alone in the process. Certain participants reported that they were isolated and lacked the emotional support and care from their family members. This was harmful to their physical and psychological health.

"Although my husband was by my side, I still value the presence of my mother accompanying me. My mother was amazing and a strong supporter of breastfeeding. I really hoped she could come to visit me after my son was born. However, in the current situation, she stays in Mainland China and cannot come. Despite being on WeChat [video message], it is not the same as having my mother by my side. I feel like [I and my baby] need her, not just for help, but for emotional support. I also struggle and feel depressed. It seems everything is becoming difficult and frustrating. On the other hand, I want to participate in peer group activities and receive face-to-face support. The lack of support for everything really makes me sad. It is not what I expected. I read a lot of breastfeeding information before my son was born. I could not, however, receive the support I thought would be available."

However, some participants recognized that staying at home with other toddlers helped reduce some pressure. Others found that although there was no need to take their older children outside, they would still need to help them with online learning (homeschool via Zoom). These daily issues intimidated participants with regard to breastfeeding. Some participants had partners working long hours outside, and who were not able to provide support and help with household chores or caring for the babies. Since the suspension of flights from the United Kingdom to Hong Kong, one participant expressed:

"My mum was not able to fly back and help me with my little son. I now have much less time to focus on breastfeeding. My partner is an A&E (Accident & Emergency) doctor who works from dawn to late night, and sometimes 24 h or more depending on how the workload in the hospital develops. I am at home with an energetic six-year-old boy, who now usually attends classes via Zoom (video message) at home because face-to-face classes are suspended. I do not have time to express my feelings and sometimes I do not even have time to breastfeed my younger son because I feel that I also need to focus and take care of my older son and simultaneously take care of all the household chores. I feel that most of the time, I am like a single mother. In the first three months after the birth of my first son, my mother and sisters returned from the UK to help me at my home. Now, due to the pandemic, I do not have family or friends to help me or to help take care of my elder son so that I can have time to focus on the baby."

3.2.2. Mothers Being Forced to Focus on Breastfeeding

During the height of the COVID-19 pandemic, compared to other participants who preferred having more or enough time for breastfeeding, several participants felt just the opposite. As they had nowhere to go and not many things to do, they could focus their attention on breastfeeding their babies. Some of them were eager to have a break and do other things to divert their attention.

"My little princess and I were afraid of being infected as if we were in confinement. My focus on breastfeeding is very strong. This, in turn, makes me resent it because it feels like my day revolves around it."

Breastfeeding is a biological norm; some people still avoid having the taboo of breastfeeding in public, and mothers are still being forced to pump in toilets or storerooms in some shopping malls in Hong Kong. Several participants try to escape complaints or unpleasant experiences of breastfeeding in public; rather, they selected breastfeeding their baby at home.

"I fear men might see. They would image my breasts to seduce . . . I do not want to breastfeed my baby uncovered in public. Now, during the pandemic, I think it is a good and the best option for me and my baby; I have had a pretty warm and free space for breastfeeding at home."

3.2.3. Mothers Going Back to "Normal" Life

Different participants had varying views on breastfeeding during the pandemic. Some participants would rather not conduct breastfeeding anywhere except at home. Some participants were concerned that they might miss the unique experience of breastfeeding and lack the opportunity to share the experience and exchange their knowledge of breastfeeding with other new mothers. One of them said that she was anxious and lost in not knowing what will happen in the future, once the COVID-19 pandemic is over.

"If there is a chance, I can breastfeed together with other like-minded mothers in public places, such as the Maternal and Child Health Center, not only in my home. Everyone can share with and coach each other on how to get into the correct position to conduct breastfeeding in various situations and different circumstances. It is a pity that there is now no such get together for happy hours and support. I feel lonely. I do not know how to breastfeed my baby with confidence in public. As such, I might give up breastfeeding earlier than I have planned."

Some participants resumed work soon after giving birth to their babies. During the pandemic, they were required to work from home. They would have to breastfeed their babies during working hours. In view of the inconvenience and disturbance that this may cause to work, this was an influencing factor for working mothers to give up breastfeeding early. The experience of one participant, who worked in the Accident and Emergency Department in a hospital, was different from those working at home. She stated that she was buried in her work and was required to wear personal protective equipment (PPE) all the time. She was tired, stressed, hot, sweaty, and dehydrated, with no time to rest. This participant could feel her engorged breasts and discomfort and had less milk.

"I work in the A&E unit, and in order to maintain infection control safety measures, I am required to wear PPE all the time. As I do not want to waste the PPE stock, I try to drink as little water as possible to avoid going to the toilet during my shift duty, and hence do not need to change my PPE. I am feeling helpless because of work affecting my breastfeeding planning. I feel like I am pumping less milk at the moment."

4. Discussion

The current study used a phenomenological approach to explore women's psychological experiences of breastfeeding during the COVID-19 pandemic, specifically in relation to how social distancing measures affected their baby feeding decisions. Two major themes demonstrated how different psychological and difficult experiences emerged in maintaining breastfeeding, alongside the impact that social distancing measures created for them.

The World Health Organization assured mothers that breastfeeding in public is safe, with suitable infection control measures during the COVID-19 pandemic [43]. However, the taboo around breastfeeding in public places in Hong Kong [20] remains. Some participants of this study reflected their worries about breastfeeding newborns while being infected with COVID-19. It is, therefore, important for policymakers to collaborate with healthcare professionals to advance information on social media that helps encourage mothers to continue breastfeeding their babies, despite the worsening COVID-19 situation.

Breastfeeding mothers have been required to face the COVID-19 pandemic and suffer from anxiety [44]; therefore, there was impeded access to healthcare services, with individuals avoiding hospitals and canceling their healthcare appointments [45,46]. The participants' dialogues in this study, as in some other studies, demonstrated that breastfeeding protects maternal and infant health in both the short- and long-term [47–52]. Moreover, breastfeeding protects against infections, providing passive and long-lasting active immunity. Both physical and psychological aspects of mothers are affected by breastfeeding, such as reducing the risk of inflammation, improving sleep distress, and reducing psychological distress [53–55]. The findings of this study also indicate concerns regarding their experiences during the COVID-19 pandemic; their mental health is safeguarded when they fulfill their breastfeeding goals [47–55]. Conversely, the mothers' feelings of grief, depression, and trauma increase if they cannot meet their breastfeeding goals.

The findings of this study also demonstrated the mothers' willingness to discontinue breastfeeding during COVID-19 due to the lack of direct support and reassurance from healthcare professionals, and their relatives. During this critical period, mothers with younger babies are likelier to face varying difficulties and feel uncomfortable with regards to breastfeeding, thus being more likely to discontinue breastfeeding [56,57]. In addition, breastfeeding mothers with older babies expressed that the lack of face-to-face inquiries and support also affected them during the pandemic [58,59]. To avoid contact with other people due to social distancing requirements, breastfeeding mothers expressed that they had negative feelings and stayed at home with limited social contact with people, resulting in declining social opportunities and support services [59]. It is vital to provide professional peer and healthcare support, and communication, during the early weeks of breastfeeding for mothers and their babies, to enhance successful breastfeeding [60–63]. During the early weeks of breastfeeding, participants of this study who particularly required care terminated breastfeeding due to an absence of practical, emotional, professional peer and healthcare support, and social gatherings. Some participants were also dissatisfied and blamed social distancing requirements during COVID-19, which affected their decision not to continue breastfeeding. Previous studies reported breastfeeding mothers had an increased risk of postnatal depression [64–67]; our analysis showed few participants planned to extend breastfeeding for a longer time. Importantly, clinicians should track the effects of breastfeeding duration on subsequent physical and mental health outcomes in this population group.

There seems to be a more pressing need for support for those women who are unable to achieve their breastfeeding goals, or who are struggling with a lack of support [68,69]. Studies reported increasing rates of perinatal depression associated with the COVID-19 lockdown in countries worldwide [64,70,71], including worry about health for both mother and baby, professional healthcare support deficits, economic burden effects, strict controls on movement, and social isolation. Policymakers must devise ways to provide holistic support to mothers, babies, and their families whenever they require it [72,73]. According to this study's findings, the experiences of participants during the COVID-19 pandemic were significantly unique and different. There was an optimistic perception, with most of the participants stating that they had an optimistic impact on their experiences of breastfeeding. They were forced to focus more on breastfeeding their baby during COVID-19 and ensuring social isolation. Participants expressed that they could access enough things for breastfeeding support, such as increasing breastfeeding time for mothers and their babies, had fewer disturbances, kept away from unpleasant opinions, and had extra communication time with supportive partners [65,74,75]. We believe that traditional beliefs and postpartum practices in mothers worldwide mainly involve direct care, dietary intake, and sufficient rest [76–79]. However, it is very important to pay attention to mothers' mental health during the current pandemic.

Some studies state that mothers living on low incomes, due to poverty caused by housing factors and lower education levels, are more likely to discontinue breastfeeding in the early weeks [80,81]. Breastfeeding mothers are required to cope with more problems and have less support within the current pandemic. The findings of our study indicated that participants without a bachelor's degree described having a more undesirable perspective of the lockdown and faced unnecessary hurdles while breastfeeding, especially those who had less support in their living environments. Housing factors, like tiny, sky-high, and dense living spaces, influenced mothers in poorer families who had fewer perceived good parenting qualities, affecting mother-baby relationships [78]. Based on the participants' experiences, the disadvantages of living circumstances and low educational qualifications both affected successful breastfeeding.

An optimistic impact was observed in participants of this study who were more privileged in their living circumstances, such as having more spacious homes, access to plenty of verdant spaces for exercise and rest, and fewer economic worries. Different components of living circumstances affect the health outcomes of breastfeeding and baby care. Past studies show that mothers having difficulty with the milk ejection reflex showed an association with stress and lactation [82–84]. While mothers with poor living circumstances experience higher levels of emotional stress regarding lactation, mothers without living space problems may perceive breastfeeding as a unique and satisfactory experience. Mothers with poor living conditions may experience, for example, the effect of postnatal depression, financial problems, emotional stress, and social isolation during breastfeeding, making the care for their baby more difficult [85,86].

Policymakers, healthcare professionals, and practitioners have been challenged to support a range of creative and resilient responses to strengthen the provision of breastfeeding for both mothers and their babies during COVID-19 [85]. To prevent transmission of the virus, and any other hurdles, behavioral support must be provided for all mothers in terms of positive and accurate information through in-person and telephone services, including telehealth formats through the internet, peer group support, and community resources. Some participants prefer to have more accurate messages through face-to-face breastfeeding support, rather than online delivery support services.

Limitations and Future Directions

This study is limited as recruitment occurred from support sites; therefore, their experiences do not necessarily represent mothers in general. The research provided strong evidence that social distancing and social isolation, due to Omicron in Spring 2022, have had an adverse cumulative health impact on breastfeeding mothers, both physically and mentally. We used telephonic and Zoom interviews to collect data, which is an increasingly common approach during the COVID-19 pandemic. Nevertheless, our sample excluded participants with significant emotional stress, or a lack of internet connection, which are important factors for discontinuing breastfeeding during the early weeks, according to our findings. While a qualitative study addresses a small group of participants, the findings of our study were not intended to generalize but to explore how mothers understood their perceived reality during the COVID-19 pandemic with regards to practical preparation for breastfeeding, taking care of their child, and supporting their families. Thus, it would be advisable to carry out similar studies in other contexts, such as for different geographic and cultural groups of mothers, to acquire a more thorough understanding of this issue.

5. Conclusions

This study used a qualitative approach to explore social support and how COVID-19 impacted mothers breastfeeding their babies during the COVID-19 pandemic in Hong Kong. An analysis of the results showed various positive and negative effects on breastfeeding mothers due to social distancing and social isolation, and different social economic factors, together with their complicated feelings particularly affecting breastfeeding mothers' feelings of guilt, anxiety, and depression. This occurrence may introduce potential risks to breastfeeding if mothers cannot meet their breastfeeding goals. The results also indicate that policymakers and healthcare professionals should implement tailored strategies to support new breastfeeding mothers, their babies, and families to better prepare them, particularly among socioeconomically disadvantaged groups, to breastfeed in places other than their homes during the pandemic. Further studies should focus on suitable psychological interventions aimed at instilling positive emotions in breastfeeding mothers, alleviating negative emotional states, and protecting their wellbeing in Hong Kong.

Author Contributions: Conceptualization, Y.-C.Y.; Data curation, Y.-C.Y.; Formal analysis, Y.-C.Y., K.-H.Y.; Investigation, Y.-C.Y., K.-H.Y., W.-K.T.; Methodology, Y.-C.Y.; Project administration, Y.-C.Y., K.-H.Y., W.-K.T.; Resources, K.-H.Y.; Software, K.-H.Y.; Validation, K.-H.Y., W.-K.T.; Writing—original draft, Y.-C.Y.; Writing—review & editing, Y.-C.Y., K.-H.Y. All authors have read and agreed to the published version of the manuscript.

Funding: This research was funded by the Institute Development Grant (IDG) of Caritas Institute of Higher Education, grant number IDG210217.

Institutional Review Board Statement: The study was conducted in accordance with the Declaration of Helsinki, and approved by the Caritas Institute of Higher Education, Research and Ethics Committee (Ref. no. HRE210136).

Informed Consent Statement: Informed consent was obtained from all subjects involved in the study.

Data Availability Statement: The interview guide has been provided in the manuscript using a table. The transcripts that contain private and confidential data, such as the wards and the sites of practice of the participants, will not be publicly available to protect the participants' privacy.

Conflicts of Interest: The authors declare no conflict of interest.

References

1. World Health Organization. WHO Coronavirus (COVID-19) Dashboard. Available online: https://covid19.who.int/ (accessed on 28 January 2022).
2. Hu, B.; Guo, H.; Zhou, P.; Shi, Z.L. Characteristics of SARS-CoV-2 and COVID-19. *Nat. Rev. Microbiol.* **2021**, *19*, 141–154. [CrossRef]
3. Nalbandian, A.; Sehgal, K.; Gupta, A.; Madhavan, M.V.; McGroder, C.; Stevens, J.S.; Cook, J.R.; Nordvig, A.S.; Shalev, D.; Sehrawat, T.S.; et al. Post-acute COVID-19 syndrome. *Nat. Med.* **2021**, *27*, 601–615. [CrossRef]
4. Song, P.; Karako, T. COVID-19: Real-time dissemination of scientific information to fight a public health emergency of international concern. *Biosci. Trends* **2020**, *14*, 1–2. [CrossRef]
5. World Health Organization. COVID-19 Public Health Emergency of International Concern (PHEIC) Global Research and Innovation Forum: Towards a Research Roadmap. Available online: https://www.who.int/publications/m/item/covid-19-public-health-emergency-of-international-concern-(pheic)-global-research-and-innovation-forum (accessed on 28 January 2022).
6. Iacobucci, G. COVID-19: UK had one of Europe's highest excess death rates in under 65s last year. *Br. Med. J.* **2021**, *372*, n799. [CrossRef]
7. Ioannidis, J.P.; Axfors, C.; Contopoulos-Ioannidis, D.G. Population-level COVID-19 mortality risk for non-elderly individuals overall and for non-elderly individuals without underlying diseases in pandemic epicenters. *Environ. Res.* **2020**, *188*, 109890. [CrossRef] [PubMed]

8. Toyoshima, Y.; Nemoto, K.; Matsumoto, S.; Nakamura, Y.; Kiyotani, K. SARS-CoV-2 genomic variations associated with mortality rate of COVID-19. *J. Hum. Genet.* **2020**, *65*, 1075–1082. [CrossRef]
9. Delahoy, M.J.; Whitaker, M.; O'Halloran, A.; Chai, S.J.; Kirley, P.D.; Alden, N.; Kawasaki, B.; Meek, J.; Yousey-Hindes, K.; Anderson, E.J.; et al. COVID-NET Surveillance Team. Characteristics and maternal and birth outcomes of hospitalized pregnant women with laboratory-confirmed COVID-19—COVID-NET, 13 States, 1 March–22 August 2020. *Morb. Mortal. Wkly. Rep.* **2020**, *69*, 1347. [CrossRef]
10. Novoa, R.H.; Quintana, W.; Llancarí, P.; Urbina-Quispe, K.; Guevara-Ríos, E.; Ventura, W. Maternal clinical characteristics and perinatal outcomes among pregnant women with coronavirus disease 2019. A systematic review. *Travel Med. Infect. Dis.* **2021**, *39*, 101919. [CrossRef]
11. Zambrano, L.D.; Ellington, S.; Strid, P.; Galang, R.R.; Oduyebo, T.; Tong, V.T.; Woodworth, K.R.; Nahabedian, J.F., III; Azziz-Baumgartner, E.; Gilboa, S.M.; et al. CDC COVID-19 Response Pregnancy and Infant Linked Outcomes Team (2020). Update: Characteristics of symptomatic women of reproductive age with laboratory-confirmed SARS-CoV-2 infection by pregnancy status—United States, January 22–October 3, 2020. *Morb. Mortal. Wkly. Rep.* **2020**, *69*, 1641. [CrossRef] [PubMed]
12. Royal College of Obstetricians & Gynaecologists. Available online: https://www.rcog.org.uk/en/guidelines-research-services/guidelines/coronavirus-pregnancy/covid-19-virus-infection-and-pregnancy/ (accessed on 31 March 2022).
13. Woodworth, K.R.; Olsen, E.O.M.; Neelam, V.; Lewis, E.L.; Galang, R.R.; Oduyebo, T.; Tong, V.T.; Woodworth, K.R.; Nahabedian, J.F., 3rd; Azziz-Baumgartner, E.; et al. CDC COVID-19 Response Pregnancy and Infant Linked Outcomes Team. Birth and infant outcomes following laboratory-confirmed SARS-CoV-2 infection in pregnancy—SET-NET, 16 jurisdictions, 29 March–14 October 2020. *Morbid. Mortal. Wkly. Rep.* **2020**, *69*, 1635. [CrossRef]
14. Barbosa-Leiker, C.; Smith, C.L.; Crespi, E.J.; Brooks, O.; Burduli, E.; Ranjo, S.; Carty, C.L.; Hebert, L.E.; Waters, S.F.; Gartstein, M.A. Stressors, coping, and resources needed during the COVID-19 pandemic in a sample of perinatal women. *BMC Pregnancy Childbirth* **2021**, *21*, 171. [CrossRef]
15. Centers for Disease Control and Prevention. Available online: https://www.cdc.gov/coronavirus/2019-ncov/downloads/cases-updates/covid-fs-Pregnancy.pdf (accessed on 28 January 2022).
16. Di Mascio, D.; Sen, C.; Saccone, G.; Galindo, A.; Grünebaum, A.; Yoshimatsu, J.; Stanojevic, M.; Kurjak, A.; Chervenak, F.; Suárez, M.J.; et al. Risk factors associated with adverse fetal outcomes in pregnancies affected by Coronavirus disease 2019 (COVID-19): A secondary analysis of the WAPM study on COVID-19. *J. Perinat. Med.* **2020**, *48*, 950–958. [CrossRef]
17. Department of Health. Breastfeeding Survey. 2019. Available online: https://www.fhs.gov.hk/english/archive/files/reports/BF_survey_2019.pdf (accessed on 30 June 2022).
18. The Government of the Hong Kong Special Administrative Region. Employment (Amendment) Ordinance 2020 Gazetted Today. Available online: https://www.info.gov.hk/gia/general/202007/17/P2020071600471.htm#:~{}:text=Employment%20(Amendment)%20Ordinance%202020%20gazetted%20today&text=The%20Government%20published%20the%20Employment,Ordinance%20(EO)%20(Cap (accessed on 30 June 2022).
19. Baby Friendly Hospital Initiative Hong Kong Association. Healthcare Facilities. Available online: https://www.babyfriendly.org.hk/en/healthcare-facilities/ (accessed on 30 June 2022).
20. 40 Per Cent of Breastfeeding Mothers Are Being Discriminated, Survey Shows UNICEF HK, in Partnership with the Government, Launches 'Breastfeeding Friendly Mall' ahead of Mother's Day. Available online: https://www.unicef.org.hk/en/40-per-cent-of-breastfeeding-mothers-are-being-discriminated-survey-showsunicef-hk-in-partnership-with-the-government-launches-breastfeeding-friendly-mall-ahead-of-mother/ (accessed on 30 June 2022).
21. Wong, K.L.; Fong, D.Y.T.; Lee, I.L.Y.; Chu, S.; Tarrant, M. Antenatal education to increase exclusive breastfeeding: A randomized controlled trial. *Obstet. Gynecol.* **2014**, *124*, 961–968. [CrossRef] [PubMed]
22. Bai, D.L.; Fong, D.Y.T.; Tarrant, M. Factors Associated with Breastfeeding Duration and Exclusivity in Mothers Returning to Paid Employment Postpartum. *Matern. Child Health J.* **2015**, *19*, 990–999. [CrossRef] [PubMed]
23. The Government of the Hong Kong Special Administrative Region. Press Releases: CHP Investigates 19725 Confirmed and 9592 Asymptomatic Additional SARS-CoV-2 Virus Cases with 27510 Cases Pending Status. Available online: https://www.info.gov.hk/gia/general/202203/03/P2022030300624.htm?fontSize=1 (accessed on 28 January 2022).
24. UK Government & Public Health England. Stay at Home: Guidance for Households with Possible or Confirmed Coronavirus (COVID-19) Infection. Available online: https://www.gov.uk/government/publications/covid-19-stay-at-homeguidance/stay-at-home-guidance-for-households-with-possible-coronaviruscovid-19-infection (accessed on 28 January 2022).
25. Brooks, S.K.; Weston, D.; Greenberg, N. Psychological impact of infectious disease outbreaks on pregnant women: Rapid evidence review. *Public Health* **2020**, *189*, 26–36. [CrossRef]
26. Caffieri, A.; Margherita, G. The psychological impact of COVID-19 on women's wellbeing during pregnancy and postpartum one year after pandemic outbreak in Italy. A Systematic review. *Mediterr. J. Clin. Psychol.* **2021**, *9*. [CrossRef]
27. Shorey, S.; Chan, V. Lessons from past epidemics and pandemics and a way forward for pregnant women, midwives and nurses during COVID-19 and beyond: A meta-synthesis. *Midwifery* **2020**, *90*, 102821. [CrossRef] [PubMed]
28. Dodgson, J.E.; Tarrant, M.; Chee, Y.O.; Watkins, A. New mothers' experiences of social disruption and isolation during the severe acute respiratory syndrome outbreak in Hong Kong. *Nurs. Health Sci.* **2010**, *12*, 198–204. [CrossRef]
29. Babetin, K. The birth of a mother: A psychological transformation. *J. Prenat. Perinat. Psychol. Health* **2020**, *34*, 410–428.

30. Makama, M.; Awoke, M.A.; Skouteris, H.; Moran, L.J.; Lim, S. Barriers and facilitators to a healthy lifestyle in postpartum women: A systematic review of qualitative and quantitative studies in postpartum women and healthcare. *Obes. Rev.* **2021**, *22*, e13167. [CrossRef]
31. Prinds, C.; Mogensen, O.; Hvidt, N.C.; Bliddal, M. First child's impact on parental relationship: An existential perspective. *BMC Pregnancy Childbirth* **2018**, *18*, 157. [CrossRef] [PubMed]
32. Papworth, R.; Harris, A.; Durcan, G.; Wilton, J.; Sinclair, C. Maternal mental health during the pandemic: A rapid evidence review of COVID-19's impact. *Cent. Ment. Health* **2021**. Available online: https://maternalmentalhealthalliance.org/mmhpandemic/ (accessed on 28 March 2022).
33. Matvienko-Sikar, K.; Meedya, S.; Ravaldi, C. Perinatal mental health during the COVID-19 pandemic. *Women Birth* **2020**, *33*, 309–310. [CrossRef]
34. Karavadra, B.; Stockl, A.; Prosser-Snelling, E.; Simpson, P.; Morris, E. Women's perceptions of COVID-19 and their healthcare experiences: A qualitative thematic analysis of a national survey of pregnant women in the United Kingdom. *BMC Pregnancy Childbirth* **2020**, *20*, 600. [CrossRef]
35. Fallon, V.; Davies, S.M.; Silverio, S.A.; Jackson, L.; De Pascalis, L.; Harrold, J.A. Psychosocial experiences of postnatal women during the COVID-19 pandemic. A UK-wide study of prevalence rates and risk factors for clinically relevant depression and anxiety. *J. Psychiatr. Res.* **2021**, *136*, 157–166. [CrossRef]
36. Mortazavi, F.; Ghardashi, F. The lived experiences of pregnant women during COVID-19 pandemic: A descriptive phenomenological study. *BMC Pregnancy Childbirth* **2021**, *21*, 193. [CrossRef]
37. Sahin, B.M.; Kabakci, E.N. The experiences of pregnant women during the COVID-19 pandemic in Turkey: A qualitative study. *Women Birth* **2021**, *34*, 162–169. [CrossRef]
38. Colaizzi, P.F. Psychological research as the phenomenologist views it. In *Existential Phenomenological Alternatives for Psychology*; Valle, R.S., King, M., Eds.; Open University Press: New York, NY, USA, 1978; pp. 48–71.
39. *NVivo (Version 12). [Computer Software]*; QSR International Pty Ltd.: Victoria, Austria, 2020.
40. Lincon, Y.S.; Guba, E.G. *Naturalistic Inquiry*; Sage: Beverly Hills, CA, USA, 1985.
41. Barbour, R.S. Checklists for improving rigour in qualitative research: A case of the tail wagging the dog? *BMJ* **2001**, *322*, 1115–1117. [CrossRef]
42. Braun, V.; Clarke, V. *Thematic Analysis: A Practical Guide*; Sage: London, UK, 2022.
43. World Health Organization. WHO Recommends Continuing Breastfeeding during COVID-19 Infection and after Vaccination. Available online: https://www.euro.who.int/en/media-centre/sections/press-releases/2021/who-recommends-continuing-breastfeeding-during-covid-19-infection-and-after-vaccination (accessed on 28 February 2022).
44. Ceulemans, M.; Hompes, T.; Foulon, V. Mental health status of pregnant and breastfeeding women during the COVID-19 pandemic: A call for action. *Int. J. Gynecol. Obstet.* **2020**, *151*, 146–147. [CrossRef]
45. Aldridge, R.W.; Lewer, D.; Katikireddi, S.V.; Mathur, R.; Pathak, N.; Burns, R.; Fragaszy, E.B.; Johnson, A.M.; Devakumar, D.; Abubakar, I.; et al. Black, Asian and Minority Ethnic groups in England are at increased risk of death from COVID-19: Indirect standardisation of NHS mortality data. *Wellcome Open Res.* **2020**, *5*, 88. [CrossRef]
46. Office for National Statistics. Coronavirus (COVID-19) Related Deaths by Ethnic Group, England and Wales: 2 March 2020 to 15 May 2020. Available online: https://www.ons.gov.uk/peoplepopulationandcommunity/birthsdeathsandmarriages/deaths/articles/coronavirusrelateddeathsbyethnicgroupenglandandwales/2march2020to10april2020 (accessed on 20 March 2022).
47. Binns, C.; Lee, M.; Low, W.Y. The long-term public health benefits of breastfeeding. *Asia Pac. J. Public Health* **2016**, *28*, 7–14. [CrossRef] [PubMed]
48. Granger, C.L.; Embleton, N.D.; Palmer, J.M.; Lamb, C.A.; Berrington, J.E.; Stewart, C.J. Maternal breastmilk, infant gut microbiome and the impact on preterm infant health. *Acta Paediatr.* **2021**, *110*, 450–457. [CrossRef] [PubMed]
49. Lyons, K.E.; Ryan, C.A.; Dempsey, E.M.; Ross, R.P.; Stanton, C. Breast milk, a source of beneficial microbes and associated benefits for infant health. *Nutrients* **2020**, *12*, 1039. [CrossRef] [PubMed]
50. Minckas, N.; Medvedev, M.M.; Adejuyigbe, E.A.; Brotherton, H.; Chellani, H.; Estifanos, A.S.; Ezeaka, C.; Gobezayehu, A.G.; Irimu, G.; Kawaza, K.; et al. Preterm care during the COVID-19 pandemic: A comparative risk analysis of neonatal deaths averted by kangaroo mother care versus mortality due to SARS-CoV-2 infection. *EClinicalMedicine* **2021**, *33*, 100733. [CrossRef]
51. Oddy, W.H. The impact of breastmilk on infant and child health. *Breastfeed. Rev.* **2002**, *10*, 5–18. [PubMed]
52. Rao, S.P.N.; Minckas, N.; Medvedev, M.M.; Gathara, D.; Prashantha, Y.N.; Estifanos, A.S.; Silitonga, A.C.; Jadaun, A.S.; Adejuyigbe, E.A.; Brotherton, H.; et al. Small and sick newborn care during the COVID-19 pandemic: Global survey and thematic analysis of healthcare providers' voices and experiences. *BMJ Glob. Health* **2021**, *6*, e004347. [CrossRef] [PubMed]
53. Browne, P.D.; Aparicio, M.; Alba, C.; Hechler, C.; Beijers, R.; Rodriguez, J.M.; Fernández, L.; de Weerth, C. Human milk microbiome and maternal postnatal psychosocial distress. *Front. Microbiol.* **2019**, *10*, 2333. [CrossRef]
54. Hahn-Holbrook, J.; Cornwell-Hinrichs, T.; Anaya, I. Economic and health predictors of national postpartum depression prevalence: A systematic review, meta-analysis, and meta-regression of 291 studies from 56 countries. *Front. Psychiatr.* **2018**, *8*, 248. [CrossRef] [PubMed]
55. Music, G. *Nurturing Natures: Attachment and Children's Emotional, Sociocultural and Brain Development*; Routledge: London, UK, 2016.

56. Balogun, O.O.; O'Sullivan, E.J.; McFadden, A.; Ota, E.; Gavine, A.; Garner, C.D.; Renfrew, M.J.; MacGillivray, S. Interventions for promoting the initiation of breastfeeding. *Cochrane Database Syst. Rev.* **2016**, *11*, CD001688. [CrossRef]
57. McFadden, A.; Gavine, A.; Renfrew, M.J.; Wade, A.; Buchanan, P.; Taylor, J.L.; Veitch, E.; Rennie, A.M.; Crowther, S.A.; Neiman, S.; et al. Support for healthy breastfeeding mothers with healthy term babies. *Cochrane Database Syst. Rev.* **2017**. [CrossRef]
58. Burns, E.S.; Duursma, L.; Triandafilidis, Z. Breastfeeding support at an Australian breastfeeding Association drop-in service: A descriptive survey. *Int. Breastfeed. J.* **2020**, *15*, 101. [CrossRef] [PubMed]
59. Lebron, C.N.; St George, S.M.; Eckembrecher, D.G.; Alvarez, L.M. "Am I doing this wrong?" Breastfeeding mothers' use of an online forum. *Matern. Child Nutr.* **2020**, *16*, e12890. [CrossRef] [PubMed]
60. Hull, N.; Kam, R.L.; Gribble, K.D. Providing breastfeeding support during the COVID-19 pandemic: Concerns of mothers who contacted the Australian Breastfeeding Association. *Breastfeed. Rev.* **2020**, *28*, 25–35.
61. Ingram, J.; Thomson, G.; Johnson, D.; Clarke, J.L.; Trickey, H.; Hoddinott, P.; Dombrowski, S.U.; Jolly, K.; ABA Study Team. Women's and peer supporters' experiences of an assets-based peer support intervention for increasing breastfeeding initiation and continuation: A qualitative study. *Health Expect.* **2020**, *23*, 622–631. [CrossRef] [PubMed]
62. McLeish, J.; Redshaw, M. Mothers' accounts of the impact on emotional wellbeing of organised peer support in pregnancy and early parenthood: A qualitative study. *BMC Pregnancy Childbirth* **2017**, *17*, 28. [CrossRef] [PubMed]
63. Thomson, G.; Ingram, J.; Clarke, J.L.; Johnson, D.; Trickey, H.; Dombrowski, S.U.; Hoddinott, P.; Darwent, K.; Jolly, K.; ABA Research Group. Exploring the use and experience of an infant feeding genogram to facilitate an assets-based approach to support infant feeding. *BMC Pregnancy Childbirth* **2020**, *20*, 569. [CrossRef] [PubMed]
64. An, R.; Chen, X.; Wu, Y.; Liu, J.; Deng, C.; Liu, Y.; Guo, H. A survey of postpartum depression and health care needs among Chinese postpartum women during the pandemic of COVID-19. *Arch. Psychiatr. Nurs.* **2021**, *35*, 172–177. [CrossRef]
65. Brown, A.; Rance, J.; Bennett, P. Understanding the relationship between breastfeeding and postnatal depression: The role of pain and physical difficulties. *J. Adv. Nurs.* **2016**, *72*, 273–282. [CrossRef]
66. Krol, K.M.; Grossmann, T. Psychological effects of breastfeeding on children and mothers. *Bundesgesundheitsblatt-Gesundh. -Gesundh.* **2018**, *61*, 977–985. [CrossRef]
67. Tanganhito, D.D.S.; Bick, D.; Chang, Y.S. Breastfeeding experiences and perspectives among women with postnatal depression: A qualitative evidence synthesis. *Women Birth* **2020**, *33*, 231–239. [CrossRef]
68. McIntyre, L.M.; Griffen, A.M.; BrintzenhofeSzoc, K. Breast is best . . . except when it's not. *J. Hum. Lact.* **2018**, *34*, 575–580. [CrossRef]
69. Stallaert, L. The nurse's role in acknowledging women's emotions of unmet breastfeeding expectations. *Nurs. Women's Health* **2020**, *24*, 319–324. [CrossRef] [PubMed]
70. Guo, J.; De Carli, P.; Lodder, P.; Bakermans-Kranenburg, M.J.; Riem, M.M. Maternal mental health during the COVID-19 lockdown in China, Italy, and the Netherlands: A cross-validation study. *Psychol. Med.* **2021**, 1–11. [CrossRef]
71. Wu, Y.; Ye, R.; Wang, Q.; Sun, C.; Ji, Y.; Zhou, H.; Chang, W. Association of COVID-19 lockdown during the perinatal period with postpartum depression: Evidence from rural areas of Western China. *Health Commun.* **2022**, 1–8. [CrossRef]
72. Douglas, M.; Katikireddi, S.V.; Taulbut, M.; McKee, M.; McCartney, G. Mitigating the wider health effects of COVID-19 pandemic response. *BMJ* **2020**, *369*, m1557. [CrossRef] [PubMed]
73. Institute of Health Visiting. First 1001 Days Movement—Joint Statement in Response to COVID-19. Available online: https://ihv.org.uk/wp-content/uploads/2020/04/200408-First-1001-Days-COVID-statement.pdf (accessed on 28 February 2022).
74. Brown, A. Breastfeeding as a public health responsibility: A review of the evidence. *J. Hum. Nutr. Diet.* **2017**, *30*, 759–770. [CrossRef]
75. Gianni, M.L.; Bettinelli, M.E.; Manfra, P.; Sorrentino, G.; Bezze, E.; Plevani, L.; Cavallaro, G.; Raffaeli, G.; Crippa, B.L.; Colombo, L.; et al. Breastfeeding difficulties and risk for early breastfeeding cessation. *Nutrients* **2019**, *11*, 2266. [CrossRef]
76. Liu, Y.Q.; Petrini, M.; Maloni, J.A. "Doing the month": Postpartum practices in Chinese women. *Nurs. Health Sci.* **2015**, *17*, 5–14. [CrossRef]
77. Malouf, R.; Henderson, J.; Alderdice, F. Expectations and experiences of hospital postnatal care in the UK: A systematic review of quantitative and qualitative studies. *BMJ Open* **2019**, *9*, e022212. [CrossRef]
78. Walker, S.; Rossi, D.M.; Sander, T.M. Women's successful transition to motherhood during the early postnatal period: A qualitative systematic review of postnatal and midwifery home care literature. *Midwifery* **2019**, *79*, 102552. [CrossRef]
79. Withers, M.; Kharazmi, N.; Lim, E. Traditional beliefs and practices in pregnancy, childbirth and postpartum: A review of the evidence from Asian countries. *Midwifery* **2018**, *56*, 158–170. [CrossRef]
80. Lubbe, W.; Botha, E.; Niela-Vilen, H.; Reimers, P. Breastfeeding during the COVID-19 pandemic–a literature review for clinical practice. *Int. Breastfeed. J.* **2020**, *15*, 82. [CrossRef]
81. Vazquez-Vazquez, A.; Dib, S.; Rougeaux, E.; Wells, J.C.; Fewtrell, M.S. The impact of the COVID-19 lockdown on the experiences and feeding practices of new mothers in the UK: Preliminary data from the COVID-19 New Mum Study. *Appetite* **2021**, *156*, 104985. [CrossRef]
82. Dewey, K.G. Maternal and fetal stress are associated with impaired lactogenesis in humans. *J. Nutr.* **2001**, *131*, 3012S–3015S. [CrossRef]

83. Grajeda, R.; Pérez-Escamilla, R. Stress during labor and delivery is associated with delayed onset of lactation among urban Guatemalan women. *J. Nutr.* **2002**, *132*, 3055–3060. [CrossRef]
84. Paul, I.M.; Downs, D.S.; Schaefer, E.W.; Beiler, J.S.; Weisman, C.S. Postpartum anxiety and maternal-infant health outcomes. *Pediatrics* **2013**, *131*, e1218–e1224. [CrossRef]
85. Ratliff, G.A.; Sousa, C.A.; Graaf, G.; Akesson, B.; Kemp, S.P. Reconsidering the role of place in health and welfare services: Lessons from the COVID-19 pandemic in the United States and Canada. *Socio-Ecol. Pract. Res.* **2022**, *4*, 57–69. [CrossRef]
86. Usher, K.; Bhullar, N.; Durkin, J.; Gyamfi, N.; Jackson, D. Family violence and COVID-19: Increased vulnerability and reduced options for support. *Int. J. Ment. Health Nurs.* **2020**, *29*, 549–552. [CrossRef]

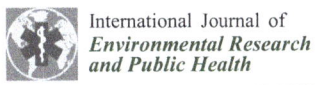

Article

Survey of Pharmacists' Knowledge, Attitudes, and Practices (KAP) concerning COVID-19 Infection Control after Being Involved in Vaccine Preparation: A Cross-Sectional Study

Nobuyuki Wakui [1,*], Mayumi Kikuchi [2], Risa Ebizuka [1], Takahiro Yanagiya [2], Chikako Togawa [1], Raini Matsuoka [1], Nobutomo Ikarashi [3], Miho Yamamura [1], Shunsuke Shirozu [1], Yoshiaki Machida [1], Kenichi Suzuki [1] and Hajime Kato [2]

[1] Division of Applied Pharmaceutical Education and Research, Hoshi University, 2-4-41 Ebara, Shinagawa-ku, Tokyo 142-8501, Japan; s171038@hoshi.ac.jp (R.E.); s181156@hoshi.ac.jp (C.T.); s181219@hoshi.ac.jp (R.M.); m-yamamura@hoshi.ac.jp (M.Y.); s-shirozu@hoshi.ac.jp (S.S.); y-machida@hoshi.ac.jp (Y.M.); kenichi-suzuki@hoshi.ac.jp (K.S.)
[2] Shinagawa Pharmaceutical Association, 2-4-2 Nakanobu, Shinagawa-ku, Tokyo 142-0053, Japan; tomato_5mk@yahoo.co.jp (M.K.); yanagiya@tnb.co.jp (T.Y.); sina89@jewel.ocn.ne.jp (H.K.)
[3] Department of Biomolecular Pharmacology, Hoshi University, 2-4-41 Ebara, Shinagawa-ku, Tokyo 142-8501, Japan; ikarashi@hoshi.ac.jp
* Correspondence: n-wakui@hoshi.ac.jp; Tel.: +81-3-5498-5760

Abstract: Vaccination is crucial for preventing the spread of COVID-19. Vaccination for COVID-19 was implemented in Japan in community units, and community pharmacists were engaged in vaccine preparation. Capturing the knowledge, attitudes, and practices (KAP) of pharmacists regarding COVID-19 infection control is important for developing future community health action strategies and plans. We conducted a cross-sectional study among 141 pharmacists who were members of a pharmacist association in the Shinagawa Ward of Tokyo (1–31 July 2021) using a Google online questionnaire. The questionnaire included demographic information and KAP questions regarding COVID-19. A correlation test was used for analyzing KAP scores. Significant correlations were found among all KAP scores. Stepwise logistic regression analysis showed "age" as a significant knowledge factor and "marriage", "pharmacist careers", "information source: official government website", and "information source: word of mouth from family and friends" as significant attitude factors. Good KAP scores were recorded in this study, indicating increased comprehension of infection control measures and increased knowledge scores, as pharmacy pharmacists were practically involved in COVID-19 infection control measures through vaccine preparation. Policymakers should understand the value of pharmacists as healthcare professionals and should enhance public health through the effective use of pharmacists.

Keywords: vaccinations; pharmacist; COVID-19; KAP; public health; infection control

1. Introduction

Severe acute respiratory syndrome caused by a novel coronavirus was first reported in China in December 2019 [1]. Later, this severe acute respiratory syndrome coronavirus 2 (SARS-CoV-2) was found to be highly contagious and resulted in life-threatening and complex respiratory illnesses [2]. The World Health Organization declared a public health emergency in January 2020, which made it an international concern [3]. Currently, the spread of SARS-CoV-2 has become a serious public health issue worldwide [4].

With the spread of SARS-CoV-2 and the unprecedented growing demand for associated healthcare, public health measures to stop the spread of infection are crucial [5]. Many people worldwide obtain information on infectious disease control by professionals through the mass media [6,7]. However, because the prevalence of COVID-19 varies widely in different regions [8,9], direct responses and guidance according to the context of each region are required. In this regard, pharmacists from all over the world are in a position to be directly or indirectly involved with patients and the local population, thus rapidly responding to public health challenges to meet local circumstances [10] and playing a key role in preventing the spread of COVID-19 [11]. Specifically, these responses include administering vaccines [12,13], educating the population regarding practices and attitudes toward preventing infection [14], participating in the supply and management of medicines [14], and actively conducting drug treatment evaluations and side effect monitoring [15]. These responses have curtailed the spread of COVID-19 and reduced the burden on medical facilities. As a result, in addition to contributing to the avoidance of healthcare disruptions [16], pharmacists provided added value to patients and the entire healthcare system and gained high confidence from the local population [17]. In Japan, pharmacists have been engaged in vaccine filling and the drug management of vaccinations for COVID-19 since June 2021. Thereby, vaccinations of local residents were efficiently carried out.

Awareness toward countermeasures is important for COVID-19 infection control, and a survey of knowledge, attitudes, and practices (KAPs) related to COVID-19 according to KAP theory [18] has been conducted on healthcare professionals in many countries [19–22]. In addition, a KAP survey for pharmacists has been reported [23–26]. However, these survey findings were conducted prior to COVID-19 vaccine development, and pharmacists' KAP information has not been reported.

The spread of the COVID-19 infection is still ongoing, and the prospects for complete convergence remain opaque. In such a situation, pharmacists play an important role through their involvement in a vaccination program to prevent the spread of the COVID-19 infection. Awareness of the KAP status for COVID-19 infection control among pharmacists after being involved with vaccinations will be informative in determining future community health action strategies and plans from the perspective of improving and promoting community public health. Therefore, we conducted a KAP survey on infection control measures for COVID-19 among pharmacists.

2. Materials and Methods

2.1. Study Design and Setting

This was a cross-sectional study conducted with pharmacists who were members of a pharmacist association in the Shinagawa Ward of Tokyo, Japan. Data collection took place between 1 July 2021, and 31 July 2021. The survey was conducted online via a web questionnaire that used a Google form. Participants responded anonymously to questions on demographics and their KAP regarding COVID-19. Of the 255 pharmacists surveyed, there were 141 respondents (a response rate of 55.3%), and all responded to all items and were included in the analysis. All participants responded anonymously (Figure 1).

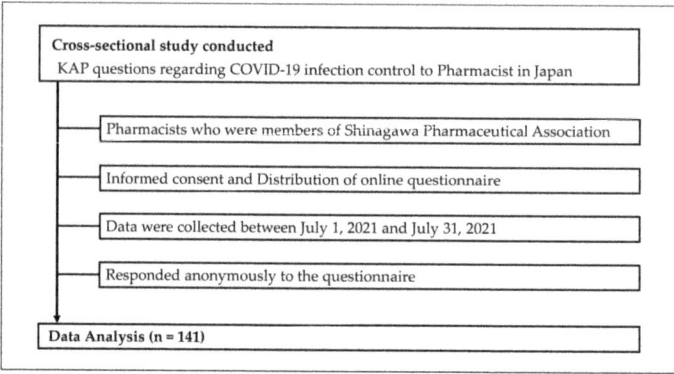

Figure 1. Flowchart of the cross-sectional study.

2.2. Content of the Survey Instrument

Data were collected from pharmacists to assess KAP on infection control measures for COVID-19. The questionnaire consisted of two parts: demographic information and KAP questions. The KAP questions assessed COVID-19 knowledge, attitudes, and practices. The knowledge section consisted of 17 questions, and participants responded to each question with a selection formula of "Yes", "No", and "Don't know". These questions assessed their level of knowledge of the clinical manifestations, transmission route, prevention, and management of COVID-19. The attitude section consisted of 16 questions that assessed attitudes regarding vaccinating against COVID-19 and preventing the spread of infection. The practice section consisted of 11 questions that assessed the measures that were taken during daily living to prevent COVID-19 infection. Regarding the items of attitudes and practices, the selection formula was "yes" or "no". In addition, as an assessment of the internal consistency of the KAP questionnaire, a reliability analysis was performed using Cronbach's alpha coefficient, which showed good reliability values of 0.80 for knowledge and 0.74 for attitudes, and an acceptable value of 0.53 for practices.

2.3. Definition of Terms

The Japanese School Education Law was revised in 2006, and pharmacy universities shifted from a 4-year system to the current 6-year system to strengthen clinical education. With this revision, only those who had been educated at a 6-year pharmacy university could take the national pharmacist examination. Therefore, some of the participants in this survey were pharmacists who graduated from a 4-year pharmacy school before the revision of the law, and some were pharmacists who graduated from a 6-year pharmacy school.

2.4. Study Variables

Demographic variables included age, sex (men and women), marital status (married and unmarried), academic background (4-year university, 6-year university, master's degree, and doctoral degree), and the information source of COVID-19. Knowledge, attitude, and practice scores were labeled as adequate knowledge, positive attitudes, and good practices, respectively, for knowledge, attitude, and practice scores based on Bloom's cutoffs and using 80% or more of the scores as the reference standard [27,28].

Knowledge scores were obtained by assigning 1 point for each correct answer, assigning 0 to an incorrect/"Don't know" answer, and summing all items. Knowledge scores ranged from 0 to 17 points, with 14 points or more labeled as adequate knowledge regarding COVID-19 and less than 14 points as inadequate knowledge.

For attitude scores, we assigned 1 point for positive attitudes and 0 points for negative attitudes for each question item and summed those items. Attitude scores ranged from 0 to 16 points, with 13 or more labeled as a positive attitude and less than 13 as a negative attitude.

For practice scores, a score of 1 was assigned if answers reflecting good practice were selected, 0 was assigned if answers reflecting bad practice were chosen, and those items were summed. Practice scores ranged from 1 to 11 points, with more than 9 points labeled as good practice and less than 9 as bad practice.

2.5. Statistical Analysis

The resulting data were encoded, validated, and analyzed using the statistical software R version 4.0.2 (R Foundation for Statistical Computing, Vienna, Austria). By setting the Google form so that it could not be finished without answers, there were 0 missing data. Numerical data were summarized with the mean and standard deviation. Categorical data were summarized by frequency and ratio. A correlation test was used to determine associations among knowledge, attitude, and practice scores. The assessment of the association between demographic variables and knowledge, attitude, and practice scores was conducted using a logistic regression analysis. A p value of less than 0.05 was considered statistically significant.

2.6. Ethical Considerations

This study was reviewed and approved by the Institutional Review Board Committee of Hoshi University (Approval No. 2021-01). Signed informed consent was obtained from all respondents, and participation was voluntary.

3. Results

3.1. Participant Information

The majority of the participants were women (65.2%) with a mean age of 44.8 years (SD: 11.9). Pharmacist career scores averaged 16.1 years (SD: 10.5), and 97 participants were married (68.8%). The academic background of the 141 participants included 93 (66.0%) bachelor's degrees in pharmacy in the fourth grade, 32 (22.7%) bachelor's degrees in pharmacy in the sixth grade, 13 (9.2%) master's degrees, and 3 (2.1%) doctoral degrees. The main sources of information on COVID-19 were 32 (22.7%) international health organizations, such as the CDC and WHO, 101 (71.6%) governmental office internet sites, 124 (87.9%) news media sources, 50 (35.5%) social media sources, 28 (19.9%) cases of word of mouth from family/friends, and 12 (8.5%) original papers (Table 1).

Table 1. Participant characteristics ($n = 141$).

Variable	
Age (years)	44.8 ± 11.9
Sex, n (%)	
Men	49 (34.8%)
Women	92 (65.2%)
Marital status, n (%)	
Married	97 (68.8%)
Unmarried	44 (31.2%)
Academic background, n (%)	
4-year university	93 (66.0%)
6-year university	32 (22.7%)
Master's degree/Doctoral degree	16 (11.3%)
Pharmacist career, n (%)	
Less than 10 years	46 (32.6%)
10 years or more and less than 20 years	39 (27.7%)
Over 20 years	56 (39.7%)
Information source of COVID-19, n (%)	
Official website and media of the WHO or CDC	32 (22.7%)
Official government website and media	101 (71.6%)
Media such as news (TV, radio, internet, magazines, and newspapers)	124 (87.9%)
Social media (Facebook, Twitter, and Instagram)	50 (35.5%)
Word of mouth from family/friends	28 (19.9%)
Original paper	12 (8.5%)
I don't remember	2 (1.4%)

3.2. Pharmacists' Knowledge of COVID-19

Table 2 shows the results regarding knowledge of COVID-19. Most respondents answered 15 of 17 knowledge items correctly (M = 14.4, SD = 2.5). Ten items had correct answer rates of over 90%. Conversely, nearly 75% of the respondents could not answer the question that included "sneezing, runny nose, stuffy nose, and headache are not common symptoms of COVID-19." Regarding the item "COVID-19 is caused by beta coronavirus", only 41.8% answered correctly, and nearly half (46.8%) answered that they did not know. Regarding the question that COVID-19 is transmitted by the ingestion of food, 70.9% of the respondents answered correctly, 17% answered incorrectly, and 12.1% answered that they did not know. On the basis of Bloom's cutoff values, 118 (83.7%) of the pharmacists were labeled as having good knowledge, with a knowledge score of 14 or higher, and 23 (16.3%) pharmacists were labeled as having inadequate knowledge, with a knowledge score of less than 14.

Table 2. Respondents' answers on COVID-19 knowledge items.

		Correct Answer	Incorrect Answer	Don't Know
K1	COVID-19 is caused by beta coronavirus.	59 (41.8%)	16 (11.3%)	66 (46.8%)
K2	COVID-19 is transmitted by food intake.	100 (70.9%)	24 (17.0%)	17 (12.1%)
K3	Common clinical symptoms of COVID-19 are fever, dry cough, dyspnea, and malaise.	128 (90.8%)	8 (5.7%)	5 (3.5%)
K4	Sneezing, runny nose, stuffy nose, and headache are less common symptoms of COVID-19.	36 (25.5%)	96 (68.1%)	9 (6.4%)
K5	PCR can be used to diagnose COVID-19.	126 (89.4%)	11 (7.8%)	4 (2.8%)
K6	Washing your hands with soap and water for at least 30 s is effective in preventing COVID-19 infection.	132 (93.6%)	6 (4.3%)	3 (2.1%)
K7	Loss of taste and smell is characteristic of COVID 19 infection.	129 (91.5%)	9 (6.4%)	3 (2.1%)
K8	Symptom-free COVID-19 patients (during the incubation period) do not spread the virus to others.	136 (96.5%)	0 (0%)	5 (3.5%)
K9	COVID-19 infection spreads through the infected person's respiratory droplets.	137 (97.2%)	1 (0.7%)	3 (2.1%)
K10	The incubation period of coronavirus is 1 to 14 days.	126 (89.4%)	8 (5.7%)	7 (5.0%)
K11	Elderly people, patients with chronic illness, DM, COPD can be severe.	137 (97.2%)	0 (0%)	4 (2.8%)
K12	Shaking hands and avoiding crowded areas and public transport can prevent COVID-19 infection.	135 (95.7%)	2 (1.4%)	4 (2.8%)
K13	Keeping social distance is effective in preventing the spread of COVID-19.	135 (95.7%)	1 (0.7%)	5 (3.5%)
K14	Antibiotics are the first-line drug if COVID-19 infection is suspected or confirmed.	121 (85.8%)	8 (5.7%)	12 (8.5%)
K15	Early response and supportive care are effective in recovering from infection, as there is no effective treatment for COVID-19.	123 (87.2%)	8 (5.7%)	10 (7.1%)
K16	Isolating and treating individuals infected with COVID-19 is an effective way to break the chain of infection.	138 (97.9%)	0 (0%)	3 (2.1%)
K17	Large-scale group activities can spread COVID-19 infection.	138 (97.9%)	0 (0%)	3 (2.1%)
	Knowledge Score	14.4 ± 2.5		

Of the questions K1–K17, "No" is the correct answer for questions K2: "COVID-19 is transmitted by food intake", K8: "Symptom-free COVID-19 patients (during the incubation period) do not spread the virus to others", and K14: "Antibiotics are the first-line drug if COVID-19 infection is suspected or confirmed". "Yes" is the correct answer for all the other questions—K1, K3, K4, K5, K6, K7, K9, K10, K11, K12, and K13.

3.3. Attitudes of Pharmacists regarding COVID-19

Table 3 shows the results regarding attitudes of COVID-19. Many respondents indicated positive attitudes for 13 of 16 items (M = 13.0, SD = 2.6). In particular, for six items, including "I would like to be vaccinated with COVID-19" (94.3%), "Pharmacists can contribute to the promotion of vaccination of local residents from the public health and social aspects" (91.5%), "Vaccination can prevent the spread of COVID-19" (94.3%), "all information regarding COVID-19 needs to be shared with other healthcare professionals" (96.5%), "it is the pharmacist's social mission to work together to curb the spread of COVID-19" (97.9%), and "I understand that this infection is very infectious" (97.9%), more than 90% of the pharmacists responded with a positive attitude. Conversely, for items related to ultimately being able to fully control COVID-19 infections (31.9%), there were fewer positive attitude responses. On the basis of Bloom's cutoff score, there were 95 (67.4%) pharmacists who were considered to have positive attitudes with an attitude score of 13 points or more, and 46 (32.6%) pharmacists who were considered to have negative attitudes with an attitude score of less than 13 points.

Table 3. Respondents' answers on COVID-19 attitudes.

		Yes	No
A1	I would like to be vaccinated with COVID-19 (answer "yes" if already vaccinated).	133 (94.3%)	8 (5.7%)
A2	I am motivated to be involved in citizens' vaccination work (such as vaccine filling).	112 (79.4%)	29 (20.6%)
A3	I don't think there is any problem even if vaccination by a pharmacist is approved as in overseas.	96 (68.1%)	45 (31.9%)
A4	If vaccination by a pharmacist is approved, I am willing to vaccinate the public.	90 (63.8%)	51 (36.2%)

Table 3. Cont.

		Yes	No
A5	If vaccination by a pharmacist is approved at a dispensing pharmacy like overseas, I think it will be a great advantage for local residents.	115 (81.6%)	26 (18.4%)
A6	If vaccination becomes possible at local pharmacies, I think it can contribute to improving the vaccination rate of local residents.	116 (82.3%)	25 (17.7%)
A7	I think pharmacists can contribute to vaccination of local residents from the public health and social aspects.	129 (91.5%)	12 (8.5%)
A8	In order to popularize antibody testing, I think it's okay for pharmacists to do antibody testing at pharmacies.	109 (77.3%)	32 (22.7%)
A9	I think that vaccination can prevent the spread of COVID-19.	133 (94.3%)	8 (5.7%)
A10	Ultimately, I think we can completely control the infection of COVID-19.	45 (31.9%)	96 (68.1%)
A11	I think healthcare professionals need to be aware of all information regarding COVID-19.	122 (86.5%)	19 (13.5%)
A12	I think all information related to COVID-19 needs to be shared with other healthcare professionals.	136 (96.5%)	5 (3.5%)
A13	I think the spread of COVID-19 can be prevented by taking the precautionary measures indicated by WHO and the government.	97 (68.8%)	44 (31.2%)
A14	I think it is necessary to use gowns, gloves, masks, and face shields when dealing with patients with COVID-19.	117 (83.0%)	24 (17.0%)
A15	I think it is the pharmacist's social mission to work together to curb the spread of COVID-19 infection.	138 (97.9%)	3 (2.1%)
A16	I understand that this infection is very infectious.	138 (97.9%)	3 (2.1%)
	Attitude score	13.0 ± 2.6	

3.4. Practices of Pharmacists regarding COVID-19

Most of the respondents answered that they were performing 10 of 11 practice items (M = 9.4, SD = 1.4). Six items, including keeping a social distance (97.9%), performing handwashing with soap routinely (97.9%), avoiding crowds (91.5%), handling possessions of patients suspected of having the coronavirus with infection prevention measures (96.5%), covering the nose and mouth with tissues and handkerchiefs when sneezing or coughing (97.2%), and ensuring that used tissues were discarded in a trash box to prevent infection (97.9%), were scored at 90% or more for good practices, and the majority also indicated good practices for other items. Conversely, items such as "I tried not to take the elevator as much as possible" (41.1%) and "I have attended workshop for COVID-19 infection prevention" (53.9%) had low values (Table 4). On the basis of Bloom's cutoff values, 111 (78.7%) of the pharmacists were labeled with good behaviors with a score of 9 or higher, and 30 (21.3%) were labeled with bad behaviors with a score of less than 9 points.

Table 4. Respondents' answers on COVID-19 practices.

		Yes	No
P1	I have attended workshop for COVID-19 infection prevention.	76 (53.9%)	65 (46.1%)
P2	I keep a social distance with others to prevent infection.	138 (97.9%)	3 (2.1%)
P3	When I touch the front door, which is touched by an unspecified number of people, I open and close it while being careful of infection.	120 (85.1%)	21 (14.9%)
P4	I wash my hands with soap routinely.	138 (97.9%)	3 (2.1%)
P5	I avoid crowds as much as possible.	129 (91.5%)	12 (8.5%)
P6	I avoid meeting friends and relatives.	125 (88.7%)	16 (11.3%)
P7	I try not to touch my eyes, nose, and mouth as much as possible.	124 (87.9%)	17 (12.1%)
P8	When dealing with the belongings of a patient suspected of having a corona infection, I take care to prevent infection.	136 (96.5%)	5 (3.5%)
P9	I try not to take the elevator as much as possible.	58 (41.1%)	83 (58.9%)
P10	When I sneeze or cough, I cover my nose and mouth with a tissue or handkerchief.	137 (97.2%)	4 (2.8%)
P11	To prevent infection, I always try to throw used tissue in the trash.	138 (97.9%)	3 (2.1%)
	Practice score	9.4 ± 1.4	

3.5. Correlations between Knowledge, Attitude, and Practice Scores

Knowledge, attitude, and practice scores showed significant associations with each other (Table 5). A strong correlation was found in the order of knowledge and attitude (r = 0.44, $p < 0.001$) > attitude and practice (r = 0.32, $p < 0.001$) > knowledge and practice (r = 0.21, $p = 0.01$).

Table 5. Correlations between knowledge, attitude, and practice scores.

	Correlation (r)	p Value
Knowledge and Attitude	0.44	<0.001
Knowledge and Practice	0.21	0.01
Attitude and Practice	0.32	<0.001

3.6. Relationship between Participants' Attributes and KAP Scores

Univariate logistic regression analysis was used to assess attribute factors associated with KAP (Table 6). The findings showed that chronological age (30 s, OR: 6.3, 95% CI: 1.6–25.1; 40 s, OR: 11.1, 95% CI: 2.5–48.8; 50 s, OR: 3.8, 95% CI: 1.1–13.3; and 60 s, OR: 16.2, 95% CI: 1.78–147.1), marital status (OR: 2.9, 95% CI: 1.2–7.3), academic background (6 years-university, OR: 0.3, 95% CI: 0.1–0.8), and pharmacist career (over 20 years, OR: 4.1, 95% CI: 1.2–13.9) were factors associated with knowledge. Marital status (OR: 0.42, 95% CI: 0.18–0.97) and source of information on COVID-19 (government official website and government official site, OR: 2.5, 95% CI: 1.2–5.3; and word of mouth from family/friends, OR: 0.4, 95% CI: 0.2–0.9) were associated with attitudes. No factors associated with practices were found (Table 6).

Table 6. Evaluation of attribute factors related to KAP using univariate logistic regression analysis.

Characteristics	Category	Good Knowledge			Good Attitude			Good Practice		
		OR	95% CI	p Value	OR	95% CI	p Value	OR	95% CI	p Value
Age	20–29 years	1			1			1		
	30–39 years	6.3	1.58–25.08	0.009	1.11	0.34–3.64	0.859	2.49	0.64–9.70	0.188
	40–49 years	11.1	2.52–48.84	0.001	1.75	0.54–5.67	0.351	1.85	0.53–6.38	0.332
	50–59 years	3.75	1.06–13.31	0.041	1.06	0.32–3.48	0.923	1.33	0.38–4.67	0.659
	60 over	16.2	1.78–147.06	0.013	1.00	0.27–3.74	1.000	2.46	0.51–11.80	0.260
Sex	Men	0.52	0.21–1.28	0.154	1.00	0.48–2.09	0.996	0.53	0.23–1.20	0.126
	Women	1			1			1		
Marital Status	Married	2.93	1.18–7.31	0.021	0.42	0.18–0.97	0.041	1.97	0.86–4.54	0.110
	Unmarried	1			1			1		
Academic background	4-year university	1			1			1		
	6-year university	0.30	0.11–0.78	0.014	0.70	0.30–1.59	0.391	1.04	0.40–2.74	0.934
	Master's degree/Doctoral degree	0.94	0.19–4.70	0.939	2.06	0.55–7.79	0.285	2.04	0.43–9.71	0.370
Pharmacist career	Less than 10 years	1			1			1		
	10 years or more and less than 20 years	1.22	0.43–3.41	0.708	2.27	0.85–6.06	0.101	1.73	0.57–5.21	0.331
	Over 20 years	4.09	1.20–13.87	0.024	0.98	0.44–2.19	0.955	1.04	0.41–2.60	0.934
Source of information on COVID-19	Official website and media of the WHO or CDC	1.48	0.46–4.71	0.509	1.99	0.79–5.02	0.145	2.19	0.70–6.83	0.176
	Official government website and media	1.8	0.71–4.58	0.215	2.48	1.16–5.31	0.019	1.35	0.57–3.21	0.498
	Media such as news (TV, radio, internet, magazines, and newspapers)	1.11	0.29–4.24	0.874	0.4	0.11–1.48	0.172	0.77	0.21–2.88	0.697
	Social media (Facebook, Twitter, and Instagram)	1.04	0.41–2.65	0.941	1.05	0.50–2.19	0.907	1.13	0.48–2.64	0.784
	Word of mouth from family/friends	0.65	0.23–1.84	0.416	0.4	0.17–0.92	0.032	0.48	0.19–1.21	0.121
	Original paper	0.35	0.09–1.26	0.108	0.97	0.28–3.39	0.956	1.39	0.29–6.70	0.684

3.7. Extraction of Factors Associated with KAP Scores by Stepwise Logistic Regression Analysis

Factors associated with KAP were extracted using stepwise multiple logistic regression analysis with factors that had a p value less than 0.20 as a result of univariate logistic regression analysis (Table 7). As a result, "age" was extracted as an important variable for knowledge. Regarding attitudes, "marriage", "academic background", "pharmacist careers", "information source: official government website", and "information source: word of mouth from family and friends" were extracted as important factors. Regarding practices, no factors showing an association were extracted.

Table 7. Extraction of attribute factors related to knowledge, attitudes, and practices by stepwise logistic regression analysis.

Characteristics	Category	Good Knowledge			Good Attitude		
		Adjusted OR	95% CI	p Value	Adjusted OR	95% CI	p Value
Age	20–29 years	1					
	30–39 years	6.3	1.58–25.08	0.009			
	40–49 years	11.1	2.52–48.84	0.001			
	50–59 years	3.75	1.06–13.31	0.041			
	60 over	16.2	1.78–147.06	0.013			
Sex	Men						
	Women						
Marital Status	Married				0.37	0.15–0.90	0.029
	Unmarried				1		
Academic background	4-year university						
	6-year university						
	Master's degree/Doctoral degree						
Pharmacist career	Less than 10 years						
	10 years or more and less than 20 years						
	Over 20 years						
Source of information on COVID-19	Official website and media of the WHO or CDC						
	Official government website and media				2.81	1.26–6.26	0.012
	Media such as news (TV, radio, internet, magazines, and newspapers)						
	Social media (Facebook, Twitter, and Instagram)						
	Word of mouth from family/friends				0.38	0.16–0.91	0.030
	Original paper						

Stepwise logistic regression analysis was performed with Age, Sex, Marital Status, Academic Background, Pharmacist Career, and Source of Information on COVID-19 as explanatory variables. As a result, Age was extracted for Good Knowledge, and Marital Status, Official Government Website and Media, and Word of Mouth from Family/Friends were extracted as important variables for Good Attitude. Variables in blank cells were not extracted as significant variables.

The odds ratios and confidence intervals for "age" in knowledge were as follows: ages in their 20 s (OR = 6.3, 95% CI = 1.58–25.08), 30 s (OR = 11.1, 95% CI = 2.52–48.84), 40 s (OR = 3.75, 95% CI = 1.06–13.31), 50 s (OR = 3.75, 95% CI = 1.06–13.31), and 60 s (OR = 16.2, 95% CI = 1.78–147.06).

The odds ratio and confidence interval for "marriage" in attitudes were OR = 0.3 and 95% CI = 0.10–0.94 for married people. The odds ratio and confidence interval for academic background were OR = 0.3 and 95% CI = 0.10–0.94 for graduating from pharmacy studies in a 6-year-university. Regarding information sources, the odds ratios and confidence intervals were OR = 2.88 and 95% CI = 1.18–7.01 for governmental official websites and media (MHLW) and OR = 0.39 and 95% CI = 0.15–1.00 for word of mouth from family/friends.

4. Discussion

In this study, we conducted a KAP survey for pharmacists involved in community vaccine preparation. The majority of the pharmacists were shown to have positive KAP, and most of the pharmacists' sources were news media (n = 124, 87.9%) and government office sites (n = 101, 71.6%). In addition, 8.5% of the pharmacists obtained information from academic journals, which was less than 10% of all participants. These results showed that conventional mass media and the internet are important information sources for pharmacists, and the current situation in which many pharmacists in Japan have not been able to obtain the latest information from academic journals was indicated. Knowledge was shown to be associated with attitudes and practices in previous KAP surveys related to COVID-19 [29–31], and in this study as well, there was a correlation among knowledge, attitudes, and practices. Our results suggested that each item of KAP was mutually influential on the others, and that all items were essential components.

Previous KAP surveys of COVID-19 infection control among Japanese pharmacists reported lower KAP scores [23]. It has also been reported that the KAP scores of pharmacists were lower than those of doctors and nurses abroad [32,33]. However, our study showed good scores for all items of KAP. Awareness and comprehension of infection control measures may have increased as pharmacists became practically involved in COVID-19 infection control measures through participating in vaccine preparation. As a result, knowledge scores may have increased. At the same time, the pharmacists' KAP scores were lower than those previously reported for doctors and nurses, possibly because the pharmacists were not involved in COVID-19 infection control. Therefore, it was considered that practices were indispensable to obtain good knowledge scores.

The aggregated results for attitude scores revealed that 90% or more pharmacists answered positively for six attitude items. Of these, almost all pharmacists answered "I would like to be vaccinated with COVID-19" and "I think that vaccination can prevent the spread of COVID-19". In addition, four items such as "I think all information related to COVID-19 needs to be shared with other healthcare professionals", "I think pharmacists can contribute to vaccination of the local residents from the public health and social aspects", "I think it is the pharmacist's social mission to work together to curb the spread of COVID-19 infection", and "I understand that this infection is very infections" had more than 90% of the pharmacists answering "I would think so". Therefore, many pharmacists indicated positive attitude scores. Conversely, only 31.9% of the pharmacists answered "I would think so" to the question "Ultimately, we can completely control COVID-19 infection", indicating the difficulty and seriousness of COVID-19 infection control.

As a result of extracting the related factors of KAP using stepwise logistic regression analysis, the related factors for knowledge and attitudes scores were extracted. Regarding knowledge scores, age was extracted as in previous studies [23], with the lowest knowledge scores for the respondents in their 20s. It may be conceivable that people in their 20s have a lower risk of becoming severely ill with COVID-19, and it is thought that the percentage of pharmacy managers who manage pharmacies is small. Conversely, regarding the attitude score, four items were extracted: "marriage", "pharmacist careers", "information source: official government website", and "information source: word of mouth from family and friends". For "marital status", the attitude scores were significantly higher in unmarried than in married individuals. This is thought to be because the percentage of women pharmacists in Japan is higher than that of men. In other words, it is conceivable that married women take more time to do housework and raise children, and it is difficult for them to be actively involved in COVID-19 infection control as a pharmacist. In addition, pharmacists with less than 10 years of experience had the most positive attitude scores in pharmacist history, and pharmacists with more than 10 years and less than 20 years had significantly lower scores. This suggested that attitude scores fluctuated according to the length of the pharmacists' career. Furthermore, the attitude scores of pharmacists who obtained information from the official website of the government were significantly high, and those of pharmacists who obtained information by word of mouth from family and friends were significantly low. These findings suggest that the presence or absence of active information collection is associated with attitude scores. As for the practice scores, as in the previous reports [19,34], no relevant vital factors were extracted, and a significant relationship was found between knowledge and attitudes. From this, we suggest that practical involvement with vaccine preparation brought about knowledge and attitude improvements.

In this study, gender was not significantly associated with KAP scores. However, a KAP survey conducted with the general public reported an association between gender and knowledge scores [35,36]. This may be due to women being more likely than men to feel anxious regarding a variety of issues [37], and because of their anxiety, they may become enthusiastic regarding collecting information on infection control. As a result, their knowledge scores may be higher. Conversely, there have been reports that no association exists between gender and knowledge in KAP surveys conducted with healthcare professionals [28,38,39]. It has been speculated that this is because healthcare workers are involved in COVID-19 infection control regardless of gender. On the other hand, a KAP survey administered to medical students reported an association between gender and knowledge scores [40]. This is probably because medical students are not yet directly involved in COVID-19 infection control as healthcare workers. Similarly, a KAP survey conducted with Japanese pharmacists during the period prior to vaccine preparation engagement, i.e., when they were not directly involved in COVID-19 infection control, showed a significant association between gender and knowledge scores [23]. From the above, we suggest that factors related to the KAP survey of COVID-19 were influenced by the practical environment of the study participants.

Regarding pharmacists' sources of information, most sources were news and government office sites, and few pharmacists obtained information from academic journals. This is a similar result to a KAP survey conducted in Japan before vaccine development [23]. Recently, the use of SNS has also been considered a useful information resource [19,41]. However, news alone does not alter the amount of information available compared to the general public, and SNS alone may be affected by erroneous information. As medical professionals involved with vaccinations need to obtain general information from the news, they also need to obtain official information distributed by the government and the latest specialized information from academic journals.

There are several limitations to this study. First, the survey was limited to pharmacists in Tokyo, and no results were obtained from pharmacists in other cities. Second, because of the cross-sectional nature of the study, a causal relationship cannot be determined. Third, the questionnaires may not correspond exactly to what the health professional thinks and does in clinical practice. Fourth, the small sample size of the study may not reflect the opinions of the entire pharmacist community. Further, the response rate was 55.3%—a little low. It is possible that some pharmacists have stopped participating in web questionnaires because they are not familiar with the operation. However, in Japan, the same information is available from media news in all regions, and in fact, pharmacists are involved in the development and manufacture of vaccines. Therefore, it is unlikely that knowledge, behaviors, and attitudes regarding infection control will vary significantly from region to region and from individual to individual. The distribution of gender and age in this study was similar to the distribution of the whole pharmacist community in Japan. Therefore, it is considered that the bias of the obtained results is small.

The points that should be emphasized in this study are that this was a cross-sectional study conducted by a Japanese pharmacist during the period when he was engaged in vaccine preparation to prevent the spread of COVID-19 in the local population. The survey was conducted at a time when the number of people infected with COVID-19 per day in Tokyo was rapidly increasing and the crisis of medical collapse was being hailed. Local pharmacists were involved in vaccine preparation, even on holidays, so that as many citizens as possible could get their first vaccination as soon as possible. In addition, community pharmacist associations actively held training sessions on vaccine preparation for pharmacists. Previously, pharmacists in Japan only dispensed prescriptions based on individual pharmacies and were not openly involved in activities such as community infection control. In view of these circumstances, the results of this study were obtained during the first practical involvement of Japanese pharmacists in community infectious disease control in a critical setting of a spreading COVID-19 infection. This can be useful information when considering the public health significance and social value of community pharmacists who were practically participating in infectious disease countermeasures, such as vaccination, not only in Japan but also globally. Indeed, pharmacists' knowledge and attitude scores under situations where practical involvement was sought were very positive. Furthermore, because more than 90% of the pharmacists replied that it is the duty of pharmacists to engage in public health, such as infection control measures, it can be said that pharmacists are very positive and highly aware of public health efforts. Moreover, as community pharmacists' knowledge, attitude, and practice scores toward COVID-19 were positive, the active utilization of pharmacists could lead to better community public health and could provide great added value to patients and the entire healthcare system. Therefore, the use of community healthcare professionals, such as pharmacists, may expand the potential of human medical resources and may consequently lead to the activation of community healthcare. It is hoped that policymakers understand the value of pharmacists as human resources and effectively utilize them for the development of public health. Furthermore, we believe that the results of this study may contribute to strengthening the role of pharmacists in communities in different parts of the world, not only in Japan.

5. Conclusions

The KAP of pharmacists on COVID-19 was very positive under situations of practical engagement in vaccination. This suggests that utilizing pharmacists may increase the professionalism of pharmacists and may provide new added value to patients and the health care system as a whole. It is hoped that policymakers will understand the value of pharmacists, who are healthcare professionals, as human resources, and make effective use of them, thus contributing to the development of public health.

Author Contributions: N.W., M.K. and R.E. designed the study. N.W., M.K., R.E., M.Y., T.Y., C.T., R.M. and H.K. collected data. N.W. and R.E. analyzed the data. N.W. wrote the manuscript. M.K., R.E., N.I., M.Y., S.S., Y.M., K.S. and H.K. critically revised the manuscript for important intellectual content. All authors have read and agreed to the published version of the manuscript.

Funding: This research received no external funding.

Institutional Review Board Statement: The study was approved by the Ethics Committee of the Hoshi University (Approval No. 2021-01).

Informed Consent Statement: Informed consent was obtained from all subjects involved in the study.

Data Availability Statement: The data are not publicly available as all participants have not consented to the public disclosure of the data online. However, the data presented in this study are available on request from the corresponding author.

Acknowledgments: We thank all the pharmacists who participated in this study.

Conflicts of Interest: The authors declare no conflict of interest.

References

1. Sharma, A.; Tiwari, S.; Deb, M.K.; Marty, J.L. Severe Acute Respiratory Syndrome coronavirus-2 (SARS-CoV-2): A Global Pandemic and Treatment Strategies. *Int. J. Antimicrob. Agents* **2020**, *56*, 106054. [CrossRef] [PubMed]
2. Zhu, N.; Zhang, D.; Wang, W.; Li, X.; Yang, B.; Song, J.; Zhao, X.; Huang, B.; Shi, W.; Lu, R.; et al. A Novel Coronavirus from Patients with Pneumonia in China, 2019. *N. Engl. J. Med.* **2020**, *382*, 727–733. [CrossRef] [PubMed]
3. PAHO. WHO Characterizes COVID-19 as a Pandemic. Available online: https://www3.paho.org/hq/index.php?option=com_content&view=article&id=15756:who-characterizes-covid-19-as-a-pandemic&Itemid=1926&lang=en (accessed on 23 June 2022).
4. WHO. WHO Director-General's Opening Remarks at the Media Briefing on COVID-19—11 March 2020. Available online: https://www.who.int/director-general/speeches/detail/who-director-general-s-opening-remarks-at-the-media-briefing-on-covid-19---11-march-2020 (accessed on 23 June 2022).
5. WHO. Considerations in Adjusting Public Health and Social Measures in the Context of COVID-19 Interim Guidance. Available online: https://www.who.int/publications/i/item/considerations-in-adjusting-public-health-and-social-measures-in-the-context-of-covid-19-interim-guidance (accessed on 23 June 2022).
6. Venegas-Vera, A.V.; Colbert, G.B.; Lerma, E.V. Positive and Negative Impact of Social Media in the COVID-19 Era. *Rev. Cardiovasc. Med.* **2020**, *21*, 561–564. [CrossRef] [PubMed]

7. Anwar, A.; Malik, M.; Raees, V.; Anwar, A. Role of Mass Media and Public Health Communications in the COVID-19 Pandemic. *Cureus* **2020**, *12*, e10453. [CrossRef]
8. Hoffmann, C.; Wolf, E. Older Age Groups and Country-Specific Case Fatality Rates of COVID-19 in Europe, USA and Canada. *Infection* **2021**, *49*, 111–116. [CrossRef]
9. Huang, Q.; Jackson, S.; Derakhshan, S.; Lee, L.; Pham, E.; Jackson, A.; Cutter, S.L. Urban-Rural Differences in COVID-19 Exposures and Outcomes in the South: A Preliminary Analysis of South Carolina. *PLoS ONE* **2021**, *16*, e0246548. [CrossRef]
10. Agomo, C.O. The Role of Community Pharmacists in Public Health: A Scoping Review of the Literature. *J. Pharm. Health Serv. Res.* **2012**, *3*, 25–33. [CrossRef]
11. Visacri, M.B.; Figueiredo, I.V.; Lima, T.M. Role of Pharmacist during the COVID-19 Pandemic: A Scoping Review. *Res. Soc. Adm. Pharm.* **2021**, *17*, 1799–1806. [CrossRef]
12. Gravlee, E.; Pittman, E.; Sparkmon, W.; Imeri, H.; Cox, H.F.; Barnard, M. COVID-19 Vaccination Engagement and Barriers among Mississippi Pharmacists. *Pharmacy* **2021**, *9*, 167. [CrossRef]
13. Mukattash, T.L.; Jarab, A.S.; Abu Farha, R.K.; Nusair, M.B.; Al Muqatash, S. Pharmacists' Perspectives on Providing the COVID-19 Vaccine in Community Pharmacies. *J. Pharm. Health Serv. Res.* **2021**, *12*, 313–316. [CrossRef]
14. Liu, S.; Luo, P.; Tang, M.; Hu, Q.; Polidoro, J.P.; Sun, S.; Gong, Z. Providing Pharmacy Services during the Coronavirus Pandemic. *Int. J. Clin. Pharm.* **2020**, *28*, 299–304. [CrossRef] [PubMed]
15. Mahmoudjafari, Z.; Alexander, M.; Roddy, J.; Shaw, R.; Shigle, T.L.; Timlin, C.; Culos, K. American Society for Transplantation and Cellular Therapy Pharmacy Special Interest Group Position Statement on Pharmacy Practice Management and Clinical Management for COVID-19 in Hematopoietic Cell Transplantation and Cellular Therapy Patients in the United States. *Biol. Blood Marrow Transplant.* **2020**, *26*, 1043–1049. [CrossRef] [PubMed]
16. Cadogan, C.A.; Hughes, C.M. On the Frontline against COVID-19: Community Pharmacists' Contribution during a Public Health Crisis. *Res. Soc. Adm. Pharm.* **2021**, *17*, 2032–2035. [CrossRef] [PubMed]
17. Mallhi, T.H.; Liaqat, A.; Abid, A.; Khan, Y.H.; Alotaibi, N.H.; Alzarea, A.I.; Tanveer, N.; Khan, T.M. Multilevel Engagements of Pharmacists during the COVID-19 Pandemic: The Way Forward. *Front. Public Health* **2020**, *8*, 561924. [CrossRef]
18. WHO. A Guide to Developing Knowledge, Attitude and Practice Surveys. Available online: https://apps.who.int/iris/bitstream/handle/10665/43790/9789241596176_eng.pdf?sequence=1 (accessed on 23 June 2022).
19. Salman, M.; Mustafa, Z.; Asif, N.; Zaidi, H.A.; Shehzadi, N.; Khan, T.M.; Saleem, Z.; Hussain, K. Knowledge, Attitude and Preventive Practices Related to COVID-19 among Health Professionals of Punjab Province of Pakistan. *J. Infect. Dev. Ctries.* **2020**, *14*, 707–712. [CrossRef]
20. Mohammed Basheeruddin Asdaq, S.; Alshrari, A.S.; Imran, M.; Sreeharsha, N.; Sultana, R. Knowledge, attitude and practices of healthcare professionals of Riyadh, Saudi Arabia towards covid-19: A cross-sectional study. *Saudi J. Biol. Sci.* **2021**, *28*, 5275–5282. [CrossRef]
21. Yi, Z.M.; Song, Z.W.; Li, X.Y.; Hu, Y.; Cheng, Y.C.; Wang, G.R.; Zhao, R.S. The Implementation of a FIP Guidance for COVID-19: Insights from a Nationwide Survey. *Ann. Transl. Med.* **2021**, *9*, 1479. [CrossRef]
22. Tsiga-Ahmed, F.I.; Amole, T.G.; Musa, B.M.; Nalado, A.M.; Agoyi, O.B.; Galadanci, H.S.; Salihu, H.M. COVID 19: Evaluating the Knowledge, Attitude and Preventive Practices of Healthcare Workers in Northern Nigeria. *Int. J. Matern. Child Health AIDS* **2021**, *10*, 88–97. [CrossRef]
23. Kambayashi, D.; Manabe, T.; Kawade, Y.; Hirohara, M. Knowledge, Attitudes, and Practices regarding COVID-19 among Pharmacists Partnering with Community Residents: A National Survey in Japan. *PLoS ONE* **2021**, *16*, e0258805. [CrossRef]
24. Hussain, I.; Majeed, A.; Saeed, H.; Hashmi, F.K.; Imran, I.; Akbar, M.; Chaudhry, M.O.; Rasool, M.F. A National Study to Assess Pharmacists' Preparedness against COVID-19 during Its Rapid Rise Period in Pakistan. *PLoS ONE* **2020**, *15*, e0241467. [CrossRef]
25. Tesfaye, Z.T.; Yismaw, M.B.; Negash, Z.; Ayele, A.G. COVID-19-related Knowledge, Attitude and Practice among Hospital and Community Pharmacists in Addis Ababa, Ethiopia. *Integr. Pharm. Res. Pract.* **2020**, *9*, 105–112. [CrossRef] [PubMed]
26. Karasneh, R.; Al-Azzam, S.; Muflih, S.; Soudah, O.; Hawamdeh, S.; Khader, Y. Media's Effect on Shaping Knowledge, Awareness Risk Perceptions and Communication Practices of Pandemic COVID-19 among Pharmacists. *Res. Soc. Adm. Pharm.* **2021**, *17*, 1897–1902. [CrossRef] [PubMed]
27. Kaliyaperumal, K. Guideline for Conducting a Knowledge, Attitude and Practice (KAP) Study. *AECS Illum.* **2004**, *4*, 7–9. [CrossRef]
28. Olum, R.; Chekwech, G.; Wekha, G.; Nassozi, D.R.; Bongomin, F. Coronavirus Disease-2019: Knowledge, Attitude, and Practices of Health Care Workers at Makerere University Teaching Hospitals, Uganda. *Front. Public Health* **2020**, *8*, 181. [CrossRef]
29. Le An, P.; Huynh, G.; Nguyen, H.T.N.; Pham, B.D.U.; Nguyen, T.V.; Tran, T.T.T.; Tran, T.D. Knowledge, Attitude, and Practice towards COVID-19 among Healthcare Students in Vietnam. *Infect. Drug Resist.* **2021**, *14*, 3405–3413. [CrossRef]
30. Desalegn, Z.; Deyessa, N.; Teka, B.; Shiferaw, W.; Hailemariam, D.; Addissie, A.; Abagero, A.; Kaba, M.; Abebe, W.; Nega, B.; et al. COVID-19 and the Public Response: Knowledge, Attitude and Practice of the Public in Mitigating the Pandemic in Addis Ababa, Ethiopia. *PLoS ONE* **2021**, *16*, e0244780. [CrossRef]
31. Yousaf, M.A.; Noreen, M.; Saleem, T.; Yousaf, I. A Cross-Sectional Survey of Knowledge, Attitude, and Practices (KAP) Toward Pandemic COVID-19 among the General Population of Jammu and Kashmir, India. *Soc. Work Public Health* **2020**, *35*, 569–578. [CrossRef]

32. Malik, U.R.; Atif, N.; Hashmi, F.K.; Saleem, F.; Saeed, H.; Islam, M.; Jiang, M.; Zhao, M.; Yang, C.; Fang, Y. Knowledge, Attitude, and Practices of Healthcare Professionals on COVID-19 and Risk Assessment to Prevent the Epidemic Spread: A Multicenter Cross-Sectional Study from Punjab, Pakistan. *Int. J. Environ. Res. Public Health* **2020**, *17*, 6395. [CrossRef]
33. Mahanta, P.; Deka, H.; Sarma, B.; Konwar, R.; Thakuria, K.D.; Kalita, D.; Singh, S.G.; Eshori, L. Knowledge, Attitude, Practice and Preparedness toward COVID-19 Pandemic among Healthcare Workers in Designated COVID Hospitals of a North-Eastern State of India. *Hosp. Top.* **2021**, 1–10. [CrossRef]
34. Limbu, D.K.; Piryani, R.M.; Sunny, A.K. Healthcare Workers' Knowledge, Attitude and Practices during the COVID-19 Pandemic Response in a Tertiary Care Hospital of Nepal. *PLoS ONE* **2020**, *15*, e0242126. [CrossRef]
35. Qutob, N.; Awartani, F. Knowledge, Attitudes and Practices (KAP) towards COVID-19 among Palestinians during the COVID-19 Outbreak: A Cross-Sectional Survey. *PLoS ONE* **2021**, *16*, e0244925. [CrossRef]
36. Zhong, B.L.; Luo, W.; Li, H.M.; Zhang, Q.Q.; Liu, X.G.; Li, W.T.; Li, Y. Knowledge, Attitudes, and Practices towards COVID-19 among Chinese Residents during the Rapid Rise Period of the COVID-19 Outbreak: A Quick Online Cross-Sectional Survey. *Int. J. Biol. Sci.* **2020**, *16*, 1745–1752. [CrossRef] [PubMed]
37. Morin, C.M.; Bjorvatn, B.; Chung, F.; Holzinger, B.; Partinen, M.; Penzel, T.; Ivers, H.; Wing, Y.K.; Chan, N.Y.; Merikanto, I.; et al. Insomnia, Anxiety, and Depression during the COVID-19 Pandemic: An International Collaborative Study. *Sleep Med.* **2021**, *87*, 38–45. [CrossRef] [PubMed]
38. Albahri, A.H.; Alnaqbi, S.A.; Alnaqbi, S.A.; Alshaali, A.O.; Shahdoor, S.M. Knowledge, Attitude, and Practice Regarding COVID-19 Among Healthcare Workers in Primary Healthcare Centers in Dubai: A Cross-Sectional Survey. *Front. Public Health* **2021**, *9*, 617679. [CrossRef] [PubMed]
39. Rivera-Lozada, O.; Galvez, C.A.; Castro-Alzate, E.; Bonilla-Asalde, C.A. Factors Associated with Knowledge, Attitudes and Preventive Practices towards COVID-19 in Health Care Professionals in Lima, Peru. *F1000Research* **2021**, *10*, 582. [CrossRef]
40. Noreen, K.; Rubab, Z.E.; Umar, M.; Rehman, R.; Baig, M.; Baig, F. Knowledge, Attitudes, and Practices against the Growing Threat of COVID-19 among Medical Students of Pakistan. *PLoS ONE* **2020**, *15*, e0243696. [CrossRef]
41. Hesaraki, M.; Akbarizadeh, M.; Ahmadidarrehsima, S.; Moghadam, M.P.; Izadpanah, F. Knowledge, Attitude, Practice and Clinical Recommendations of Health Care Workers towards COVID-19: A Systematic Review. *Rev. Environ. Health* **2021**, *36*, 345–357. [CrossRef]

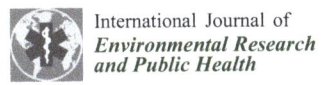

Article

Impact of COVID-19 on Urban Mobility and Parking Demand Distribution: A Global Review with Case Study in Melbourne, Australia

Biruk G. Mesfin [1], Daniel(Jian) Sun [2] and Bo Peng [3,*]

[1] State Key Laboratory of Ocean Engineering, School of Naval Architecture, Ocean and Civil Engineering, Shanghai Jiao Tong University, No. 800 Dongchuan Road, Min-Hang District, Shanghai 200240, China; birukgmesfin@sjtu.edu.cn
[2] Smart City and Intelligent Transportation Interdisciplinary Center, College of Future Transportation, Chang'an University, Wei-Yang District, Xi'an 710021, China; jiansun@chd.edu.cn
[3] School of International and Public Affairs, Shanghai Jiao Tong University, No. 1954 Huashan Road, Xu-Hui District, Shanghai 200092, China
* Correspondence: bpeng@sjtu.edu.cn; Tel.: +86-21-6193-3047

Abstract: The tremendous impact of the novel coronavirus (COVID-19) on societal, political, and economic rhythms has given rise to a significant overall shift from pre- to post-pandemic policies. Restrictions, stay-at-home regulations, and lockdowns have directly influenced day-to-day urban transportation flow. The rise of door-to-door services and the demand for visiting medical facilities, grocery stores, and restaurants has had a significant impact on urban transportation modal demand, further impacting zonal parking demand distribution. This study reviews the overall impacts of the pandemic on urban transportation with respect to a variety of policy changes in different cities. The parking demand shift was investigated by exploring the during- and post-COVID-19 parking policies of distinct metropolises. The detailed data related to Melbourne city parking, generated by the Internet of things (IoT), such as sensors and devices, are examined. Empirical data from 2019 (16 March to 26 May) and 2020 (16 March to 26 May) are explored in-depth using explanatory data analysis to demonstrate the demand and average parking duration shifts from district to district. The results show that the experimental zones of Docklands, Queensbery, Southbanks, Titles, and Princess Theatre areas have experienced a decrease in percentage change of vehicle presence of 29.2%, 36.3%, 37.7%, 23.7% and 40.9%, respectively. Furthermore, on-street level analysis of Princess Theatre zone, Lonsdale Street, Exhibition Street, Spring Street, and Little Bourke Street parking bays indicated a decrease in percentage change of vehicle presence of 38.7%, 56.4%, 12.6%, and 35.1%, respectively. In conclusion, future potential policymaking frameworks are discussed that could provide further guidance in stipulating epidemic prevention and control policies, particularly in relation to parking regulations during the pandemic.

Keywords: COVID-19; urban mobility; parking demand; IoT parking sensors; explanatory data analysis; parking policies

Citation: Mesfin, B.G.; Sun, D.; Peng, B. Impact of COVID-19 on Urban Mobility and Parking Demand Distribution: A Global Review with Case Study in Melbourne, Australia. *Int. J. Environ. Res. Public Health* **2022**, *19*, 7665. https://doi.org/10.3390/ijerph19137665

Academic Editors: Sachiko Kodera and Essam A. Rashed

Received: 29 April 2022
Accepted: 14 June 2022
Published: 23 June 2022

Publisher's Note: MDPI stays neutral with regard to jurisdictional claims in published maps and institutional affiliations.

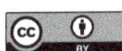

Copyright: © 2022 by the authors. Licensee MDPI, Basel, Switzerland. This article is an open access article distributed under the terms and conditions of the Creative Commons Attribution (CC BY) license (https://creativecommons.org/licenses/by/4.0/).

1. Introduction

Since the primary case of COVID-19 was recorded in Wuhan, China, on 9 December 2019, there has been an alarming and rapid spread of the virus to every corner of the globe, highly catalyzed by the international passenger and cargo air transport network serving major cities in East Asia, the United States, and elsewhere [1]. Owing to the emergency, daily routines in cities throughout the world were chaotic during the first six months of 2020. The normal lives of people in many countries ceased as the pandemic crisis worsened. The human toll has been extensive due to the exponentially increasing number of cases and deaths around the world. Social distancing, stay-at-home regulations, and various other social restrictions have brought about a tremendous shift from the previously defined standards of human social interaction, such as greetings and hugging [2]. On the economic front, the endemic, epidemic, and then the pandemic has caused many businesses to delay or cease operations. Importing and exporting in most countries throughout the world have been highly disrupted due to the pandemic's impact on the aviation industry [3–5], maritime industry [6], regional railway systems [7] and urban mobility [8]. In the manufacturing industry, sectors have been advised by the World Health Organization (WHO) to concentrate on producing medical supplies for fighting the pandemic, which has resulted in both collaborations and disputes regarding global transactions that involve medical supplies such as masks, gloves, and ventilators [9]. In regard to global politics, the pandemic's impact has been dependent on nations' health security strategy and emergency response capacity. The political impact has expanded due to significant global political decisions regarding emergency flight cancellations throughout the world. The status quo has impacted the aviation industry greatly, with 90% of passenger flights being cancelled [5]. In China, a number of airlines discontinued flights to and from the epicenter of the virus (Wuhan) and then across the entire country to avoid an escalation of the situation from epidemic to pandemic status. Moreover, following a loss of revenue, airlines throughout the world reacted to these changes by shifting from passenger to cargo flights, such as Ethiopian Airlines [10] and United Airlines [11].

As the pandemic impacted socioeconomic status, the political focus moved from the global to urban scale, with urban mobility being one of the most highly affected sectors. Modal travel shifts occurred, mainly on account of social distancing and contact-free policies. Urban mass transportation, such as car-sharing, ride-sharing, and ride-hailing, has been the most severely affected service types. Ride-sharing and taxi-hailing services, as well as urban electric commercial vehicles have been on the rise in recent years owing to AI-driven smart applications, and management and is favored due to a variety of factors, including minimized travel costs, traffic congestion, emissions and energy issues [12–14]. However, in the aftermath of the pandemic; for example, the ride-sharing market is predicted to have lost a quota share of 50% to 60% during 2020 [15], but this is anticipated to rise by 70% to 80% with new countermeasures, such as barriers between drivers and passengers to adhere to social distancing restrictions.

Acute social restrictions in several highly impacted cities with stay-at-home restrictions have resulted in the emergence of more door-to-door delivery services to satisfy the basic living requirements of those who cannot leave home. Moreover, panic buying and the fear of contamination during the crisis have encouraged many consumers to download smart applications from service providers such as grocery stores and restaurants. This app-based evolution has resulted in many grocery stores recording their highest ever daily revenues at the end of March 2020, with consumer spending up by 87.4% [16]. The nature of droplet transmission means that the most effective virus prevention is contact avoidance, which has led to mass-gathering restrictions for theaters, bars, sports clubs, and schools, while trips to pharmacies, grocery stores, and restaurants have increased. The shift of travel destination followed by parking demand shift forced the reshaping of parking facilities in order to satisfy the demand. Parking garages have been used as major emergency preparedness spaces and temporary medical centers. When considering vacant garages to micro-mobility maintenance disruptions and lay-offs, reacting to the demands of the public and ensuring the safety of core workers have been essential. To this end, different parking policies have been introduced, from the lessening of parking restrictions and penalties to fee adjustments.

The parking service providers highly affected by the pandemic include metropolises, academic institutions, and air terminals. Parking-related income is noteworthy for small cities, contributing to more than 30% of the yearly budget income, and there has been an estimated 90% income loss in this sector [17]. The question arises as to how countries will quantify and counter such socioeconomic and political disturbance. To investigate the impact of the pandemic on different sectors, a number of data-driven studies have been carried out globally. One of such interest is the MOBIS-COVID19 study [18], a joint project of ETH Zurich and the University of Basel, using mobile phone GPS tracking data from 3700 participants to examine the impact of COVID-19 in Switzerland. Conversely, on designing countermeasure frameworks, recent studies and approaches, such as avoid–shift–improve [ASI] [19] and the PASS approach [20], in which "P", "A", "S", and "S" correspond to different stages of the pandemic comprising categorical targets of transportation users and service providers, as well as governments, have been utilized.

This study assesses the impact of COVID-19 via the visualized Melbourne dataset, released by the city data administration to promote understanding on the impact of COVID-19 on city mobility. The visualizing and comparing of on-street car parking sensor data for the two preferred periods, between 16 March and 26 May 2019 and 16 March and 26 May 2020 are carried out to quantify the impact of COVID-19 on different business districts and socioeconomic classes for better assessing the impact of COVID-19. The remaining part of the paper is structured as follows: Section 2 reviews the impact range of COVID-19 and analyzes the impact on urban mobility; Section 3 focuses on analyzing the impact of the pandemic on parking demand and revenue; Section 4 visualizes the parking demand variation during the pandemic via the case study approach, using Melbourne CBD parking data; Section 5 provides conclusions and future research recommendations.

2. Impact of COVID-19 on Urban Mobility

From world-wide expert survey results, Zhang et al. [21] presented significant impacts of COVID-19 on transport and logistics. Following the disturbance, many cities have enforced dynamic policy approaches to minimize the negative impact of the pandemic on the general public. The major approaches to reduce the risk of the pandemic include providing contactless mobility modes and creating open spaces, such as pedestrian space, cycle ways, and open street developments. A few summarized examples are provided in Table 1 to illustrate cities impacted by the pandemic and forced to shift mobility policy measures and responses.

Table 1. Summary for mobility policy measures and responses.

City, Country	Measures and Responses
Paris, France [22]	The COVID-19 pandemic accelerated/prioritized the implementation of Paris Mayor Anne Hidalgo's 2024 vision for 650 km of cycle.
Milan, Italy [23]	35 km of streets were repurposed and made open for active modes of transportation, and a 30 km/h speed limit was introduced.
Bogota, Colombia [24]	The Colombian capital has opened 76 km of temporary bicycle lanes, and 22 km of the new lanes were opened on 17 March 2020 by repurposing vehicle lanes.
Budapest, Hungary [25]	Bike lanes were added at the edges of multi-lane streets.
Brussels, Belgium [26]	The government has created 40 km of new cycle paths and turned the city center into a 20 km long walkable area.
Auckland, New Zealand [27]	The first authorities to fund pop-up bike lanes, widened sidewalks and related infrastructures during lockdown.
Helsinki and Espoo, Finland [28]	The COVID-19 outbreak forced the city to open the bike season earlier than the previous year with a total of 351 bike stations (242 in Helsinki and 109 in Espoo).

3. Impact of COVID-19 on Parking Demand and Revenue

The parking system is a direct replica of the urban mobility disturbance by COVID-19. For instance, the parking demand to access essential destination's parks increased during the pandemic [29], while on the other side, parking demand to public gathering places such as stadiums, theaters, malls, etc., dropped. Since the flare-up of COVID-19, the USD 131B parking industry has had difficulty, mostly in hotels and aviation vicinities, encountering a drop of 50–70% commuter parking movement and more than 95% accommodation revenue losses daily [30]. In addition, a reduction in income occurred from parking authorization with fewer parkers and from communities halting or unwinding authorization [31]. A small known reality is that municipalities' budgets intensely depend on parking-related incomes. Some detailed illustrations are presented in Table 2, for indicating the dependence of cities on parking revenue [17].

Table 2. Municipalities budget from parking-related revenues (in United States Dollars, 2019–2020 fiscal year).

Cities	Total Parking Related Revenue	Parking Tax	Fees, Fines, and Citations
San Francisco	USD 439.7M	USD 85.5M	USD 354.2M
New York	USD 1.1B+	USD 300M	USD 785M
Chicago	USD 299.7M	USD 134M	USD 25.1M

3.1. COVID-19 Impact on On-Street Parking

To demonstrate the extent of the on-street parking affected by the pandemic, two studies are reviewed in this section: the smart parking system developers Smarking [17], which was carried out by a random sampling of 511 zones over the US (averaging 136 parking spaces), and IEM [32], which was studied on 650 installed PrestoSense parking sensors in different parts of Geneva, Switzerland.

The Smarking [17] survey showed a decrease in parking on the street at 80–90% since the US national emergency statement issued on Friday, 13 March 2020. Before and after the COVID-19 outbreak, the annual dynamics of parking activities have changed a lot: a year-over-year increase in 10%, to 80–90% decrease, compared to the same period last year (See Figure 1). Similarly, the peak daily occupancy of on-street parking spaces surveyed across the country shows that the pattern before and after Friday, 13 March has changed significantly.

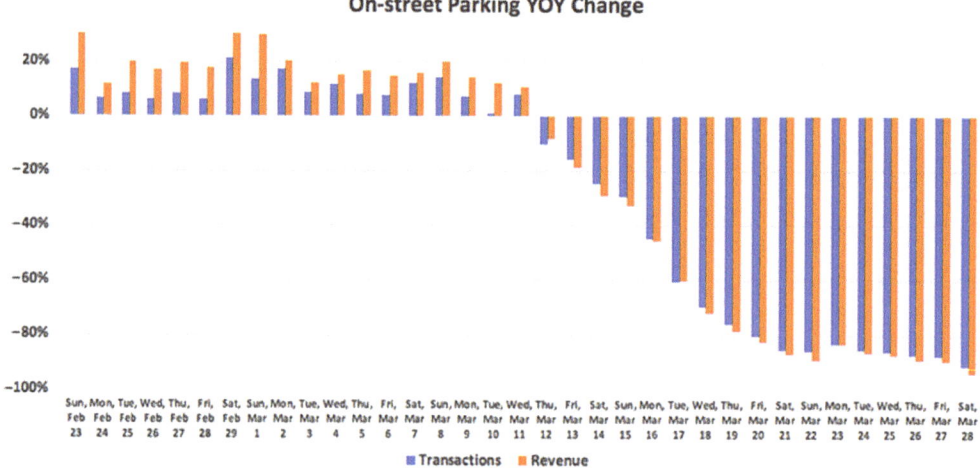

Figure 1. On-street parking year-over-year (YOY) change (from a random sample of 511 zones/blocks across the US).

Conversely, IEM [32] studied data from 650 PrestoSense parking monitoring sensors installed in different regions of Geneva, Switzerland, to illustrate how the parking patterns on the streets have changed in areas where semi-confinement was announced. This study focused on parking demand (in terms of occupancy and turnover) fluctuation before and after the emergency declaration date of 16 March 2020. The state of emergency was declared between 16 March and 11 May 2020, in which the semi-confinement period spanned from 16 March to April, and the progressive de-confinement period spanned from April to 11 May 2020.

During the semi-confinement period, parking restrictions such as vehicle parking control were suspended in Geneva. To analyze the policy shift impact, the PrestoSense vehicle detection sensors were installed in on-street parking bays of residential areas, offices and cultural areas to detect vehicle occupancy and the parking duration of a parked vehicle.

The on-street parking demand comparison assessment was performed between residential areas versus offices and cultural areas. In residential complexes, before the semi-confinement period, the parking usage in residential areas showed an average occupancy level of 82% (see Figure 2a) with an average car turnover rate of 7.2 per day; here, the turnover rate is defined as the average number of vehicles using the same parking space at a certain time gap. In the same area during the semi-confinement period, an increase in the occupancy level to 93.4% (see Figure 2b) and a decrease in car turnover rates to 3.2 cars per day was clearly observed.

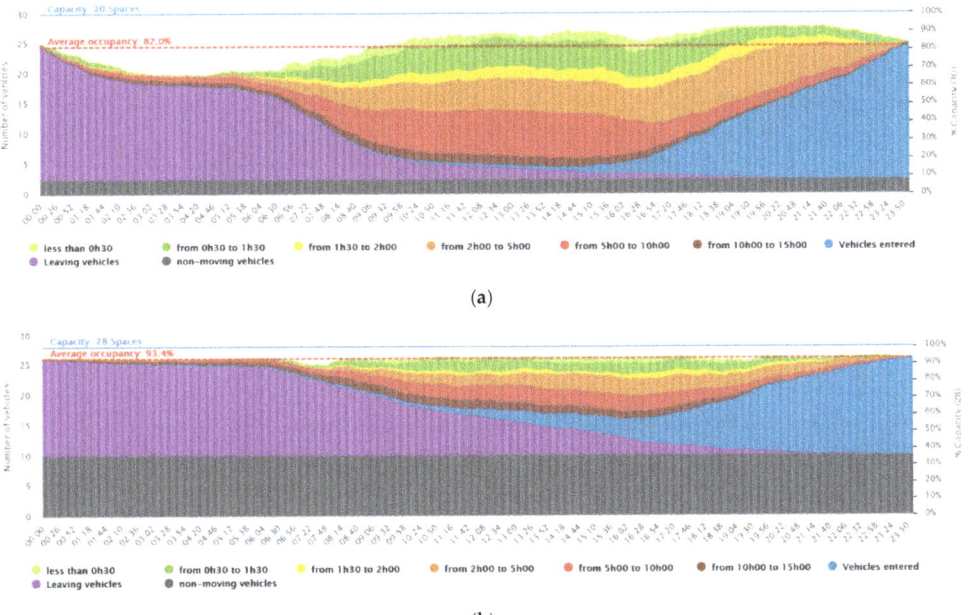

Figure 2. Average occupancy of the selected residential area (Rue des Pâquis, Geneve): (**a**) before the confinement period (between 5 January and 5 February 2020), and (**b**) during the confinement period (between 1 and 30 April 2020).

Meanwhile, in office and cultural sites, before the semi-confinement period, an average occupancy level of 39.3% (see Figure 3a), and car turnover rate of 5.7 cars per parking space per day was observed, whereas in the same area during the semi-confinement period, a substantial drop in occupancy levels to 26.6% (see Figure 3b) and a decrease in car turnover rates to 1.7 per parking space per day was marked.

3.2. COVID-19 Impacts on Off-Street Parking

A study [17] under this topic was reviewed to show the impact of COVID-19 on off-street parking garages. During the investigation, a collection of 935 off-street parking locales, consisting of both private and city-owned parking garages was studied. The results show a comparative drift from on-street parking prior to the COVID-19 emergency: 10% YOY increment (see Figure 4). Then, after 13 March 2020, the parking demand dropped dramatically by about 90%.

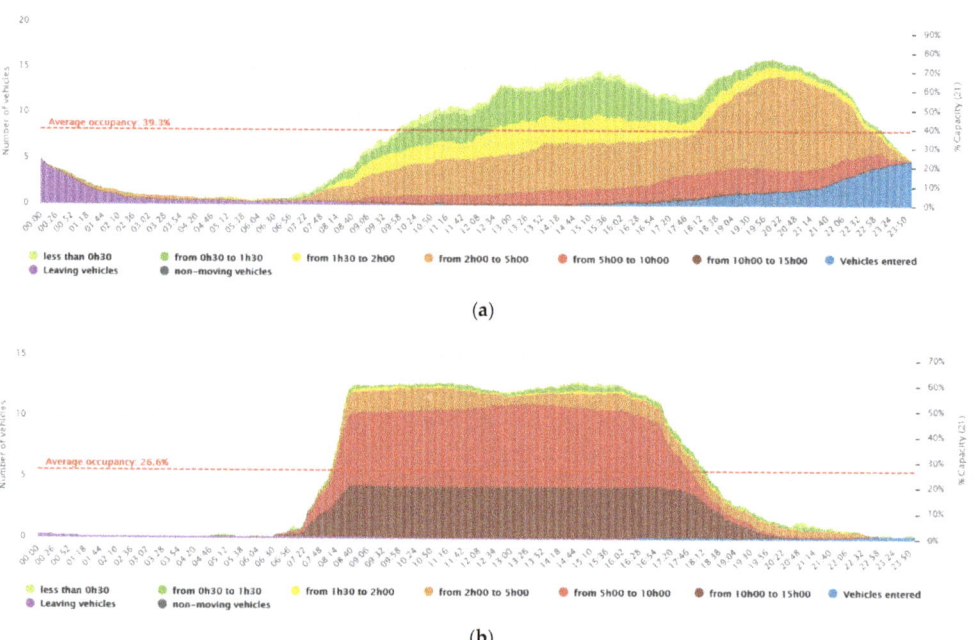

Figure 3. Average occupancy of the selected Office and Cultural site (Bd. Du théâtre, Geneve): (**a**) before the confinement period (between 5 January and 5 February 2020), and (**b**) during the confinement period (between 1 and 30 April 2020).

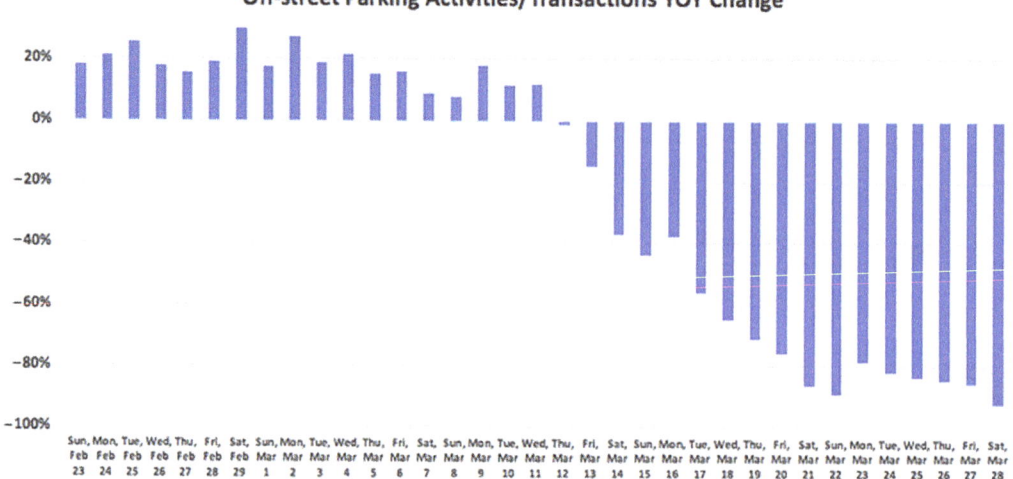

Figure 4. Off-street parking activities YOY change (from a random sample of 511 zones/blocks across the USA).

4. Case Study: Melbourne City, Australia

To investigate the impact of COVID-19 on parking demand distribution on different types of urban areas and streets, this study used the parking data from Melbourne CBD parking bays, Australia, visualized to illustrate how the parking demand on different central districts was shifted by the pandemic. The in-ground parking sensors recorded vehicle arrival and departure times (from 1 January to 1 May 2020), which were released upon customer request to grasp the strike of COVID-19 on city movement. On-street car parking sensor data for 2019 [33] and from January–May, 2020 [34] were obtained to visualize the impact variation of COVID-19 on parked vehicle volume and average parking duration. Visualizing these parking sensors data will help to illustrate how the parking demand in terms of parking volume and average parking duration on different central districts is shifted by the pandemic during the state of emergency. The state of emergency was declared by the Minister for Health on 16 March 2020, under section 198 (1) of the Public Health and Wellbeing Act 2008 (Act) throughout the state of Victoria due to the serious threat to public health in Victoria due to the novel coronavirus 2019 [35].

On this case study, Melbourne city areas and streets were selected and analyzed to assess how the city areas and streets are impacted negatively with respect to parking demand after the first stage of the state of emergency dated from 16 March 2020. The assessment area selection criteria included the high shift in parking volume after the state of emergency versus the rest of the areas listed on the dataset, and the authors think the picked areas for analysis, named as Docklands, Queensbery, South banks, Titles, and Princess Theatre will illustrate the image for the high impact of COVID-19 on parking demand distribution. Further, at street-level impact analysis, streets of Princess Theatre were evaluated with respect to parking volume and parking duration indicators. The streets of Princess Theatre were chosen for analysis since this area shows a higher shift in parking demand out of the five selected areas.

The impact assessment and comparison were conducted between two periods, 16 March–26 May 2020 versus 16 March–26 May 2019. The parking demand indicators are parking volume, in terms of vehicles present, and average parking duration. The sensors read whether there is a parked vehicle or not, in which the data are given by (false, true) or (0, 1). The sum of the values "true" or "1" gives the total number of vehicles present or parked at a certain location during a certain period. The average parking duration was obtained by dividing the parking load (vehicle-minutes) by the total number of vehicles present during the entire duration of the assessment (Equation (1)). It can also be calculated as the sum of parking duration of all vehicles divided by the total number of vehicles parked during the survey period.

$$\text{Average Parking duration (minutes)} = \frac{\text{Parking load (veh. minutes)}}{\text{Parking volume (veh.)}} \quad (1)$$

The authors believe that the study area (Figure 5) is planned to present the interior CBD of Melbourne. The black dots in Figure 5b show the on-street parking bays in the selected experimental areas of Melbourne streets [36].

4.1. Areal Based IMPACT Analysis

Parking volume comparison: After the state of emergency, the vehicles present in on-street parking bays showed a significant decrease. For almost two months from 16 March to 26 May 2020, Docklands, Queensbery, Southbanks, Titles, and Princess Theatre areas showed a decrease in percentage change of vehicles present of 29.2%, 36.3%, 37.7%, 23.7%, and 40.9%, respectively, compared to the same period of the previous year from 16 March to 26 May 2019. Princess Theatre appeared to have the highest fall in parking volume percentage change from the picked experimental areas. As presented in Table 3 and Figure 6, the on-street parking spot demand decreased relatively within these periods, mainly due to the state of emergency restrictions, including the advice to stay home.

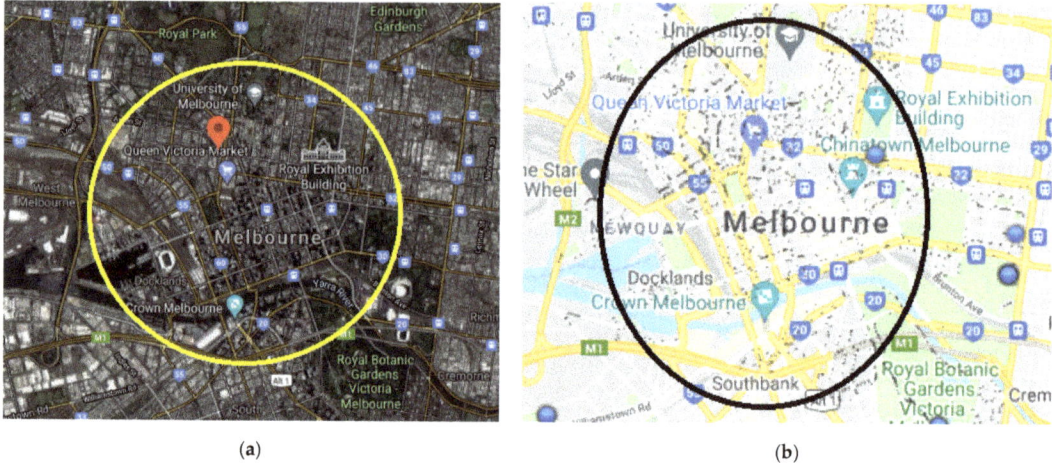

(a) (b)

Figure 5. Study area: (**a**) Melbourne CBD, VIC, Australia; (**b**) on-street parking bays.

Table 3. Area level comparisons of parking volume in terms of number of vehicles present between two periods (16 March to 26 May 2019 versus 16 March to 26 May 2020).

Area	Number of Vehicles Present		Percentage Change
	16 March–26 May 2019	16 March–26 May 2020	
Docklands	482,426	341,538	−29.2%
Queensbery	330,106	210,257	−36.3%
Southbanks	243,897	151,845	−37.7%
Titles	184,969	141,161	−23.7%
Princess Theatre	178,102	105,273	−40.9%

Average parking duration comparison: After the state of emergency from 16 March to 26 May 2020, the average parking duration of on-street parking bays showed a significant increase. As shown in Table 4 and Figure 7, Docklands, Queensbery, Southbanks, Titles, and Princess Theatre areas showed an increase in percentage change of average parking duration of 45.3%, 17.9%, 64.5%, 38.2% and 89.3%, respectively, compared to the same period of the previous year from 16 March to 26 May 2019. Princess Theatre appeared to have the highest increase in average parking duration percentage change from the picked experimental areas. Referring to Tables 3 and 4, Princess Theatre is the area that experienced the highest drop in vehicles present, with −40.9%, and the highest increase in percentage change of average parking duration, with +89.3%. This is mainly due to the socio-economic nature of the Princess Theatre area, which is famous for being an entertainment and gathering site [37]. The reason for the high shift in parking demand of this kind of areas was the state of emergency and restriction on gathering activities. Technically, the average parking duration (in min.) is defined as the ratio of total vehicle hours to the number of vehicles parked, i.e., parking load in Veh. min over parking presence (in Veh.). Therefore, mathematically, as a vehicle parking presence decreases with a wider gap than the parking load, the average parking duration may increase in a significant range.

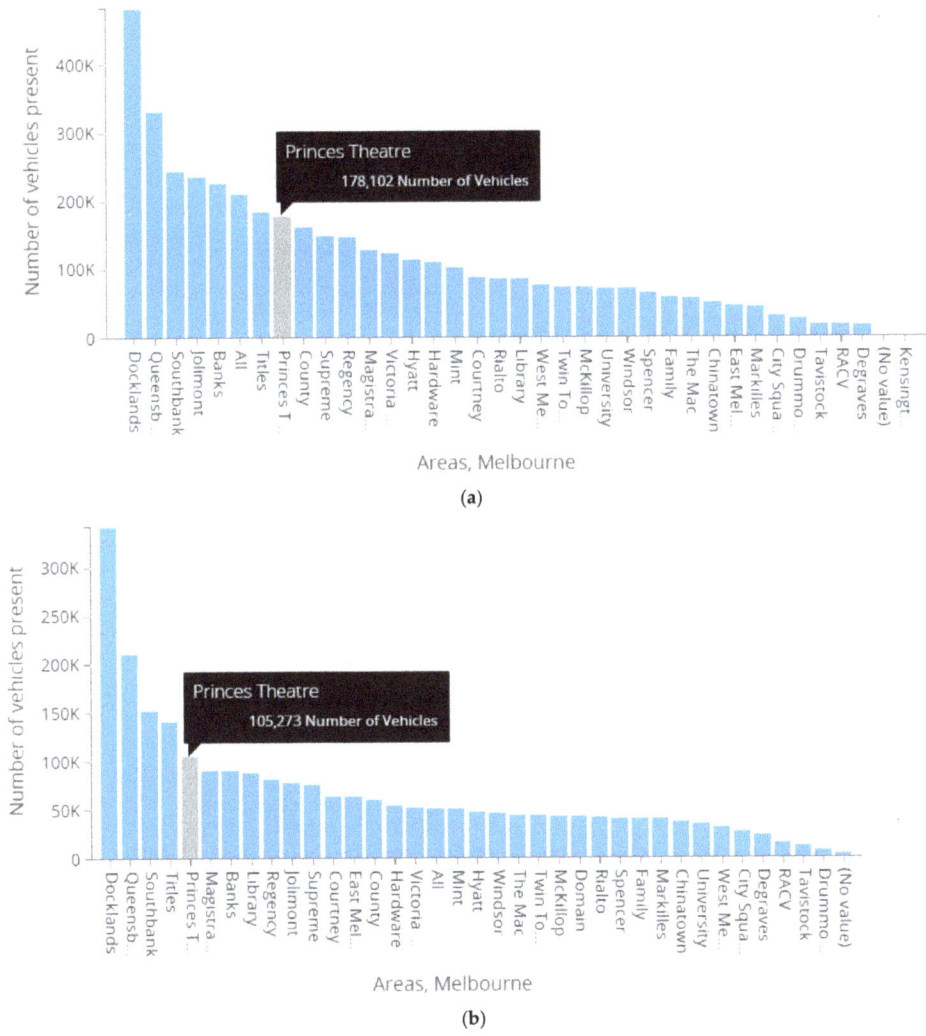

Figure 6. Bar graph representation of Princess Theatre's area parking volume in terms of vehicles present between two periods: (**a**) 16 March to 26 May 2019 versus (**b**) 16 March to 26 May 2020.

Table 4. Area level comparisons of the average parking duration change in minutes between periods (16 March to 26 May 2019 versus 16 March to 26 May 2020).

Area	Average Parking Duration (min)		Percentage Change
	16 March–26 May 2019	16 March–26 May 2020	
Docklands	48.65	70.71	45.3%
Queensbery	90.15	106.29	17.9%
Southbanks	76.51	125.88	64.5%
Titles	39.51	54.61	38.2%
Princess Theatre	36.18	68.5	89.3%

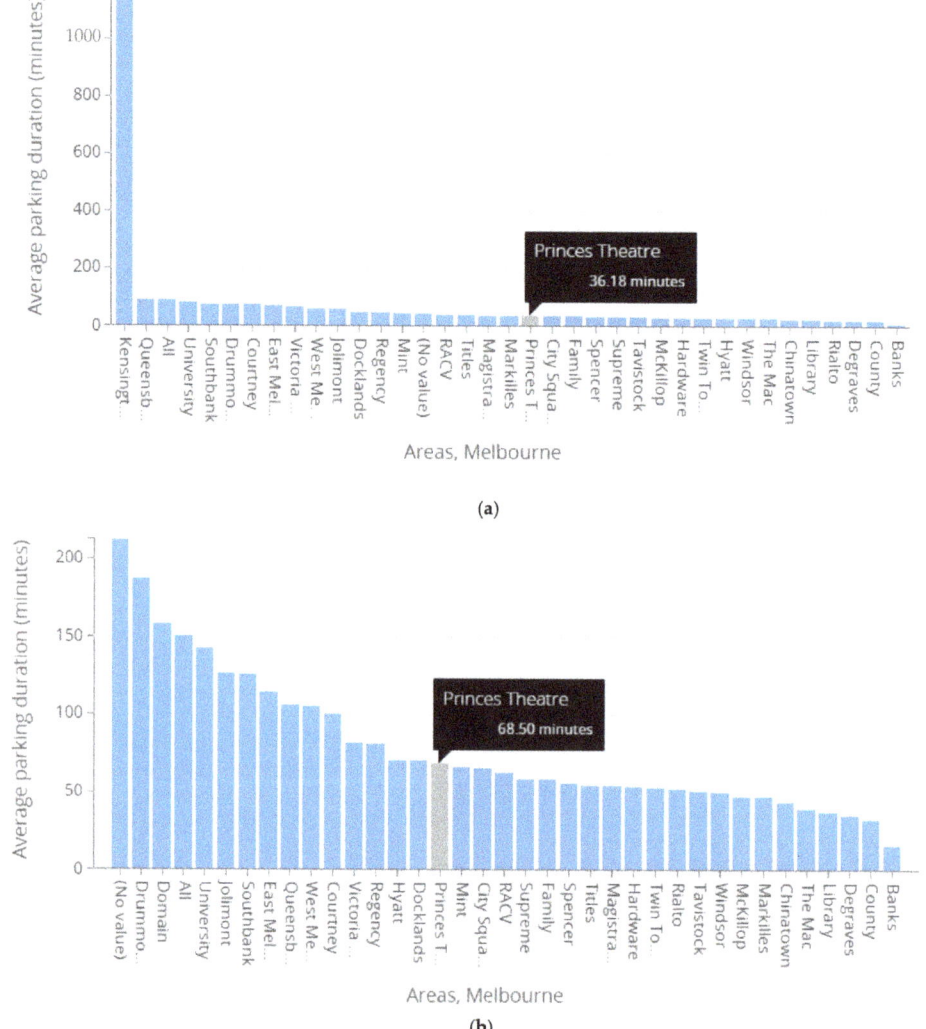

Figure 7. Bar graph representation, referring to the Princess Theatre area average parking duration between two periods: (**a**) 16 March to 26 May 2019 versus (**b**) 16 March to 26 May 2020.

4.2. Street Level Impact Analysis

For this part of the impact assessment, the streets circling Princess Theatre area (Lonsdale Street, Exhibition Street, Spring Street, and Little Bourke Street) were selected for parking demand visualization.

Parking volume comparison: After the state of emergency, the vehicles present in on-street parking bays showed a significant decrease. For almost two months from 16 March to 26 May 2020, Lonsdale Street, Exhibition Street, Spring Street, and Little Bourke Street parking bays showed a decrease in percentage change of vehicles present of 38.7%, 56.4%, 12.6%, and 35.1%, respectively, compared to the same period of the previous year from 16 March to 26 May 2019.

Exhibition Street appeared to have the highest fall in parking volume percentage change from the streets around Princess Theatre. As presented in Table 5, Exhibition Street, with a 56.4% drop in parking volume, lost the proportion of vehicles present within the area, from 27% to 20%. This is mainly because Exhibition Street is famous for being home to many heritage buildings, such as the Victorian Heritage Register [38], which are classified as one of Melbourne's visiting sites, and which was highly impacted by the COVID-19 state of emergency measures.

Table 5. Street level comparisons of the parking volume in terms of the change in number of vehicles present between two periods (16 March to 26 May 2019 versus 16 March to 26 May 2020).

Princess Theatre Streets	Number of Vehicles Present		Percentage Change
	16 March–26 May 2019	16 March–26 May 2020	
Lonsdale street	112,863	69,166	−38.7%
Exhibition street	47,299	20,630	−56.4%
Spring street	8040	9054	−12.6%
Little Bourke street	9900	6423	−3.51%

Average parking duration comparison: After the state of emergency from 16 March to 26 May 2020, the average parking duration of the selected streets' on-street parking bays showed a significant increase. As shown in Table 6, Lonsdale, Exhibition, Spring, and Little Bourke streets showed an increase in percentage change of average parking duration of 84%, 103.6%, 153.4%, and 58.3%, respectively, compared to the same period of the previous year from 16 March to 26 May 2019.

Table 6. Street level comparisons of the average parking duration change, in minutes, between two periods (16 March to 26 May 2019 versus 16 March to 26 May 2020).

Princess Theatre Streets	Average Parking Duration (min)		Percentage Change
	16 March–26 May 2019	16 March–26 May 2020	
Lonsdale Street	35.42	65.18	84%
Exhibition Street	37.19	75.71	103.6%
Spring Street	29.17	73.93	153.4%
Little Bourke Street	45.45	71.96	58.3%

Spring Street appeared to have the highest increment in average parking duration percentage change from the streets around Princess Theatre, and Little Bourke Street with a 58.3% increment in average parking duration lost the proportion of average parking duration in the area, from 31% to 25%. This is mainly because Little Bourke Street is famous for its department stores and many boutiques [39], in which most of them were closed in relation to the COVID-19 state of emergency measures, having a direct impact on the interest of on-street parking from visitors.

5. Conclusions

As presented in the previous section, the parking volume and average parking duration were highly impacted due to the COVID-19 state of emergency in Melbourne city. Areal/zonal-based impact analysis, from 16 March to 26 May 2020, in Docklands, Queensbery, Southbanks, Titles, and Princess Theatre areas showed a decrease in percentage change of vehicles present of 29.2%, 36.3%, 37.7%, 23.7%, and 40.9%, respectively, compared to the same period of the previous year from 16 March to 26 May 2019. Then, considering the average parking duration as a parameter, Docklands, Queensbery, Southbanks, Titles, and Princess Theatre areas showed an increase in percentage change of average parking duration of 45.3%, 17.9%, 64.5%, 38.2%, and 89.3%, respectively, within same period.

Furthermore, the street-level impact analysis of the Princess Theatre area, Lonsdale Street, Exhibition Street, Spring Street, and Little Bourke Street parking bays showed a decrease in percentage change of vehicles present of 38.7%, 56.4%, 12.6%, and 35.1%, respectively. With the same parametrical comparisons as the zonal analysis, Lonsdale, Exhibition, Spring, and Little Bourke streets showed an increase in percentage change of average parking duration of 84%, 103.6%, 153.4%, and 58.3%, respectively. The variation in the impact of the pandemic might come from a different basis. The social, infrastructural, and institutional nature of the urban areas and streets might have been impacted by the pandemic regarding parking demand sensitivity.

Quantifying the impact throughout the urban area might be useful for implementing different types of parking policies and interventions and to further help maximizing the performance of COVID-19 urban mobility measures. The massive declines on intercity transportation brought the direct drop in parking demand. Cities are scrambling to recover not only the lost parking revenues, but also the significant reduction in fees and fines. As parking is one of the significant incomes of most municipalities, the decline in income has resulted in tremendous challenges to support their health care system.

Analyzing the mitigation measures and preparing for the coming "new normal" [40,41] may assist in understanding the opportunities behind the risks regarding parking industries. When dealing with policies and measures during the pandemic, it is critical to understand the interrelationship between jobs and food access, housing, public health, and mobility. The pandemic is an opportunity for private and public parking transit operators to advance mobility and parking needs and to strengthen economic resilience, particularly for the most vulnerable populations with equity and accessibility concepts.

The parking industry response implementation from COVID-19 might include three basic creative approaches of adaptiveness, pivoting needs, and replacing the lost revenue approach [30]. Parking lots have been adapted to be used as COVID-19 screening and as real-time tracking platforms that support the city's requirements with all the parking KPIs and the most up-to-date information accessible for the governmental task forces. The common topics on pivoting demands are that the industry should repurpose, be agile, and be adaptable during this time. A few ways for pivoting the needs in times of instability to preserve the quality of the parking and mobility programs can be framed as operational and financial sections. In operational prioritizing: moving all customer support to a virtual environment, transitioning enforcement staff to assist with healthcare operations, and renegotiating travel contracts to lower rates and move transport drivers to on-demand benefits. In financial prioritizing: plan and finance the year into smaller fiscal budgets rather than completing the full budget process (due to the flexible nature of the pandemic impact) and arrange to prioritize socio-economic zones based on needs targeting equity, accessibility, and vulnerability. In addition, a fast recovery plan to support the potential revenue loss has to be developed and implemented as early as possible. Financial models are required to understand the revenue impacts on the ground, with varying possibilities on the expected saturation curve and with further extension for the coming years. Understanding the pandemic projection, the estimated saturation line, and the nation's health institutions' capacity helps to design an acceptable and successful financial recovery plan.

Planners and specialists witness new opportunities to sustain their projects, which mainly push for smart working and reduce unnecessary labor intensity. The COVID-19 pandemic may require to examine the operations holistically and to be smarter about our future programs. Some potential positive outcomes are becoming more virtual and customer friendly, expanding and exploring new technologies, and aligning parking pricing models with the true cost of our parking and mobility programs. Following this, the COVID-19 impact on parking policy change in relation with the demand shift of commercial ridesharing vehicles can be modeled by discrete decision models, which introduce a behavioral framework regarding a commercial vehicle parking choice [42]. With additional considerations regarding the expected future COVID-19 factors, the model may be used for capturing pick and delivery vehicles regarding parking policy sensitivity.

Future CITY-20's studies of post-COVID-19 parking and urban space trends are divided into three categories: **Smart Parking and Curb Management, Artificial Intelligence** and **Data Driven Technology**, and **Autonomous Vehicles (AVs)**. Smart parking management and enforcement ethos can cure almost all parking problems during the emergency period of the pandemic. Real-time IoT parking solutions and management are expected to be used in future applications to optimize parking operation and management [43,44]. COVID-19 has also expedited the improvement in artificial intelligence in numerous diverse aspects representing a lessening of human contact or nearness, which furthermore may be regarded as a catalyst for the advancement of open source information and data. For instance, recent publications such as [45–47] have mined and structured big data to forecast and predict this and other illnesses. The rise of AVs may be placed in public transportation services, which may serve as an advanced arrangement to defend the transit workforce.

Author Contributions: Conceptualization, B.G.M. and D.S.; methodology, B.G.M.; formal analysis, B.G.M.; resources, D.S.; data curation, B.G.M.; writing—original draft preparation, B.G.M.; writing—review and editing, D.S.; visualization, B.G.M.; supervision, D.S. and B.P.; project administration, B.P.; funding acquisition, D.S. and B.P. All authors have read and agreed to the published version of the manuscript.

Funding: This research was funded in part by the National Nature Science Foundation of China (71971138, 52172319), the National Social Science Foundation of China (21AZD047) and the Social Science Foundation of Shanghai (2020BZZ001, 2021BGL012), and the APC was funded by (21AZD047). Any opinions, findings and conclusions or recommendations expressed in this paper are those of the authors and do not necessarily reflect the views of the sponsors.

Conflicts of Interest: The authors declare no conflict of interest. The funders had no role in the design of the study; in the collection, analyses, or interpretation of data; in the writing of the manuscript, or in the decision to publish the results.

Abbreviations

AI	artificial intelligence
APP	smart mobile/computer/Android/TV applications
AV	autonomous vehicles
CBD	Central Business District
COVID-19	Coronavirus disease 2019
EIT	European Institute of Innovation and Technology
IATA	International Air Transport Association
ICAO	International Civil Aviation Organization
IEM	Ingenierie Electronique et Monetique
IoT	Internet of Things
MOBIS	Mobility Behaviour In Switzerland
TUMI	Transformative Urban Mobility Initiative
WHO	World Health Organization
YOY	year-over-year

References

1. Zhang, Y.; Zhang, A.; Wang, J. Exploring the roles of high-speed train, air and coach services in the spread of COVID-19 in China. *Transp. Policy* **2020**, *94*, 34–42. [CrossRef] [PubMed]
2. Chinazzi, M.; Davis, J.T.; Ajelli, M.; Gioannini, C.; Merler, M.L.S.; Piontti, A.P.Y.; Mu, K.; Rossi, L.; Sun, K.; Viboud, C.; et al. The effect of travel restrictions on the spread of the 2019 novel coronavirus (COVID-19) outbreak. *Science* **2020**, *368*, 395–400. [CrossRef] [PubMed]
3. IATA. COVID-19 Impact on Asia-Pacific Aviation Worsens. 2020. Available online: https://www.iata.org/en/pressroom/pr/2020-0-24-01/ (accessed on 2 February 2021).
4. ICAO. Economic Impacts of COVID-19 on Civil Aviation. 2020. Available online: https://www.icao.int/sustainability/Pages/Economic-Impacts-of-COVID-19.aspx (accessed on 2 February 2021).
5. Mazareanu, E. Coronavirus: Impact on the Aviation Industry Worldwide—Statistics & Facts. Statista. 2020. Available online: https://www.statista.com/topics/6178/coronavirus-impact-on-the-aviation-industry-worldwide/ (accessed on 2 February 2021).
6. Teoh, P. The Impact of the COVID-19 Pandemic on Shipping. 2020. Available online: https://www.maritime-executive.com/editorials/the-impact-of-the-covid-19-pandemic-on-shipping (accessed on 2 February 2021).

7. Citroën, P. COVID-19 and Its Impact on the European Rail Supply Industry. 2020. Available online: https://www.globalrailwayreview.com/article/98741/covid19-european-rail-supply-industry/ (accessed on 2 February 2021).
8. EIT. COVID-19: What Is Happening in the Area of Urban Mobility. 2020. Available online: https://eit.europa.eu/news-events/news/covid-19-what-happening-area-urban-mobility (accessed on 2 February 2021).
9. WHO. Shortage of Personal Protective Equipment Endangering Health Workers Worldwide. 2020. Available online: https://www.who.int/news/item/03-03-2020-shortage-of-personal-protective-equipment-endangering-health-workers-worldwide (accessed on 2 February 2021).
10. Ahlgren, L. Ethiopian Airlines Adapting Passenger Aircraft for Cargo Use. 2020. Available online: https://theworldnews.net/et-news/ethiopian-airlines-adapting-passenger-aircraft-for-cargo-use (accessed on 2 February 2021).
11. Rivero, N. The Pandemic has Turned United Airlines into a Thriving Freight Company. Available online: https://qz.com/2062867/the-pandemic-turned-united-airlines-into-a-freight-company/ (accessed on 24 May 2022).
12. Sun, D.J.; Ding, X. Spatiotemporal evolution of ridesourcing markets under the new restriction policy: A case study in Shanghai. *Transp. Res. Part A Pract. Policy* **2019**, *130*, 227–239. [CrossRef]
13. Chen, F.; Yin, Z.; Ye, Y.; Sun, D.J. Taxi Hailing Choice Behavior and Economic Benefit Analysis of Emission Reduction Based on Multi-mode Travel Big Data. *Transp. Policy* **2020**, *97*, 73–84. [CrossRef]
14. Sun, D.J.; Zheng, Y.; Duan, R. Energy Consumption Simulation and Economic Benefit Analysis for Urban Electric Commercial-Vehicles. *Transp. Res. Part D Transp. Environ.* **2021**, *103083*, 1–16. [CrossRef]
15. MarketsandMarkets. COVID-19 Impact on Ride Sharing Market by Service Type, Data Service, and Region—Forecast to 2021. 2021. Available online: https://www.marketsandmarkets.com/Market-Reports/covid-19-impact-on-ride-sharing-market-15098676.html (accessed on 2 February 2021).
16. Dishman, L. The Delivery App Landscape Is Changing and Sustaining Businesses during COVID-19. 2020. Available online: https://www.uschamber.com/co/good-company/launch-pad/coronavirus-pandemic-food-delivery-businesses (accessed on 2 February 2021).
17. Smarking. Real Time Market Observation #2: COVID-19 Impact on US Municipal Parking. 2020. Available online: https://www.smarking.com/post/real-time-market-observation-2-covid-19-impact-on-us-municipal-parking (accessed on 2 February 2021).
18. MOBIS. MOBIS-COVID-19—Institute for Transport Planning and Systems, ETH Zurich. 2020. Available online: https://www.ivt.ethz.ch/en/research/mobis-covid19.html (accessed on 2 February 2021).
19. TUMI. The COVID-19 Outbreak and Implications to Sustainable Urban Mobility—Some Observations. 2020. Available online: https://www.transformative-mobility.org/news/the-covid-19-outbreak-and-implications-to-public-transport-some-observations (accessed on 2 February 2021).
20. Zhang, J. Transport Policymaking that Accounts for COVID-19 and Future Public Health Threats: A PASS Approach. *Transp. Policy* **2020**, *99*, 405–418. [CrossRef] [PubMed]
21. Zhang, J.; Hayashi, Y.; Frank, L.D. COVID-19 and Transport: Findings from a World-Wide Expert Survey. *Transp. Policy* **2021**, *103*, 68–85. [CrossRef] [PubMed]
22. Reid, C. Paris to Create 650 Kilometers of Post-Lockdown Cycleways. Available online: https://www.forbes.com/sites/carltonreid/2020/04/22/paris-to-create-650-kilometers-of-pop-up-corona-cycleways-for-post-lockdown-travel/?sh=2004910e54d4 (accessed on 30 July 2021).
23. Laker, L. Milan Announces Ambitious Scheme to Reduce Car Use After Lockdown, Italy. The Guardian. Available online: https://www.theguardian.com/world/2020/apr/21/milan-seeks-to-prevent-post-crisis-return-of-traffic-pollution (accessed on 30 July 2021).
24. Wray, S. Bogotá Expands Bike Lanes to Curb Coronavirus Spread—Smart Cities World. Available online: https://www.smartcitiesworld.net/news/news/bogota-expands-bike-lanes-overnight-to-curb-coronavirus-spread-5127 (accessed on 30 July 2021).
25. Municipality of Budapest. Temporary Bike Lanes Will Help Traffic during the Pandemic—Koronavírus Budapest—EN. Available online: https://koronavirus.budapest.hu/en/2020/04/06/temporary-bike-lanes-will-help-traffic-during-the-pandemic/ (accessed on 30 July 2021).
26. Todts, W. Think Global, Act Local to Transform Cities but also the Planet. Transport & Environment. Available online: https://www.transportenvironment.org/newsroom/blog/think-global-act-local-transform-cities-also-planet (accessed on 30 July 2021).
27. Reid, C. New Zealand First Country to Fund Pop-Up Bike Lanes, Widened Sidewalks during Lockdown. Available online: https://www.forbes.com/sites/carltonreid/2020/04/13/new-zealand-first-country-to-fund-pop-up-bike-lanes-widened-sidewalks-during-lockdown/?sh=4de4f08d546e (accessed on 30 July 2021).
28. City of Helsinki. City Bike Season to Start in Helsinki Earlier than Last Year. Available online: https://www.hel.fi/uutiset/en/helsinki/city-bike-season-to-start (accessed on 30 July 2021).
29. Geng, D.C.; Innes, J.; Wu, W.; Wang, G. Impacts of COVID-19 pandemic on urban park visitation: A global analysis. *J. For. Res.* **2020**, *1*, 3. [CrossRef] [PubMed]
30. Smarking. Real Time Market Observation: COVID-19 Impact on the US Parking Industry. 2020. Available online: https://www.smarking.com/post/real-time-market-observation-covid-19-impact-on-the-us-parking-industry (accessed on 8 February 2021).

31. Elsey, J.; Reedstrom, C.; Taxman, D. Curbing COVID-19: How the Parking Industry Is Responding and Adapting. Kimley-Horn. 2020. Available online: https://www.kimley-horn.com/curbing-covid19-parking-impact/ (accessed on 2 February 2021).
32. IEM. How the COVID-19 Pandemic Affected Parking Behavior—IEM. 2020. Available online: https://www.iemgroup.com/2020/07/01/how-the-covid-19-pandemic-affected-parking-behaviour/ (accessed on 8 February 2021).
33. City of Melbourne. On-Street Car Parking Sensor Data—2019, Open Data. Socrata. 2020. Available online: https://data.melbourne.vic.gov.au/Transport/On-street-Car-Parking-Sensor-Data-2019/7pgd-bdf2 (accessed on 2 November 2020).
34. City of Melbourne. On-Street Car Parking Sensor Data—2020 (Jan—May), Open Data. Socrata. 2020. Available online: https://data.melbourne.vic.gov.au/Transport/On-street-Car-Parking-Sensor-Data-2020-Jan-May-/4n3a-s6rn (accessed on 2 November 2020).
35. Premier of Victoria. State of Emergency Declared in Victoria Over COVID-19. 2020. Available online: https://www.premier.vic.gov.au/state-emergency-declared-victoria-over-covid-19 (accessed on 30 June 2021).
36. City of Melbourne. On-Street Parking Bays, Open Data. Socrata. 2020. Available online: https://data.melbourne.vic.gov.au/Transport/On-street-Parking-Bays/crvt-b4kt (accessed on 30 June 2021).
37. Princess Theatre. 2020. Available online: https://tomelbourne.com.au/princess-theatre/ (accessed on 30 June 2021).
38. Victoria State Government. 63 Exhibition Street: Melbourne Planning Permit Application No. 2014003155. 2020. Available online: https://www.planning.vic.gov.au/__data/assets/pdf_file/0028/108694/11-2014003155-63-Exhibition-St,-Melbourne.pdf (accessed on 30 June 2021).
39. Little Bourke Street, Melbourne. 2019. Available online: https://www.gpsmycity.com/attractions/little-bourke-street-23991.html (accessed on 30 June 2021).
40. Albani, M. COVID-19: There Is No Returning to Normal after the Crisis, World Economic Forum. 2020. Available online: https://www.weforum.org/agenda/2020/04/covid-19-three-horizons-framework/ (accessed on 2 February 2021).
41. Nian, G.; Peng, B.; Sun, D.J.; Ma, W.; Peng, B. Impact of COVID-19 on urban mobility during post-epidemic period in megacities: From the perspectives of taxi travel and social vitality. *Sustainability* **2020**, *12*, 7954. [CrossRef]
42. Chiara, G.D.; Cheah, L.; Azevedo, C.L.; Ben-Akiva, M.E. A policy-sensitive model of parking choice for commercial vehicles in urban areas. *Transp. Sci.* **2020**, *54*, 606–630. [CrossRef]
43. Ni, X.-Y.; Sun, D.J. An Agent-Based Simulation Model for Parking Variable Message Sign Location Problem. *Transp. Res. Rec.* **2018**, *2672*, 135–144. [CrossRef]
44. Sun, D.J.; Ni, X.-Y.; Zhang, L. A Discriminated Release Strategy for Parking Variable Message Sign Display Problem Using Agent-based Simulation. *IEEE Trans. Intell. Transp. Syst.* **2016**, *17*, 38–47. [CrossRef]
45. Allam, Z.; Jones, D.S. On the Coronavirus (COVID-19) Outbreak and the smart city network: Universal data sharing standards coupled with artificial intelligence (AI) to benefit urban health monitoring and management. *Healthcare* **2020**, *8*, 46. [CrossRef] [PubMed]
46. Li, L.; Yang, Z.; Dang, Z.; Meng, C.; Huang, J.; Meng, H.; Wang, D.; Chen, G.; Zhang, J.; Peng, H.; et al. Propagation analysis and prediction of the COVID-19. *Infect. Dis. Model.* **2020**, *5*, 282–292. [CrossRef] [PubMed]
47. Rashidi, T.H.; Shahriari, S.; Azad, A.K.M.; Vafaee, F. Real-time time-series modelling for prediction of COVID-19 spread and intervention assessment. *medRxiv* **2020**. [CrossRef]

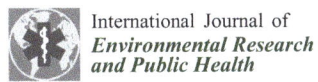

Article

Psychological and Physical Changes Caused by COVID-19 Pandemic in Elementary and Junior High School Teachers: A Cross-Sectional Study

Nobuyuki Wakui [1,*], Nanae Noguchi [1], Kotoha Ichikawa [1], Chikako Togawa [1], Raini Matsuoka [1], Yukiko Yoshizawa [1], Shunsuke Shirozu [1], Kenichi Suzuki [1], Mizue Ozawa [2], Takahiro Yanagiya [2] and Mayumi Kikuchi [2]

[1] Division of Applied Pharmaceutical Education and Research, Faculty of Pharmaceutical Sciences, Hoshi University, 2-4-41 Ebara, Shinagawa-ku, Tokyo 142-8501, Japan; s181180@hoshi.ac.jp (N.N.); s181012@hoshi.ac.jp (K.I.); s181156@hoshi.ac.jp (C.T.); s181219@hoshi.ac.jp (R.M.); y-yoshizawa@satsuki-ph.com (Y.Y.); s-shirozu@hoshi.ac.jp (S.S.); kenichi-suzuki@hoshi.ac.jp (K.S.)

[2] Shinagawa Pharmaceutical Association, 2-4-2 Nakanobu, Shinagawa-ku, Tokyo 142-0053, Japan; mitziozza1965@gmail.com (M.O.); yanagiya@tnb.co.jp (T.Y.); tomato_5mk@yahoo.co.jp (M.K.)

* Correspondence: n-wakui@hoshi.ac.jp; Fax: +81-5498-5760

Abstract: This study aimed to determine psychological and physical differences in elementary and junior high school teachers during COVID-19. This questionnaire-based cross-sectional study was conducted among 427 teachers in Tokyo, Japan (between 15 and 30 October 2020). The questionnaire explored school type (elementary and middle schools), sex, age, and COVID-19 changes (psychological changes, physical changes, impact on work, and infection control issues perceived to be stressed). Post hoc tests for *I cannot concentrate on work at all*, found a significant difference for *no change–improved* and *male teacher in elementary school female teacher in junior high school* ($p = 0.03$). Regarding *stress situation due to implementation of COVID-19 infection control*, there were significant differences for *disinfection work by teachers* between *male teachers in elementary school female teachers in junior high school* ($p = 0.04$) and *female teachers in elementary school female teachers in junior high school* ($p = 0.03$). COVID-19 produced differences in psychological and physical changes between male and female teachers in elementary and junior high schools. Some experienced psychological and physical stress, whereas others showed improvement. Given that teachers' mental health also affects students' educational quality, it is important to understand and improve teachers' psychological and physical circumstances and stress.

Keywords: COVID-19; elementary teacher; junior high school teacher; psychological change; physical changes

Citation: Wakui, N.; Noguchi, N.; Ichikawa, K.; Togawa, C.; Matsuoka, R.; Yoshizawa, Y.; Shirozu, S.; Suzuki, K.; Ozawa, M.; Yanagiya, T.; et al. Psychological and Physical Changes Caused by COVID-19 Pandemic in Elementary and Junior High School Teachers: A Cross-Sectional Study. *Int. J. Environ. Res. Public Health* **2022**, *19*, 7568. https://doi.org/10.3390/ijerph19137568

Academic Editors: Sachiko Kodera and Essam A. Rashed

Received: 23 May 2022
Accepted: 20 June 2022
Published: 21 June 2022

Publisher's Note: MDPI stays neutral with regard to jurisdictional claims in published maps and institutional affiliations.

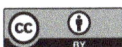

Copyright: © 2022 by the authors. Licensee MDPI, Basel, Switzerland. This article is an open access article distributed under the terms and conditions of the Creative Commons Attribution (CC BY) license (https://creativecommons.org/licenses/by/4.0/).

1. Introduction

A new type of coronavirus occurred in Wuhan City, Hubei Province, China, in December 2019, [1] which was later named SARS-CoV-2 [2,3]. SARS-CoV-2 rapidly spread worldwide, and the World Health Organization (WHO) declared a pandemic in March 2020 due to the spread of COVID-19 caused by SARS-CoV-2 [4]. Subsequent lockdown restrictions occurred throughout the world, which introduced significant changes and confusion to daily life [5,6]. Currently, the total number of infected people worldwide is more than 560 million, and the number of deaths is more than 6 million [7].

In Japan, an emergency declaration was issued for the first time in April 2020 [8], and the government requested that restaurants and schools should close and working from home was encouraged [9,10]. A new way of life was proposed to reduce the spread of infection, and a comprehensive behavioral change was required [11]. Specifically, basic infection control measures, such as hand washing and physical distance [12,13], as well as routine infection control measures, such as thorough avoidance of three Cs (closed spaces, crowded places, close-contact settings) [14] and a reduction in human contact by 80%, were implemented [15]. Such measures were also introduced in many parts of the world [16,17], which is a stressor for many people [18].

A new method of education in schools was introduced to ensure the rights of children to receive an education [19]. Specifically, in addition to basic infection control measures, restrictions included eating silently and the promotion of online classes [19]. However, it has been recognized that these restrictions impose a physical and mental burden on teachers managing the learning environment of students [20], which affects the mental health of teachers [21].

In previous studies, education has been considered as one of the highly stressful occupations [22]; moreover, occupational stress affects mental and physical health, and increases the risk of developing conditions, such as depression [23]. Indeed, teachers have a higher risk of developing depression compared with other occupations [24], and the development of burnout syndrome due to accumulated stress has also been reported [25]. During the COVID-19 pandemic, teachers may be more highly stressed than previously [26] as they are required to take various measures to prevent the spread of infection in addition to their own personal safety [27].

In a survey conducted in Greece in 2020, changes were found in teachers' mind and body related to COVID-19, and results showed that many teachers felt anxious due to the COVID-19 pandemic [28]. Compared with before the pandemic, mental changes were associated with decreased QOL [29], increased stress [30], and increased burnout [30,31]. There are some reports that female faculty are more likely to develop fear, depression, stress disorders and depression in comparison of sex [32]. In terms of physical changes, worsening of diet, sleep, and alcohol consumption have also been reported [6,17,18].

However, these reports have not analyzed the differences between elementary school teachers and junior high school teachers, and the stress situation of teachers by school type has not been clarified. Teachers are required to provide support for elementary school pupils and junior high school pupils in accordance with the students' developmental stage; hence, the nature of their work and the way they interact with pupils should differ [33]. This has led to the possibility that the stress status of teachers involved in teaching during the COVID-19 pandemic can vary widely between elementary and junior high schools. Therefore, it is of crucial public health importance to clarify the stress situation of teachers by school type to improve teachers' mental health [34].

Therefore, this study conducted a cross-sectional survey of elementary and junior high school teachers to clarify the physical and psychological differences during the COVID-19 pandemic.

2. Materials and Methods
2.1. Study Design and Participants

This was a cross-sectional study conducted among elementary and junior high school teachers in the Shinagawa Ward of Tokyo, Japan. The questionnaire (see Supplementary Materials) was designed to be answered in about 10 min. The participants included elementary and junior high school teachers in Shinagawa Ward, Tokyo. Data were collected for over 16 days between 15 October 2020 and 30 October 2020. Questionnaires were distributed to teachers of 18 elementary schools and 11 junior high schools selected randomly, and collection was by mail. Teachers who participated in the study responded anonymously to the questionnaire. Study participants provided informed written consent and participants participated in the study voluntarily (Figure 1).

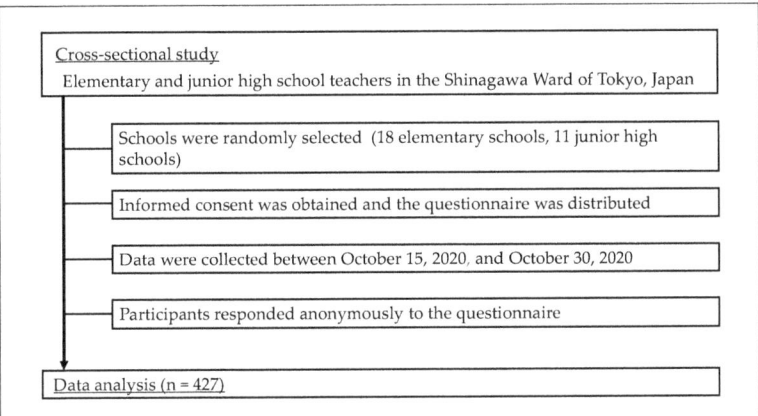

Figure 1. Flow-chart of the cross-sectional study.

2.2. Survey Items

The questionnaire consisted of five sections, one for demographic data (age, sex, type of school), and four sections asked about the impact of COVID-19 (psychological changes, physical changes, impact on work, and stressed relating to infection control items).

Of the four sections of the questionnaire, the psychological change, physical change, and impact on work sections were prepared using items related to this study from the Disaster Reliever Mental Health Manual prepared in Japan [35]. The "infection countermeasure matter that causes stress" question item was made to be the matter for which the implementation is required in the infection countermeasure guideline for school education [36]. All the questions in the four sections investigating the impact of COVID-19 were closed questions.

In terms of psychological change, 13 items were investigated, including, feeling high, irritation, anger, indignation, regret, anxiety, chagrin, impotent feelings, depression, no sense of reality, no sense of time, emotions are paralyzed, unable to concentrate on work at all, and no longer wanting to engage with others.

Six physical changes were investigated: insomnia/nightmares, palpitations, standing dizziness, sweating, dyspnea, and digestive symptoms. The following four items were investigated regarding the effect on work: excessively immersed in the work, reduction in thinking ability, lower concentration ability, and lower work efficiency. These items were measured at three levels: more improved than before, same as before, more deteriorated than before.

As for the infection countermeasures that felt stress, nine items were surveyed, namely always wearing a mask, body temperature and health status, disinfection work by teachers, social distancing, activity restriction during class, using face shields, prohibition or restriction of play and conversation, eating without talking/no refills, and not allowing children to serve. These items were measured at two levels—feeling stressed and not feeling stressed. Subsequently, it was investigated whether there were significant differences between the types and sex of schools according to these questionnaire responses.

2.3. Sample Size

An online sample size calculator, Raosoft® was used to set the sample size. Sample sizes were calculated using 50% response rate, 95% confidence interval, 5% error margin, and the population of teachers in elementary and middle schools in Tokyo as approximately 49,000 [37] (elementary school, $n = 33,912$, junior high school Rao soft, n = 15,340). As a result, the sample size recommended was 382. Therefore, the number of participants surveyed in this study was 427, which included an adequate sample size.

2.4. Statistical Analysis

Free statistical software R version 4.0.5 (R Core Team, R Foundation for Statistical Computing, Vienna, Austria) was used for statistical analysis. Pairwise elimination was used to exclude missing data from the analysis if any of the two variables had missing data, to use as much data as possible. Categorical data were tabulated with frequency and percentage, and continuous data were tabulated with mean ± SD. Differences in characteristics by school type and sex were assessed by Fisher's exact test. In addition, for items with significant differences, multiple comparison tests of proportions were performed using the Hochberg methods. The level of significance in all tests was set at $p < 0.05$.

2.5. Ethical Considerations

The study was conducted with the approval of the Ethics Committee of the Hoshi University (approval no. 2020-05). The study was conducted in accordance with the Declaration of Helsinki Ethical Guidelines for Medical Research Involving Human Subjects. All participants provided written informed consent.

3. Results

3.1. Demographic Features

There were 427 participants, of whom 305 (71.4%) were elementary school teachers and 122 (28.6%) were junior high school teachers (Table 1). A total of 418 participants responded to sex—157 (37.6%) males and 261 (62.4%) females. A total of 403 participants responded to age—92 (22.8%) in their 20 s, 139 (34.5%) in their 30 s, 79 (19.6%) in their 40 s, 64 (15.9%) in their 50 s, and 29 (7.2%) in their 60 s.

Table 1. Participants' characteristics (n = 427).

Variables	
School Type (n = 427)	
Elementary school	305 (71.4 %)
Junior high school	122 (28.6 %)
Sex (n = 418)	
Male	157 (37.6 %)
Female	261 (62.4 %)
Age (n = 403)	
20–29 years	92 (22.8%)
30–39 years	139 (34.5%)
30–49 years	79 (19.6%)
50–59 years	64 (15.9%)
>60 years	29 (7.2%)

3.2. Changes in Psychological Conditions before and after School Closure Due to COVID-19

Changes in psychological status before and after school closures are presented in Table 2. Fischer's exact test revealed significant differences in the item "I cannot concentrate on work at all" ($p = 0.02$). In addition, when multiple comparison tests were performed as a post hoc test for I cannot concentrate on work at all, a significant difference was found in the part of no change–improved and male teacher in elementary school female teacher in junior high school ($p = 0.03$). Regarding the significant difference found in the item "I cannot concentrate on work at all," junior high school teachers (males, 9.2%; females, 11.1%) had a higher response rate than elementary school teachers (males, 0%; females, 3.9%), indicating that they had improved. Furthermore, female teachers had a higher response rate to improvement than male teachers.

Table 2. Changes in psychological conditions before and after school closures due to COVID-19.

	Elementary School		Junior High School		p-Value
	Male Teacher	Female Teacher	Male Teacher	Female Teacher	
Feeling high (n = 409)					0.82
Improved	11 (12.2%)	20 (9.9%)	7 (10.8%)	4 (7.7%)	
No Change	63 (70.0%)	143 (70.8%)	49 (75.4%)	35 (67.3%)	
Deteriorated	16 (17.8%)	39 (19.3%)	9 (13.8%)	13 (25.0%)	
Irritation (n = 410)					0.06
Improved	3 (3.4%)	24 (11.8%)	11 (16.9%)	4 (7.5%)	
No Change	66 (74.2%)	129 (63.5%)	40 (61.5%)	31 (58.5%)	
Deteriorated	20 (22.5%)	50 (24.6%)	14 (21.5%)	18 (34.0%)	
Anger (n = 408)					0.42
Improved	3 (3.4%)	22 (10.9%)	7 (10.8%)	4 (7.7%)	
No Change	73 (82.0%)	146 (72.3%)	47 (72.3%)	38 (73.1%)	
Deteriorated	13 (14.6%)	34 (16.8%)	11 (16.9%)	10 (19.2%)	
Indignation (n = 409)					0.10
Improved	3 (3.4%)	17 (8.4%)	5 (7.7%)	2 (3.8%)	
No Change	71 (79.8%)	155 (76.4%)	50 (76.9%)	33 (63.5%)	
Deteriorated	15 (16.9%)	31 (15.3%)	10 (15.4%)	17 (32.7%)	
Anxiety (n = 411)					0.73
Improved	9 (10.1%)	26 (12.8%)	6 (9.2%)	8 (14.8%)	
No Change	55 (61.8%)	106 (52.2%)	40 (61.5%)	29 (53.7%)	
Deteriorated	25 (28.1%)	71 (35.0%)	19 (29.2%)	17 (31.5%)	
Chagrin (n = 411)					0.24
Improved	7 (7.9%)	24 (11.8%)	10 (15.4%)	8 (14.8%)	
No Change	69 (77.5%)	135 (66.5%)	44 (67.7%)	31 (57.4%)	
Deteriorated	13 (14.6%)	44 (21.7%)	11 (16.9%)	15 (27.8%)	
Impotent feeling (n = 409)					0.33
Improved	6 (6.7%)	16 (8.0%)	8 (12.3%)	4 (7.4%)	
No Change	67 (75.3%)	149 (74.1%)	50 (76.9%)	35 (64.8%)	
Deteriorated	16 (18.0%)	36 (17.9%)	7 (10.8%)	15 (27.8%)	
Depression (n = 412)					0.499
Improved	4 (4.4%)	19 (9.4%)	8 (12.3%)	5 (9.3%)	
No Change	63 (70.0%)	129 (63.5%)	45 (69.2%)	34 (63.0%)	
Deteriorated	23 (25.6%)	55 (27.1%)	12 (18.5%)	15 (27.8%)	
NSOR (n = 411)					0.86
Improved	8 (8.8%)	26 (12.9%)	10 (15.4%)	5 (9.4%)	
No Change	72 (79.1%)	146 (72.3%)	47 (72.3%)	41 (77.4%)	
Deteriorated	11 (12.1%)	30 (14.9%)	8 (12.3%)	7 (13.2%)	
NSOT (n = 412)					0.89
Improved	5 (5.5%)	19 (9.4%)	7 (10.8%)	5 (9.3%)	
No Change	77 (84.6%)	161 (79.7%)	51 (78.5%)	42 (77.8%)	
Deteriorated	9 (9.9%)	22 (10.9%)	7 (10.8%)	7 (13.0%)	
EAP (n = 412)					0.40
Improved	3 (3.3%)	9 (4.4%)	6 (9.2%)	5 (9.4%)	
No Change	82 (90.1%)	173 (85.2%)	53 (81.5%)	42 (79.2%)	
Deteriorated	6 (6.6%)	21 (10.3%)	6 (9.2%)	6 (11.3%)	
ICCOW (n = 413)					0.02
Improved	0 (0%)	8 (3.9%)	6 (9.2%)	6 (11.1%)	
No Change	78 (85.7%)	169 (83.3%)	49 (75.4%)	39 (72.2%)	
Deteriorated	13 (14.3%)	26 (12.8%)	10 (15.4%)	9 (16.7%)	
NLWTEWO (n = 412)					0.50
Improved	3 (3.3%)	13 (6.4%)	5 (7.7%)	4 (7.5%)	
No Change	74 (82.2%)	153 (75.0%)	54 (83.1%)	41 (77.4%)	
Deteriorated	13 (14.4%)	38 (18.6%)	6 (9.2%)	8 (15.1%)	

p-values were derived from Fisher's exact test analysis. Abbreviations: NSOR = No sense of reality; NSOT = No sense of time; EAP = Emotions are paralyzed; ICCOW = I cannot concentrate on work at all; NLWTEWO = No longer wanting to engage with others.

3.3. Changes in Physical Symptoms before and after School Closure Due to COVID-19

Changes in physical conditions before and after school closure are presented in Table 3. Fischer's exact test showed significant differences for insomnia/nightmares ($p = 0.009$) and standing dizziness ($p = 0.03$). Regarding insomnia/nightmares, many female teachers of elementary (18.0%) and junior high schools (18.5%) answered that physical symptoms had deteriorated. Moreover, at the same time, a small number of female teachers responded that their insomnia/nightmare symptoms had improved (elementary female teacher: 7.8%, junior high school female teacher: 9.3%). Regarding standing dizziness, many female teachers in junior high school answered that it had deteriorated. In addition, a multiple comparisons test was performed for insomnia/nightmares and standing dizziness as a post hoc test, and no significant differences were found.

Table 3. Changes in physical symptoms before and after school closures due to COVID-19.

	Elementary School		Junior High School		p-Value
	Male Teacher	Female Teacher	Male Teacher	Female Teacher	
Insomnia/nightmares (n = 413)					0.009
Improved	1 (1.1%)	16 (7.8%)	2 (3.2%)	5 (9.3%)	
No Change	82 (90.1%)	152 (74.1%)	56 (88.9%)	39 (72.2%)	
Deteriorated	8 (8.8%)	37 (18.0%)	5 (7.9%)	10 (18.5%)	
Palpitations (n = 413)					0.13
Improved	1 (1.1%)	12 (5.9%)	1 (1.6%)	0 (0%)	
No Change	86 (94.5%)	173 (84.4%)	59 (92.2%)	48 (90.6%)	
Deteriorated	4 (4.4%)	20 (9.8%)	4 (6.2%)	5 (9.4%)	
Standing dizziness (n = 414)					0.03
Improved	1 (1.1%)	16 (7.8%)	2 (3.1%)	0 (0%)	
No Change	85 (93.4%)	169 (82.4%)	57 (89.1%)	46 (85.2%)	
Deteriorated	5 (5.5%)	20 (9.8%)	5 (7.8%)	8 (14.8%)	
Sweating (n = 414)					0.83
Improved	1 (1.1%)	7 (3.4%)	1 (1.6%)	1 (1.9%)	
No Change	85 (93.4%)	182 (88.8%)	56 (87.5%)	49 (90.7%)	
Deteriorated	5 (5.5%)	16 (7.8%)	7 (10.9%)	4 (7.4%)	
Dyspnea (n = 414)					0.93
Improved	1 (1.1%)	5 (2.4%)	1 (1.6%)	0 (0%)	
No Change	87 (95.6%)	190 (92.7%)	59 (92.2%)	51 (94.4%)	
Deteriorated	3 (3.3%)	10 (4.9%)	4 (6.2%)	3 (5.6%)	
Digestive symptoms (n = 414)					0.55
Improved	1 (1.1%)	7 (3.4%)	0 (0%)	1 (1.9%)	
No Change	85 (93.4%)	176 (85.9%)	58 (90.6%)	48 (88.9%)	
Deteriorated	5 (5.5%)	22 (10.7%)	6 (9.4%)	5 (9.3%)	

p-Value derives from Fischer's exact test analysis.

3.4. Impact of COVID-19 on Work before and after School Closure

The impact of COVID-19 on work before and after school closures presented in Table 4. Fischer's exact test showed no significant differences among all four items. In sex comparisons, a greater proportion of female respondents stated that they had deteriorated in lowering of concentration ability compared with male teachers. In the comparison between the types of school, a large proportion of junior high school teachers answered that all four items deteriorated. In terms of lowering of work efficiency, >15% of the teachers indicated that they had deteriorated, especially junior high school teachers who indicated that they had deteriorated to a greater extent than elementary school teachers.

Table 4. Impact of COVID-19 on work before and after school closures.

	Elementary School		Junior High School		p-Value
	Male Teacher	Female Teacher	Male Teacher	Female Teacher	
EIITW (n = 406)					0.37
Improved	6 (6.7%)	18 (9.0%)	4 (6.2%)	6 (11.5%)	
No Change	76 (85.4%)	154 (77.0%)	54 (83.1%)	36 (69.2%)	
Deteriorated	7 (7.9%)	28 (14.0%)	7 (10.8%)	10 (19.2%)	
LOTTA (n = 408)					0.80
Improved	7 (7.9%)	13 (6.5%)	5 (7.7%)	3 (5.6%)	
No Change	70 (78.7%)	154 (77.0%)	50 (76.9%)	38 (70.4%)	
Deteriorated	12 (13.5%)	33 (16.5%)	10 (15.4%)	13 (24.1%)	
LOTCA (n = 403)					0.79
Improved	6 (6.8%)	11 (5.6%)	3 (4.6%)	4 (7.4%)	
No Change	66 (75.0%)	151 (77.0%)	53 (81.5%)	37 (68.5%)	
Deteriorated	16 (18.2%)	34 (17.3%)	9 (13.8%)	13 (24.1%)	
LOTWE (n = 406)					0.31
Improved	1 (1.1%)	11 (5.5%)	3 (4.6%)	3 (5.7%)	
No Change	73 (83.0%)	150 (75.0%)	46 (70.8%)	36 (67.9%)	
Deteriorated	14 (15.9%)	39 (19.5%)	16 (24.6%)	14 (26.4%)	

Abbreviations: EIITW = Excessively immersed in the work; LOTTA = Lowering of the thinking ability; LOTCA = Lowering of the concentration ability; LOTWE = Lowering of the work efficiency. p-values were derived from Fisher's exact test analysis.

3.5. Stress Causes for Teachers Associated with COVID-19 Infection Control

The stress situation due to COVID-19 infection countermeasures is presented in Table 5. Fischer's exact test showed significant differences in four items, namely, always wearing mask ($p = 0.04$), disinfection work by teachers ($p = 0.03$), activity restriction during class ($p = 0.05$), and prohibition or restriction of play and conversation ($p = 0.04$). In addition, when the multiple comparison tests were carried out as a post hoc test for the four items that showed significant differences, there were two significant differences in faculty disinfection work, between the two combination parts of male teachers in elementary school and female teachers in junior high school ($p = 0.04$) and female teachers in elementary school and female teachers in junior high school ($p = 0.03$).

Table 5. Stress causes for teachers associated with COVID-19 infection control.

	Elementary School		Junior High School		p-Value
	Male Teacher	Female Teacher	Male Teacher	Female Teacher	
AWM (n = 413)					0.04
No	29 (31.9%)	50 (24.6%)	27 (41.5%)	12 (22.2%)	
Yes	62 (68.1%)	153 (75.4%)	38 (58.5%)	42 (77.8%)	
BTAHSG (n = 413)					0.54
No	67 (73.6%)	144 (70.9%)	52 (80.0%)	41 (75.9%)	
Yes	24 (26.4%)	59 (29.1%)	13 (20.0%)	13 (24.1%)	
DWBT (n = 412)					0.03
No	42 (46.2%)	91 (45.0%)	25 (38.5%)	13 (24.1%)	
Yes	49 (53.8%)	111 (55.0%)	40 (61.5%)	41 (75.9%)	
Social distance (n = 413)					0.71
No	59 (64.8%)	138 (68.0%)	43 (66.2%)	40 (74.1%)	
Yes	32 (35.2%)	65 (32.0%)	22 (33.8%)	14 (25.9%)	
ARDC (n = 413)					0.05
No	23 (25.3%)	74 (36.5%)	28 (43.1%)	24 (44.4%)	
Yes	68 (74.7%)	129 (63.5%)	37 (56.9%)	30 (55.6%)	
UFS (n = 413)					0.08
No	68 (74.7%)	143 (70.4%)	56 (86.2%)	40 (74.1%)	
Yes	23 (25.3%)	60 (29.6%)	9 (13.8%)	14 (25.9%)	

Table 5. Cont.

	Elementary School		Junior High School		p-Value
	Male Teacher	Female Teacher	Male Teacher	Female Teacher	
POROPAC (n = 413)					0.04
No	35 (38.5%)	99 (48.8%)	36 (55.4%)	33 (61.1%)	
Yes	56 (61.5%)	104 (51.2%)	29 (44.6%)	21 (38.9%)	
EWTNR (n = 413)					0.42
No	42 (46.2%)	113 (55.7%)	32 (49.2%)	26 (48.1%)	
Yes	49 (53.8%)	90 (44.3%)	33 (50.8%)	28 (51.9%)	
DNLCR (n = 413)					0.62
No	70 (76.9%)	153 (75.4%)	48 (73.8%)	45 (83.3%)	
Yes	21 (23.1%)	50 (24.6%)	17 (26.2%)	9 (16.7%)	

Abbreviations: AWM = Always wearing mask; BTAHSG = Body temperature and health status grasping; DWBT = Disinfection work by teachers; ARDC = Activity restriction during class; UFS = Using face shield; POROPAC = Prohibition or restriction of play and conversation; EWTNR = Eat without talking /no refills; DNLCR = Do not let children serve. p-values were derived from Fisher's exact test analysis.

4. Discussion

In Japan, the number of teachers suffering psychologically and physical increased more than twice over the 10-year period from 2002 to 2011, with an actual number of more than 5000 [38]. Worldwide, teachers' occupational mental health problems are serious [24], and main teachers' reasons for leaving are mental illness resulting from stress disorders and depression. Changes in schools due to COVID-19 have been linked with increased stress for faculty staff. This study assessed psychological and physical changes in teachers by school type and sex during the COVID-19 pandemic. The results showed significant differences in psychological symptom changes for *I cannot concentrate on work at all*, and in physical symptom changes for *insomnia/nightmares* and *standing dizziness*. Additionally, there were significant differences between males and females in elementary and junior high school teachers in the items of *always wearing a mask, disinfection work by teachers, activity restriction during class, and prohibition or restriction of play and conversation in stressful situations* resulting from the implementation of COVID-19 infection control measures. Furthermore, multiple comparison tests were performed on items for which a significant difference was found. As a result, two significant differences were found. The first was in the combination of elementary school male teachers–junior high school female teachers and improved–unchanged in *I cannot concentrate on work at all*. The second was in terms of stress—there was a significant difference between elementary school male teachers–junior high school female teachers and elementary school female teachers–junior high school female teachers in *disinfection work* by teachers.

The significant differences in the combination of female teachers in elementary school female teachers in male schools and improved–no change in *I cannot concentrate on work at all* of the psychological change may be attributed to the fact that the perceived stress and burden of elementary and middle school faculty was alleviated by COVID-19 spread. Previous investigations have reported that junior high school teachers are stressed by instructing students in club activities, and that elementary school teachers are stressed by the implementation of executive officials and committees [39]. Almost all students in junior high schools in Japan belong to clubs, and teachers provide guidance to students outside hours every day, including in holidays. In reality, junior high school teachers provide club activities even at the expense of holidays, and this is regarded as a cause of stress for teachers in Japan. With this in mind, it is possible that the burden on junior high school teachers was greatly reduced by the limitations on club activities due to the spread of COVID-19.

In Japan, more females than males work and are responsible for housework and parenting, and the decrease in teaching time for division activities requiring out-of-hours work is believed to directly affect the reduction in the burden on female teachers in junior high schools. Worldwide, it has also been reported that the burden of female teachers who are compatible with home and work is substantial [40,41], and the results of this survey may be transferrable to other countries.

In terms of physical changes, Fischer's exact test showed significant differences in two items, *insomnia/nightmares* and *standing dizziness*. However, all post hoc tests for multiple comparisons showed no significant differences. In terms of *insomnia/nightmares*, elementary and junior high school female teachers showed higher improved response rates than male teachers. In contrast, there was a higher number of female teachers who responded that their *insomnia/nightmares* had deteriorated. Regarding this, the causes of *insomnia/nightmares* is believed to be stress, and females are more likely to feel psychological stresses, such as anxiety, than males. Therefore, while COVID-19 induces stress due to changes, at the same time, the reduction in workload may reduce stress. Regarding *standing dizziness*, the response rate of the participants who answered that the *standing dizziness* deteriorated was higher in middle school teachers than the elementary school teachers. For females, 0% of junior high school teachers and 7.8% of elementary school teachers responded that *standing dizziness* had improved, with the percentages of value differing by 7.8%. This may be because club activities are a major burden for junior high school teachers, and furthermore, female find balancing work with housework and childcare is stressful. However, some teachers answered that they improved in all items, and it is suggested that there some positive aspects to the spread of COVID-19.

No significant differences were found between school type and teacher sex in changes in *impact on work*. When checking each item, about 70% of teachers answered that there was no change in all items. Moreover, regardless of the sex and school type, approximately 10–20% of teachers responded that they had deteriorated in terms of *decreased thinking, concentration*, and *lowering of the work efficiency*, and a small percentage of teachers responded that they had improved. From this, it is suggested that the deterioration of thinking ability, concentration, and work efficiency occurred in some school teachers irrespective of the type of school and sex because anxiety [27] was newly generated by COVID-19.

The Fischer's exact test found significant differences in the items always wearing a mask, disinfection work by teachers, activity restriction during class, and prohibition or restriction of play and conversation in the stress situation resulting from the implementation of COVID-19 infection countermeasure. Furthermore, the results of the multiple comparison test revealed significant differences in teacher disinfection work. In always wearing a mask, a higher proportion of females felt stressed compared with males. This may be because make-up adheres to the mask and make-up is spoiled [42]; in addition, hairstyles do not last well under the moisture from wearing the mask [43], and females report feeling stress from this.

Regarding disinfection work by teachers, a higher proportion of junior high school teachers reported feeling stressed compared with elementary school teachers. In addition, the percentage of females who answered that they were feeling stressed was higher than males. This is thought to be due in part to the fact that junior high schools have club activities and the range of activities is wider than that of elementary schools; therefore, the range of disinfection by teachers is also wider. In addition, generally, more females are more sensitive than males about their appearance and hands, consequently, the continuous use of disinfectants, which can cause rough hands [44], may make females more sensitive and susceptible to stress than in males. Moreover, given that females have lower physical strength than young males, they are more likely to feel the burden considering that the disinfection range is broad, including desks, chairs, rockers, and other items [36], which takes time and effort because carrying equipment, such as cleaning tools, can be a heavy burden.

Regarding the items of activity restriction during class and prohibition or restriction of play and conversation, a higher proportion of elementary school teachers felt stressed compared with junior high school teachers. Additionally, the percentage of males feeling stressed was higher than that of females. This is thought to have led to the burden and stress among elementary school teachers because there are more children in elementary school who are mentally younger than those in junior high school, and it is difficult to take command. Male elementary school teachers can be more stressed than female teachers because male teachers are more in charge of instructing students. Male teachers, in particular, often yell to discipline their students, which can be a reason for stress [45]. Equally, a number of teachers felt they had improved in some items, and it can be said that the spread of COVID-19 is not only bad but also that it has had a positive effect in some areas.

There are several limitations to this study. First, Fisher's exact test showed significant differences, whereas the multiple comparison test showed that some of them did not significantly differ. As 18 tests were performed for a single item in this study's multiple testing, it is possible that a so-called type 2 error occurred. Second, this study is aimed at teachers in Tokyo, and the opinions of teachers in other areas are not reflected. Thirdly, this study did not perform model analysis. Accordingly, the current study tested and reported the distribution of the results obtained during the COVID-19 pandemic and epidemic and the differences between them. Some of the dependent variables included herein had three levels, so all analyses were performed in a unified manner using Fisher's exact test for ease of interpretation. Given that this survey found significant differences between the levels, further research considering the use of models, such as logistic regression analysis, can be considered in order to evaluate the factors. Nonetheless, this study is the first to assess differences in elementary and junior high schools among teachers and psychological and physical differences between sex due to the COVID-19 pandemic.

The emphasized point of our study is that previous reports have only assessed the relationship between sexes [29] or school differences [46] and psychological and physical effects, and no survey like this one has previously been conducted. In addition, it is interesting to evaluate not only the rate of increasing stress due to the spread of COVID-19 but also the rate of improvement. In fact, statistically significant differences between male and female teachers in elementary and junior high schools were also observed in the rate of improvement in this study. Reports evaluating the percentage of points that were improved by COVID-19 spread are unusual and remarkable. Even after COVID-19 has ended, it will be important to conduct surveys to assess the differences in improvements and deterioration between schools and sex, as well as overall improvement and deterioration, and to evaluate the causes objectively.

Teachers play an important role not only in their studies but also in the development of children's mental health, as experts in education in daily contact with students and children [47]. Teachers' mental health also affects students' educational quality, so it is important to understand and improve teachers' psychological and physical situations and stress. While the spread of COVID-19 has increased the stressors of many teachers, it is also possible that the work has been streamlined. It is recommended that administrative personnel involved in education and members of local educational committees conduct surveys such as this on a regular basis and assess the results to understand the mental health of faculty members and to strive to improve the working environment.

5. Conclusions

COVID-19 resulted in differences in psychological and physical changes between male and female teachers in elementary and junior high schools. While most teachers showed no change, some experienced psychological and physical stress, whereas others experienced improvement. Policymakers of administrative and educational committees should conduct surveys like this on teachers on a regular basis to understand the psychological and physical stress situations of teachers in a multidimensional manner as well as to decide the policy for the improvement.

Supplementary Materials: The following supporting information can be downloaded at: https://www.mdpi.com/article/10.3390/ijerph19137568/s1, COVID-19 questionnaire survey.

Author Contributions: N.W. and M.K. designed the study. N.N., K.I., C.T., R.M., M.O., T.Y. and M.K. collected data. N.W. and N.N. analyzed the data. N.W. wrote the manuscript. N.N., Y.Y., S.S., K.S. and M.K. critically revised the manuscript for important intellectual content. All authors have read and agreed to the published version of the manuscript.

Funding: This research did not receive any external funding.

Institutional Review Board Statement: The study was approved by the Ethics Committee of the Hoshi University (approval no: 2020-05).

Informed Consent Statement: Informed consent was obtained from all subjects involved in the study.

Data Availability Statement: The data is not publicly available as all participants have not consented to the public disclosure of the data online. However, the data presented in this study are available on request from the corresponding author.

Acknowledgments: We thank all the teachers who participated in this study.

Conflicts of Interest: The authors declare no conflict of interest.

References

1. WHO. Origin of SARS-CoV-2 Virus. Available online: https://www.who.int/emergencies/diseases/novel-coronavirus-2019/origins-of-the-virus (accessed on 15 May 2022).
2. Gorbalenya, A.E.; Baker, S.C.; Baric, R.S.; de Groot, R.J.; Drosten, C.; Gulyaeva, A.A.; Haagmans, B.L.; Lauber, C.; Leontovich, A.M.; Neuman, B.W.; et al. Severe acute respiratory syndrome-related coronavirus: The species and its viruses–A statement of the Coronavirus Study Group. *bioRxiv* **2020**. [CrossRef]
3. Coronaviridae Study Group of the International Committee on Taxonomy of Viruses. The species severe acute respiratory syndrome-related coronavirus: Classifying 2019-nCoV and naming it SARS-CoV-2. *Nat. Microbiol.* **2020**, *5*, 536–544. [CrossRef] [PubMed]
4. Cucinotta, D.; Vanelli, M. WHO declares COVID-19 a pandemic. *Acta Biomed.* **2020**, *91*, 157–160. [CrossRef] [PubMed]
5. Di Renzo, L.; Gualtieri, P.; Pivari, F.; Soldati, L.; Attinà, A.; Cinelli, G.; Leggeri, C.; Caparello, G.; Barrea, L.; Scerbo, F.; et al. Eating habits and lifestyle changes during COVID-19 lockdown: An Italian survey. *J. Transl. Med.* **2020**, *18*, 229. [CrossRef] [PubMed]
6. Ruiz-Roso, M.B.; de Carvalho Padilha, P.; Mantilla-Escalante, D.C.; Ulloa, N.; Brun, P.; Acevedo-Correa, D.; Arantes Ferreira Peres, W.; Martorell, M.; Aires, M.T.; de Oliveira Cardoso, L.; et al. Covid-19 confinement and changes of adolescent's dietary trends in Italy, Spain, Chile, Colombia and Brazil. *Nutrients* **2020**, *12*, 1807. [CrossRef] [PubMed]
7. WHO. WHO Coronavirus (COVID-19) Dashboard. Available online: https://covid19.who.int/ (accessed on 15 May 2022).
8. Cabinet Secretariat. Japan, Countermeasures against COVID-19. Available online: https://corona.go.jp/news/pdf/kinkyujitai_sengen_0407.pdf (accessed on 15 May 2022).
9. Ministry of Internal Affairs and Communications-Japan. Active Utilization of Telework as a Countermeasure against New Coronavirus Infectious Diseases. Available online: https://www.soumu.go.jp/main_sosiki/joho_tsusin/telework/02ryutsu02_04000341.html (accessed on 15 May 2022).
10. Ministry of Internal Affairs and Communications-Japan. Impact of COVID-19 on Society. Available online: https://www.soumu.go.jp/johotsusintokei/whitepaper/ja/r02/pdf/n2300000.pdf (accessed on 15 May 2022).
11. Ministry of Health, Labour and Welfare in Janan. Practical Example of "New Lifestyle". Available online: https://www.mhlw.go.jp/stf/seisakunitsuite/bunya/0000121431_newlifestyle.html (accessed on 15 May 2022).
12. Ministry of Health, Labour and Welfare in Japan. to Prevent New Coronavirus Infection. Available online: https://www.mhlw.go.jp/stf/covid-19/kenkou-iryousoudan.html#h2_1 (accessed on 15 May 2022).
13. Cabinet Secretariat. Japan, Initiatives to Prevent the Spread of Infection. Available online: https://corona.go.jp/proposal/ (accessed on 15 May 2022).
14. Ministry of Health, Labour and Welfare in Janan. Avoid the "Three Cs"! Available online: https://www.mhlw.go.jp/content/3CS.pdf (accessed on 15 May 2022).
15. Ministry of Health, Labour and Welfare in Janan. Announced "10 Points to Reduce Contact with People by 80%". Available online: https://www.mhlw.go.jp/stf/seisakunitsuite/bunya/0000121431_00116.html (accessed on 15 May 2022).
16. Górnicka, M.; Drywień, M.E.; Zielinska, M.A.; Hamułka, J. Dietary and lifestyle changes during COVID-19 and the subsequent lockdowns among polish adults: A cross-sectional online survey PLifeCOVID-19 study. *Nutrients* **2020**, *12*, 2324. [CrossRef]
17. Rawat, D.; Dixit, V.; Gulati, S.; Gulati, S.; Gulati, A. Impact of COVID-19 outbreak on lifestyle behavior: A review of studies published in India. *Diabetes Metab. Syndr.* **2021**, *15*, 331–336. [CrossRef]
18. Werner, A.; Kater, M.J.; Schlarb, A.A.; Lohaus, A. Sleep and stress in times of the COVID-19 pandemic: The role of personal resources. *Appl. Psychol. Health Well Being* **2021**, *13*, 935–951. [CrossRef]
19. Ministry of Education, Culture, Sports, Science and Technology in Japan. Guidelines for Sustainable School Management in Response to the Novel Coronavirus Disease. Available online: https://www.mext.go.jp/content/20220401-mxt_kouhou01-000004520_02.pdf (accessed on 15 May 2022).

20. Panisoara, I.O.; Lazar, I.; Panisoara, G.; Chirca, R.; Ursu, A.S. Motivation and continuance intention towards online instruction among teachers during the COVID-19 pandemic: The mediating effect of burnout and technostress. *Int. J. Environ. Res. Public Health* **2020**, *17*, 8002. [CrossRef]
21. Palma-Vasquez, C.; Carrasco, D.; Hernando-Rodriguez, J.C. Mental health of teachers who have Teleworked due to COVID-19. *Eur. J. Investig. Health Psychol. Educ.* **2021**, *11*, 515–528. [CrossRef]
22. Johnson, S.; Cooper, C.; Cartwright, S.; Donald, I.; Taylor, P.; Millet, C. The experience of work-related stress across occupations. *J. Manag. Psychol.* **2005**, *20*, 178–187. [CrossRef]
23. Desouky, D.; Allam, H. Occupational stress, anxiety and depression among Egyptian teachers. *J. Epidemiol. Glob. Health* **2017**, *7*, 191–198. [CrossRef] [PubMed]
24. Kidger, J.; Brockman, R.; Tilling, K.; Campbell, R.; Ford, T.; Araya, R.; King, M.; Gunnell, D. Teachers' wellbeing and depressive symptoms, and associated risk factors: A large cross-sectional study in English secondary schools. *J. Affect. Disord.* **2016**, *192*, 76–82. [CrossRef] [PubMed]
25. Chennoufi, L.; Ellouze, F.; Cherif, W.; Mersni, M.; M'rad, M.F. Stress et épuisement professionnel des enseignants tunisiens [Stress and burnout among Tunisian teachers]. *Encéphale* **2012**, *38*, 480–487. (In French) [CrossRef] [PubMed]
26. Santamaría, M.D.; Mondragon, N.I.; Santxo, N.B.; Ozamiz-Etxebarria, N. Teacher stress, anxiety and depression at the beginning of the academic year during the COVID-19 pandemic. *Glob. Ment. Health* **2021**, *8*, e14. [CrossRef]
27. Wakui, N.; Abe, S.; Shirozu, S.; Yamamoto, Y.; Yamamura, M.; Abe, Y.; Murata, S.; Ozawa, M.; Igarashi, T.; Yanagiya, T.; et al. Causes of anxiety among teachers giving face-to-face lessons after the reopening of schools during the COVID-19 pandemic: A cross-sectional study. *BMC Public Health* **2021**, *21*, 1050. [CrossRef]
28. Stachteas, P.; Stachteas, C. The psychological impact of the COVID-19 pandemic on secondary school teachers. *Psychiatriki* **2020**, *31*, 293–301. [CrossRef]
29. Lizana, P.A.; Vega-Fernadez, G.; Gomez-Bruton, A.; Leyton, B.; Lera, L. Impact of the COVID-19 pandemic on teacher quality of life: A longitudinal study from before and during the health crisis. *Int. J. Environ. Res. Public Health* **2021**, *18*, 3764. [CrossRef]
30. Kotowski, S.E.; Davis, K.G.; Barratt, C.L. Teachers feeling the burden of COVID-19: Impact on well being, stress, and burnout. *Work* **2022**, *71*, 407–415. [CrossRef]
31. Minihan, E.; Adamis, D.; Dunleavy, M.; Martin, A.; Gavin, B.; McNicholas, F. COVID-19 related occupational stress in teachers in Ireland. *Int. J. Educ. Res.* **2022**, *3*, 100114. [CrossRef]
32. McLean, C.P.; Asnaani, A.; Litz, B.T.; Hofmann, S.G. Gender differences in anxiety disorders: Prevalence, course of illness, comorbidity and burden of illness. *J. Psychiatr. Res.* **2011**, *45*, 1027–1035. [CrossRef] [PubMed]
33. Ministry of Education, Culture, Sports, Science and Technology in Japan. Characteristics of Each Child's Developmental Stage and Issues to be Emphasized. Available online: https://www.mext.go.jp/b_menu/shingi/chousa/shotou/053/shiryo/attach/1282789.htm (accessed on 15 May 2022).
34. Silva, D.F.O.; Cobucci, R.N.; Lima, S.C.V.C.; de Andrade, F.B. Prevalence of anxiety, depression, and stress among teachers during the COVID-19 pandemic: A PRISMA-compliant systematic review. *Medicine* **2021**, *100*, e27684. [CrossRef] [PubMed]
35. National Information Center of Stress and Disaster Mental Health. Mental and Physical Reactions That Can Occur to Disaster Supporters. Available online: https://saigai-kokoro.ncnp.go.jp/document/medical_personnel02_2.html (accessed on 15 May 2022).
36. Ministry of Education, Culture, Sports, Science and Technology in Japan. Hygiene Management Manual for New Coronavirus Infectious Diseases in Schools-New Lifestyles in Schools. Available online: https://www.mext.go.jp/a_menu/coronavirus/mext_00029.html (accessed on 15 May 2022).
37. Tokyo Metropolitan Board of Education. Tokyo Compulsory Education Elementary and Junior High School Overview. Available online: https://www.kyoiku.metro.tokyo.lg.jp/administration/statistics_and_research/academic_report/files/report2020/gaiyou-shouchuugimu.pdf (accessed on 15 May 2022).
38. Toyokeiai Online, the Harsh Reality of "Teachers" Who Suffer from 5000 People Every Year. Available online: https://toyokeizai.net/articles/-/390826 (accessed on 15 May 2022).
39. Ministry of Health, Labour and Welfare in Janan. White Paper on Prevention of Death from Overwork (Text). 2018. Available online: https://www.mhlw.go.jp/wp/hakusyo/karoushi/18/index.html (accessed on 15 May 2022).
40. Dogra, P.; Kaushal, A. Underlying the triple burden effects on women educationists due to COVID-19. *Educ. Inf. Technol.* **2022**, *27*, 209–228. [CrossRef] [PubMed]
41. Solís García, P.; Lago Urbano, R.; Real Castelao, S. Consequences of COVID-19 confinement for teachers: Family-work interactions, technostress, and perceived organizational support. *Int. J. Environ. Res. Public Health* **2021**, *18*, 11259. [CrossRef] [PubMed]
42. Yokoyama, E.; Udodaira, K.; Nicolas, A.; Yamashita, E.; Maudet, A.; Flament, F.; Velleman, D. A preliminary study to understand the effects of mask on tinted face cosmetics. *Skin Res. Technol.* **2021**, *27*, 797–802. [CrossRef]
43. Times, P.R. "Mask Swell" Becomes a New Enemy? How to Solve Your Worries by "Frizz Type" Taught by a Popular Hairdresser! Available online: https://prtimes.jp/main/html/rd/p/000000484.000024101.html (accessed on 15 May 2022).
44. Kuo, F.L.; Yang, P.H.; Hsu, H.T.; Su, C.Y.; Chen, C.H.; Yeh, I.J.; Wu, Y.H.; Chen, L.C. Survey on perceived work stress and its influencing factors among hospital staff during the COVID-19 pandemic in Taiwan. *Kaohsiung J. Med. Sci.* **2020**, *36*, 944–952. [CrossRef]
45. Sargent, P. *Real Man or Real Teacher?: Contradictions in the Lives of Men Elementary School Teachers*; Men's Studies Press: Harriman, NY, USA, 2001; p. 248.

46. Ji, Y.; Wang, D.; Riedl, M. Analysis of the correlation between occupational stress and mental health of primary and secondary school teachers. *Work* **2021**, *69*, 599–611. [CrossRef]
47. Halladay, J.; Bennett, K.; Weist, M.; Boyle, M.; Manion, I.; Campo, M.; Georgiades, K. Teacher–student relationships and mental health help seeking behaviors among elementary and secondary students in Ontario Canada. *J. Sch. Psychol.* **2020**, *81*, 1–10. [CrossRef]

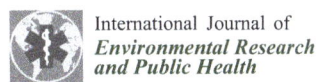

Article

The Control of Metabolic CO$_2$ in Public Transport as a Strategy to Reduce the Transmission of Respiratory Infectious Diseases

Marta Baselga [1], Juan J. Alba [1,2] and Alberto J. Schuhmacher [1,3,*]

1. Institute for Health Research Aragón (IIS Aragón), 50009 Zaragoza, Spain; mbaselga@iisaragon.es (M.B.); jjalba@unizar.es (J.J.A.)
2. Department of Mechanical Engineering, University of Zaragoza, 50018 Zaragoza, Spain
3. Fundación Agencia Aragonesa para la Investigación y el Desarrollo (ARAID), 500018 Zaragoza, Spain
* Correspondence: ajimenez@iisaragon.es

Abstract: The global acceptance of the SARS-CoV-2 airborne transmission led to prevention measures based on quality control and air renewal. Among them, carbon dioxide (CO$_2$) measurement has positioned itself as a cost-efficiency, reliable, and straightforward method to assess indoor air renewal indirectly. Through the control of CO$_2$, it is possible to implement and validate the effectiveness of prevention measures to reduce the risk of contagion of respiratory diseases by aerosols. Thanks to the method scalability, CO$_2$ measurement has become the gold standard for diagnosing air quality in shared spaces. Even though collective transport is considered one of the environments with the highest rate of COVID-19 propagation, little research has been done where the air inside vehicles is analyzed. This work explores the generation and accumulation of metabolic CO$_2$ in a tramway (Zaragoza, Spain) operation. Importantly, we propose to use the indicator ppm/person as a basis for comparing environments under different conditions. Our study concludes with an experimental evaluation of the benefit of modifying some parameters of the Heating–Ventilation–Air conditioning (HVAC) system. The study of the particle retention efficiency of the implemented filters shows a poor air cleaning performance that, at present, can be counteracted by opening windows. Seeking a post-pandemic scenario, it will be crucial to seek strategies to improve air quality in public transport to prevent the transmission of infectious diseases.

Keywords: airborne; CO$_2$; collective transport; SARS-CoV-2; tramway; filtration; infectious diseases; epidemiology; public health; COVID-19

Citation: Baselga, M.; Alba, J.J.; Schuhmacher, A.J. The Control of Metabolic CO$_2$ in Public Transport as a Strategy to Reduce the Transmission of Respiratory Infectious Diseases. *Int. J. Environ. Res. Public Health* **2022**, *19*, 6605. https://doi.org/10.3390/ijerph19116605

Academic Editors: Sachiko Kodera and Essam A. Rashed

Received: 26 April 2022
Accepted: 27 May 2022
Published: 28 May 2022

Publisher's Note: MDPI stays neutral with regard to jurisdictional claims in published maps and institutional affiliations.

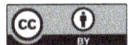

Copyright: © 2022 by the authors. Licensee MDPI, Basel, Switzerland. This article is an open access article distributed under the terms and conditions of the Creative Commons Attribution (CC BY) license (https://creativecommons.org/licenses/by/4.0/).

1. Introduction

Public health strategies are modulated by adjusting to the development of knowledge about the transmission routes of COVID-19. The viral transmission of SARS-CoV-2 human–human has been described from direct respiratory dissemination and indirect dissemination. On the one hand, direct respiratory dissemination, where the symptomatic or asymptomatic patient expels contaminated particles in respiratory events, and, on the other hand, indirect dissemination or via fomites, where transmission is due to contact with contaminated surfaces. On the other hand, it is possible to differentiate between the droplet and bioaerosol models with indirect dissemination. While droplets predominate in close contact, bioaerosols can be transmitted through the air over time and distance [1]. Regarding this pandemic, the scientific community has redefined the concept of bioaerosol, extending its consideration to airborne particles smaller than 100 μm, based on evidence and common factors related to the aerodynamics of the particles [1,2]. The spread patterns of SARS-CoV-2 could not be explained by traditional epidemic models, where homogeneity in the transmission is assumed [3]. As recognized by the WHO in April 2021 [4], a predominance airborne way has been suggested compared to other propagation models [1,5].

The size of the SARS-CoV-2 virion varies between 70 and 90 nanometers [6,7], and an average concentration of the virus in the sputum of 7.0×10^6 copies/mL and a maximum of

2.35×10^9 copies/mL [8]. Consequently, the viral load occupies 2.14×10^6% del bioaerosol on average. With this value, Lee [9] estimated a theoretical minimum and initial aerosol size of 4.7 µm to contain SARS-CoV-2. However, experimental bioaerosol sampling studies suggest the presence of the virus in smaller particle sizes (even < 0.25 µm) [10–13]. Despite numerous factors influencing the airborne transmission of pathogens, such as dynamics or their aerial persistence, contagion events can only be explained by a medium and long-distance airborne transmission model [5]—for example, among small animals [14,15], from viral superspreading events [16], in the long-distance transmission where infected individuals do not come into contact direct [17], by asymptomatic individuals transmission rates [18], and by the prevalence of spread in closed spaces [19]. Specifically, a superspreading event affected public transportation. Shen et al. [20] reported a massive infection of 24/68 (35.3%) people from a single infected individual while being transported in a bus with air recirculation and poor ventilation.

At the pandemic's beginning, this route of contagion was dismissed, and more attention was paid to contagion by droplets and fomites. Consequently, there was controversy about whether asymptomatic infected individuals could be transmitters of SARS-CoV-2. However, currently, it has been estimated that 44% (CI95; 30–57%) of secondary cases were infected during the incubation period [21], where the individuals were asymptomatic. The global acceptance of the COVID-19 airborne spread allowed an improvement in the preventive methods, including new techniques for epidemiological management, such as the measurement of exhaled carbon dioxide (CO_2) as an indicator of the risk of contagion [2,22].

Carbon dioxide measurement began to be used in the 19th century to design ventilation systems in architecture [23]. In the pre-pandemic period, CO_2 measurement helped improve academic performance in schools and colleges [24] and, sporadically, control infectious diseases [25]. Due to the COVID-19 pandemic, CO_2 measurement has become one of the preferred preventive strategies to reduce the risk of contagion by aerosols [22,26,27]. The direct measurement of aerosols to determine the risk of contagion by SARS-CoV-2 is highly complex and expensive since it requires highly specialized equipment. While there are handheld instruments or simple sensors to direct measure of aerosol concentrations, these instruments present different limitations such as they can not discriminate human-exhaled versus environmental aerosols; usually, they cover a limited range of particle diameter and hardly measure the submicronic particles. To overcome these hurdles, the CO_2 level has been suggested as an indirect indicator of respiratory infectious diseases' transmission [22]. CO_2 is co-expired with bioaerosols that may contain SARS-CoV-2 in infected people [28–30]. Its quantification provides an idea of indoor air renewal and establishes the risk of infection as it depends on the viral load [31]. Consequently, the measurement of indoor CO_2 is suggested as a reasonable ventilation proxy for respiratory infectious disease. Through its reading, it is possible to determine what percentage of the air has been exhaled by another individual (y) according to the expression $y = C_e\, x + C_a(1 - x)$, where C_e corresponds to the concentration of CO_2 in exhaled air (estimated at 40,000 ppm), C_a to ambient CO_2 concentration, and x to the fraction of exhaled air. For example, if we assume a basal value is 440 ppm (fresh air outdoors), a group of people manages to increase it to 2300 ppm. In that case, the approximate percentage of air that those individuals have already breathed will be around 4.7%.

Despite the ventilation rates being known to influence the concentration of microorganisms in the environment [32], the increase in the exhalation rate of aerosols depending on CO_2 has been poorly explored [30]. The concentration of airborne particles and the level of CO_2 cannot be directly related due to a disparity between the bioaerosols generated and the respiratory activity [28]. For example, aerosol generation during forced vocalization or coughing is not comparable to emission rates during respiration [33]. Thus, two different scenarios (for example, a library versus a gym) with similar CO_2 levels have to be interpreted individually.

To date, COVID-19 superspreading events have been reported indoors [34–40]. Thus, the use of air renewal proxy indoors is crucial for maintaining spaces with a low risk of contagion by aerosols. Many countries are making high economic investments to equip schools with CO_2 meters [41,42]. In addition, other isolated initiatives have successfully implemented this methodology in shopping centers [43], collective transport [44–46], offices [47], or university and school classrooms [47–52]. Specifically, a recent study in Italy reported an 82% reduction in secondary COVID-19 infections in schools where they controlled air renewal from CO_2 measurements [53].

Currently, CO_2 concentration limits have been proposed as a reference to minimize COVID-19 spreading. Usually, it is set between 700 and 1000 ppm regardless of the event [54,55]. Urban collective transport is one of the policies designed to promote sustainable cities [56]. To prevent respiratory infectious diseases spread, it is important to analyze the risk involved in every specific means of transport. References on the emission of bioaerosols in collective transport are scarce despite being the environment with the second-highest transmission rate of SARS-CoV-2. Lan et al. [57] point to 18% of cases in the transport sector, only behind the health sector (22%) in the transmission rate of COVID-19 disease. Before the pandemic, some reports pointed to metabolic CO_2 concentrations of up to 3700 ppm in buses [58–61], suggesting poor air renewal. However, due to the pandemic, it has been possible to reduce it to <800 ppm by implementing simple ventilation measures [45]. The operating conditions of the subways require reinforcement of artificial ventilation, for which values close to 1000 ppm have been found [44,62,63].

Trams have similar characteristics to buses since they circulate outside, and the contribution of natural ventilation can substantially favor air renewal. However, no specific information on air quality in trams has been reported. This work evaluates the accumulation of metabolic CO_2 in the Zaragoza Tram (Spain) in circulation under different conditions. On the one hand, the objective was to analyze the concentration of CO_2 in different events (e.g., weekend versus midweek, with and without air recirculation or with different weather conditions). To compare air renewal regardless of the event, the ppm/person indicator was used. However, secondary air purification methods that affect contagion risk, such as added air filtration, must also be considered. Then, the performance of the installed filtration system is analyzed against the concentration of submicron aerosols (such as the airborne virus SARS-CoV-2). The work concludes with suggestions for measuring CO_2 and recommendations to reduce the risk of contagion in collective transport.

2. Materials and Methods

2.1. Measurement of Metabolic CO_2

The metabolic CO_2 level was measured using Aranet 4 Pro meters (Aranet Wireless Solutions España SL, Madrid, Spain), with technical characteristics shown in Table 1. The increase in CO_2 (ΔCO_2) was determined according to Equation (1):

$$\Delta CO_2 = CO_{2,indoors} - CO_{2,outdoors} \qquad (1)$$

Table 1. Technical characteristics of the Aranet 4 Pro meters.

Parameters measured	CO_2	<9999 ppm
	Temperature	0–50 °C
	Relative humidity	0–85%
	Atmospheric pressure	0.3–1.1 atm
Sensor type	N-DIR (Non-Dispersive Infrarred)	
Communication technology	Bluetooth (−12–4 dBm)	
Sampling frequency	1 min	
Precision	±50 ppm (CO_2)	
Dimensions/Weight	70 × 70 × 24 mm/104 g	

The Urbos 3 tram models (CAF, Beasain ES) have a total length of 33 m, a width of 2.65 m, and a height of 3.2 m. They have a capacity of 200 seats, of which 54 are seats. Travelers wore a mask at all times, and the windows remained partially open during all routes. Eight CO_2 meters were installed at a 2.25 m height at different points of the Tram, according to the distribution of Figure 1a. The objective was to obtain realistic and uniform measurements, representative of the level of exposure experienced by an average user without running the risk that the measurement would be altered due to the direct exhalation of the passengers. As shown in Figure 1b, the meters were installed on grab bars, for which it was necessary to manufacture anti-vandal housings with holes to guarantee air transfer.

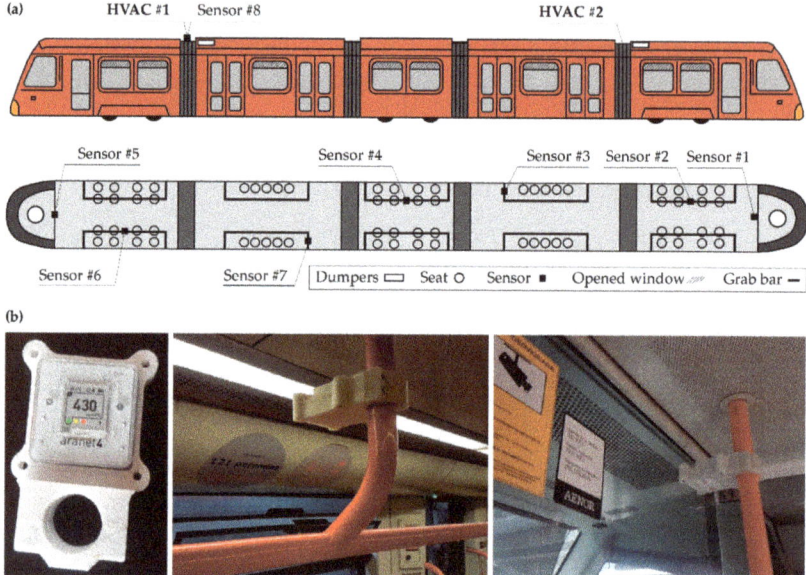

Figure 1. Schematic representation (**a**) of the meters distribution in the Tram and (**b**) installed sensors in the Tram. Where, # refers to the meter ID.

2.2. Probability of Contagion Determination by the CO_2 Level

The CO_2 measurement was used as a tool to determine the risk of contagion. This was possible thanks to the theoretical model updated by Peng and Jiménez [22] and the Aireamos consortium [31].

The risk of airborne indoors transmission (for one person in one hour) P was described from an alternative equation to that of Wells–Riley [64] (Equation (2)), enunciated by Rudnick et al. [65] (Equation (3)):

$$P = 1 - e^{-n} \qquad (2)$$

$$P = 1 - \exp\left(\frac{Itqf}{n}\right) R \qquad (3)$$

where I is the number of infected people in a space, t is the exposure time measured in hours, q is the number of pathogens spread per hour, f is the fraction re-inhaled ($[C - C_0]/C_a$), n is the number of people exposed to the infectious individual, and R is the particle retention efficiency, that is, the fraction of retained aerosols by the PPE from the exposed individual. In turn, C is the concentration of CO_2 indoors, C_0 outside, and C_a the concentration exhaled during respiration, defined in parts per million (ppm). The value of n corresponds to the infectious dose inhaled by a susceptible person. However, Rudnick et al. [65] assumed some conditions for the model's description: (1) the indoor air is thoroughly mixed, so the infectious aerosol generated can be found anywhere in the space. (2) The external concentration of CO_2 remains constant during the event. (3) Removal of viral aerosols due to virus survival, filtration, or other mechanisms is negligible compared to ventilation.

Peng and Jiménez [22] applied another alternative to the Wells–Riley formulation regarding the COVID-19 pandemic. The authors derived analytical expressions for the probability of infection indoors through the concentration of CO_2. The expected value of $\langle n \rangle$ can be calculated for an uninfected person, assuming the probability that the individual is immune η_{in} according to Equation (4):

$$\langle n \rangle = (1 - \eta_{in}) C_p B D (1 - m_{in}) \tag{4}$$

where C_p corresponds to the average number of viruses (quantos.m^3), B to the respiratory rate of the susceptible person (m^3 h^{-1}) that will vary depending on the activity carried out at that time, D the event duration (h), and m_{in} the filtration efficiency of the mask during inhalation. Consequently, assuming no pre-existence of viral aerosols before the event, the analytical expression for the expected value of C_p can be described by Equation (5):

$$C_p = \frac{\eta_{in}(N-1)E_p(1-m_{ex})}{V}\left(\frac{1}{\lambda} - \frac{1-e^{-\lambda D}}{\lambda^2 D}\right) \tag{5}$$

where N is the number of occupants, E_p is the exhalation rate of SARS-CoV-2 per infected person (quantos.h^{-1}), m_{ex} is the filtration efficiency of the mask during exhalation, V is the volume of air in the space (m^3), and λ the global rate constant of virus infectivity loss (h^{-1}), including all those mechanisms that may affect virus survival (filtration, ventilation, etc.). Assuming that the increase in CO_2 (ΔCO_2) of the indoor air concerning that of the outdoor air is only produced by human activity, it can be described as follows (Equation (6)):

$$n_{\Delta CO2} = \Delta C_{p.CO2} B D \tag{6}$$

where the CO_2 increment volume and the CO_2 exhalation rate per person mixing ratio (ΔCO_2), in m^3.h^{-1}, can be described as (Equation (7)), where λ_0 corresponds at ventilation rate (h^{-1}):

$$\Delta C_{p.CO2} = \frac{N E_{p.CO2}}{V}\left(\frac{1}{\lambda_0} - \frac{1-e^{-\lambda_0 D}}{\lambda_0^2 D}\right) \tag{7}$$

As a result of this model, Peng and Jiménez [22] propose an acceptable probability of infection limit of $p = 0.01\%$. Although it does not imply safety in any situation, since with high N and/or D and/or the event occurs many times, the probability of infection for the susceptible person is understated.

2.3. Studied Routes of the Zaragoza Tram

Eighty-eight round trips (44 complete trips) with an average of ~40 min each were analyzed. As shown in Figure 2, each complete path stops at 42 stations. The routes included in stations #7–#10/#33–#36, and #10–#16/#27–#33 correspond to the university area and the city center, respectively.

The CO_2 meters were installed for three months in the vehicle. We hypothesized that the variation in the meteorological data obtained during the study days could translate into variations in the Tram's ventilation capacity. The variables of interest for five reference days of December 2020 are shown in Table 2. According to data provided by the Zaragoza weather station, the average wind speed value in December was 3.25 ($\pm$1.65) m/s, so it can be considered that on days B, C, and D, the values of wind speed and maximum gusts were low. Low wind speed was an unfavorable condition for the natural ventilation of the Tram.

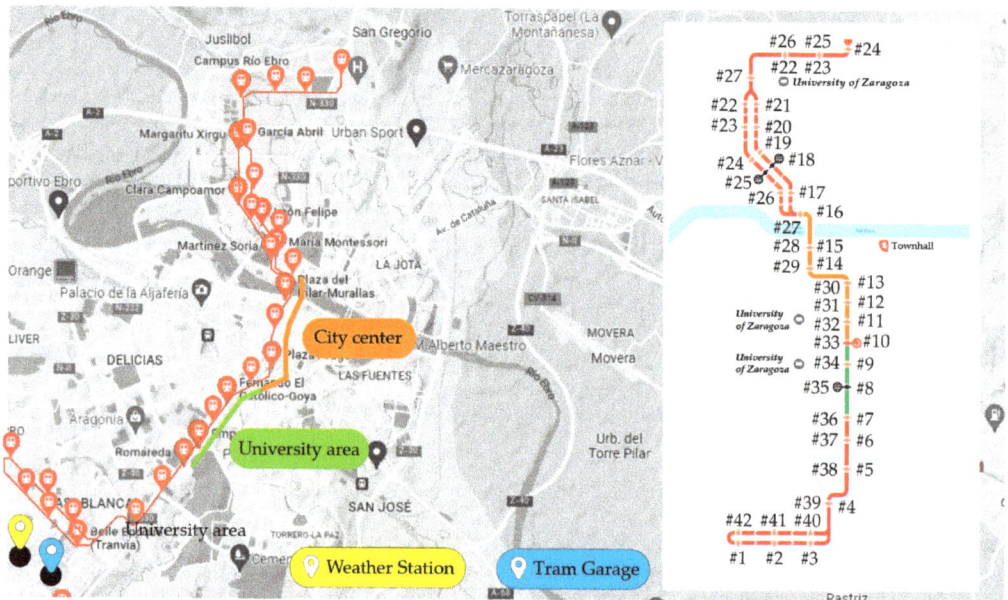

Figure 2. Route of the Zaragoza Tram. Where, # refers to the station ID.

Table 2. Meteorological variables of the reference days A, B, C, D, and E. Information prepared by the Agencia Estatal de Meteorología of Spain (data collected at the Valdespartera Station, Zaragoza Spain, 23 December 2020).

Day	T_{aver}	T_{min}	T_{max}	D_w	$W_{s,aver}$	$W_{s,max}$	P_{max}	P_{min}
A	9.6 °C	6.1 °C	13.1 °C	30°	3.1 m/s	8.9 m/s	996.8 atm	990.0 atm
B	8.2 °C	4.4 °C	11.9 °C	16°	1.7 m/s	6.1 m/s	996.8 atm	990.0 atm
C	5.4 °C	3.3 °C	7.4 °C	10°	1.9 m/s	5.0 m/s	998.2 atm	996.0 atm
D	7.9 °C	3.8 °C	12.0 °C	16°	1.9 m/s	5.6 m/s	994.7 atm	990.8 atm
E	8.9 °C	6.2 °C	11.6 °C	31°	4.7 m/s	11.1 m/s	994.9 atm	992.4 atm

T_{aver}: temperature (average); T_{min}: temperature (minimum); T_{max}: temperature (maximum); D_W: wind direction; $W_{s,aver}$: wind speed (average); $W_{s,max}$: wind speed (maximum); P_{max}: atmospheric pressure (maximum); and P_{min}: atmospheric pressure (minimum).

2.4. Determination of Filtration Efficiency against Submicron Particles and Filters' Pressure Drop

The filter's performance was studied in-vitro to assess its effectiveness against submicron particle sizes, as is the case with the SARS-CoV-2 virus and other respiratory viruses. The filter used during the tests was specially implemented due to the current COVID-19 pandemic (Coarse 75% according to UNE-EN ISO 16890, Merak Long Life Filter, Madrid SP). As depicted in Figure 1, two filters were arranged in two HVAC units installed in the Tram, which drive a total flow of 2800–3300 m^3/h, with an air ratio of 1:3 fresh/return air.

As shown in Figure 3a, NaCl aerosols were produced using a Topas-ATM226 generator with a saline solution of sodium chloride (3 wt.% NaCl in distilled water). Microdroplets were evaporated using a tubular silica air dryer to produce solid particles. The particle size distribution (Figure 3b) inside the cabin was measured using an SMPS TSI 3936 composed of an electrostatic classifier (DMA TSI 3081) and a condensation particle counter (CPC TSI 3782). An 0.6 L/min flow rate drags the particles. The filter was placed between bronze discs sealed with Teflon tape, with 30 × 20 mm Teflon washers on each side. The desired flow rate was adjusted variating the exposed filter area (2.05, 4.1, and 8.1 mm). The measurements lasted 120 s and were made in duplicate. Measurements were made passing through a free tube between measurements to calculate relative efficiency according to Equation (8), where C_{up} stands for concentration upstream and C_{down} stands for concentration downstream. The retention efficiency is expressed in global efficiency as 'global number of particles':

$$\eta = 100 \times \frac{C_{up} - C_{down}}{C_{up}} \quad (8)$$

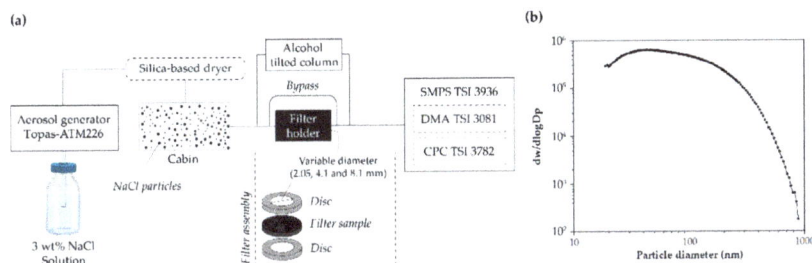

Figure 3. Performance test. (**a**) Diagram of the equipment used to characterize the filters and (**b**) particle concentration distribution for efficiency determination measurements in the range 0.1–1.0 µm.

According to Bernoulli's principle, the pressure drop was carried out using alcohol columns connected to the free ends of the tubes. Measurements were also made with a 0.6 L/min volumetric flow rate.

2.5. Statistic Analysis

The statistical analysis of the data has been carried out using the R-UCA v.4.0.2 software (University of Cadiz Spain, 2017) [66]. Mean comparisons were made with the Student's *t*-test at a 99% confidence interval (CI99).

3. Results

3.1. CO_2 Levels along the Route Are Closely Related to Occupancy

As shown in Figure 4a,b, the increase in the CO_2 concentration inside the Tram gradually increases as it approaches the city's downtown area #33–#36 and #27–#33 stations; approximately, at minutes 20 and 70 on the outward and return routes, respectively. The CO_2 increase corresponds to the difference between the Tram indoor values concerning the external reference value (atmospheric) registered with sensor #8. Analyzing the increment makes it possible to determine the global CO_2 concentration corresponding to metabolic CO_2 to rule out possible external contamination. The calculated ppm/person ratio (Figure 4c) suggests a concentration of ΔCO_2 in the final areas of the route associated with an accumulation of CO_2 in the vehicle, which begins to be evident after driving through the city center. It may be explained because the number of travelers increases in the city center and accumulates CO_2 not recirculated at subsequent stops. On average, the Tram doors open for 16.6 ± 3.6 s at each stop.

ΔCO_2 concentration is closely related to tram occupancy (Figure 5a), although there is some dispersion associated with external variables (Figure 5b). In absolute CO_2 values, the maximum average was 835 ± 232 ppm, reaching a maximum value of 1229 ppm. In contrast, the lowest average was 541 ± 82 ppm. The pattern of ΔCO_2 concentration on weekdays compared to weekend days is different, although it follows similar trends. As shown in Tables S1 and S2, the average of the trips made on weekends in the morning was 565 ± 318 ppm; in the afternoon, it was 580 ± 323 ppm, and, at night, it was 602 ± 330 ppm. On weekdays, an average of 592 ± 319 ppm was obtained in the morning, 595 ± 324 ppm in the afternoon, and 541 ± 292 ppm at night.

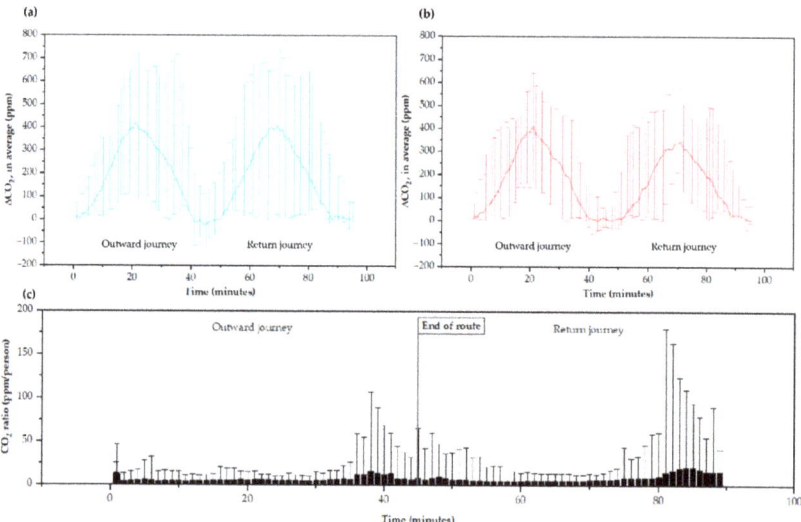

Figure 4. CO_2 increment average levels (**a**) in all weekday and (**b**) in all weekend routes, and (**c**) ppm/person ratio average and maximum gap along routes. The error bars in (**a**,**b**) correspond to the difference between the maximum/minimum data and the average data of all studied routes.

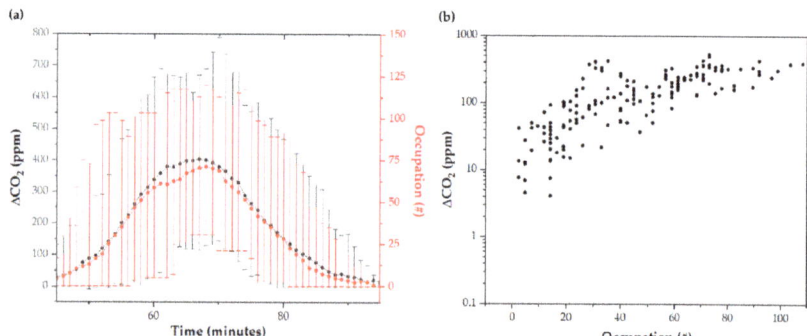

Figure 5. ΔCO_2 increment and tram occupancy as (**a**) a function of time, and as (**b**) a function of tram occupancy. The error bars correspond to the difference between the maximum/minimum data and the average data of all the studied routes.

3.2. CO_2 Levels Distribution Is Similar at Different Points Inside the Tram

ΔCO_2 dispersion measurements at the different points of the Tram were assessed using the records from each sensor, as shown in Figure 6. Passenger occupancy is rarely uniform along the Tram, and differences in the capacity distribution can lead to spatially disparate values. The average Relative Standard Deviation (RSD) was determined to determine the homogeneity of the CO_2 distribution in the Tram. The RSD of 0.09 ± 0.02 suggested that the measurements were relatively homogeneous, although accumulation tendencies are typically observed in the central area of the Tram.

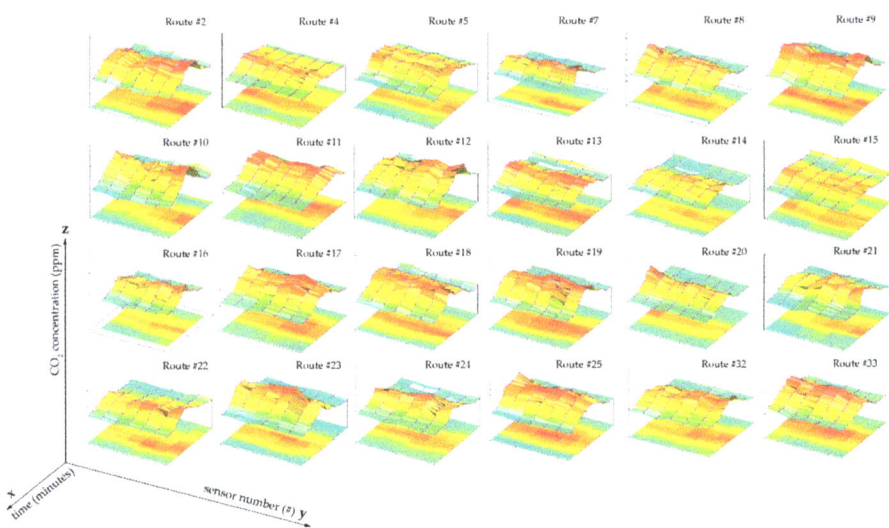

Figure 6. Distribution of ΔCO_2 in the Tram (z-axis) as a function of time (x-axis) and ΔCO_2 measures (y-axis) on routes #2, #4–#25, and #32–#33, where there is homogeneity in the CO_2 measurement along the tram and a strong relationship with occupancy.

3.3. Improving the Air Renewal by the Closing of the Air Return

To study the influence of the return of air from inside the Tram to the air conditioning equipment, we worked with the data obtained through Sensors #3 and #7, located just below the grilles of the air return ducts. Days C and D were selected as a reference for the study due to the similarity between meteorological variables. The ΔCO_2 varies when the air return is closed, as deduced in Figure 7. From the analyses carried out, the extreme values at the beginning and end of the route corresponding to the accumulation of gas in the Tram have been removed, offering a more realistic view of the internal atmosphere during the tour. Under these conditions, the average ppm/person rate without return was 3.5 ± 0.1 (Sensor #3) and 5.1 ± 0.1 ppm (Sensor #7) without air return, and 4.9 ± 0.7 (Sensor #3) and 6.0 ± 0.4 (Sensor #7) with air return. A reduction in ΔCO_2 between 9% and 36% can be seen concerning air return ΔCO_2 levels.

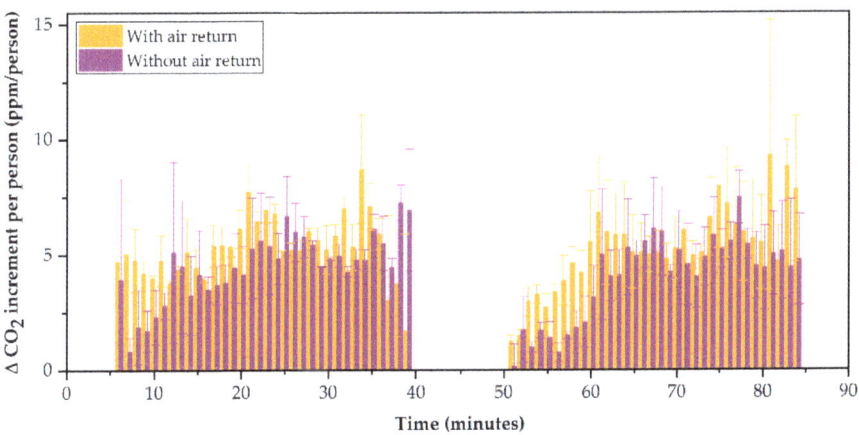

Figure 7. Registered ppm/person values depending on the air return.

3.4. Wind Speed Contributes to Increasing Ventilation Rates

The days were divided depending on the wind speed into Set A (Day A and E) and Set B (Day B to D). Sets were made to assess whether the weather plays a crucial role in the ventilation. The objective of this section is to compare the ventilation pattern on days with different weather, with special attention to the average wind and gusts and the average temperature. The average weather conditions of interest for the days of each Set are shown in Table 3. In Set A, the average wind speed was 3.9 ± 1.1 m/s, while, in Set B, it was 1.8 ± 0.1 m/s, with maximum gusts of 10.0 ± 1.6 m/s and 5.6 ± 0.6 m/s, respectively. Figure 8a,b represent the ppm/person index for Set A and Set B, respectively. In addition, 88.4% of the ppm/person indices was higher in Set B than Set A. It was found that the means of the data from Set B were significantly lower than those from Set A using a hypothesis contrast (CI99; −3.26−−1.38). Limits are harmful in the CI, confirming that higher data on Set A. A Student's t-test shows that the average ΔCO_2 concentration increases on days with lower wind speeds are higher. However, the difference between the ppm/person index in Set B compared to Set A is 2.3 ± 3.3 ppm, compared to averages of 5.2 ± 3.7 ppm (Set A) and 7.5 ± 3.0 ppm (Set B), which represents a reduction of between 31 and 44%. These data suggest that the weather can substantially affect the recirculation of air inside the Tram, as shown in Figure 8.

Table 3. Meteorological variables of the reference Sets A and B. Information prepared by the Agencia Estatal de Meteorología of Spain (data collected at the Valdespartera Station, Zaragoza Spain, 23 December 2020).

Day	T_{aver}	T_{min}	T_{max}	D_w	$W_{s,aver}$	$W_{s,max}$
Set A	9.6 ± 0.5 °C	6.1 °C	13.1 °C	30 ± 0.5°	3.9 ± 1.1 m/s	11.1 m/s
Set B	7.2 ± 1.5 °C	3.3 °C	12.0 °C	14 ± 3.5°	1.8 ± 0.1 m/s	6.1 m/s

T_{aver}: temperature (average); T_{min}: temperature (minimum); T_{max}: temperature (maximum); D_W: wind direction; $W_{s,aver}$: wind speed (average) and; $W_{s,max}$: wind speed (maximum).

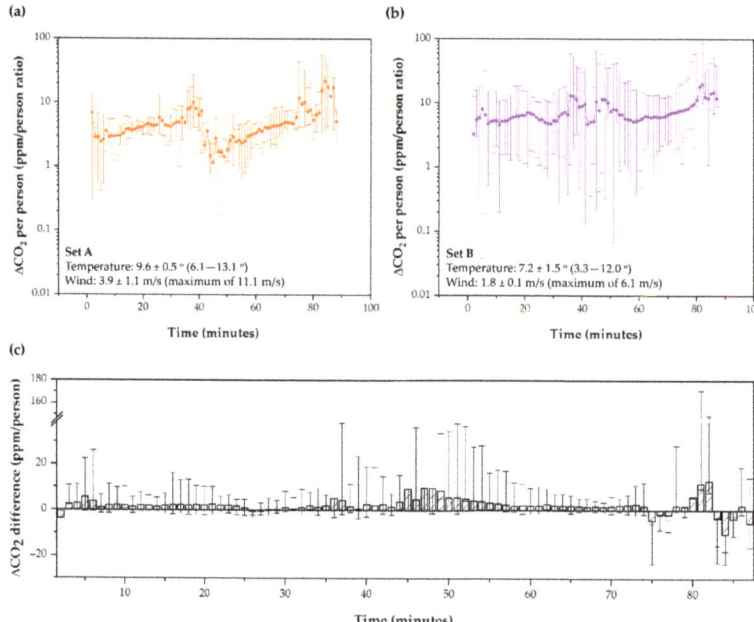

Figure 8. ΔCO_2 per person ratio (ppm/person) in (**a**) Set A, and in (**b**) Set B depending on time; (**c**) difference between Set B and Set A depending on time.

3.5. Tram Speed Does Not Influence the Indoor Ventilation Rate

Tram speed while circulating did not seem to have a substantial effect on the reduction of ΔCO_2 (Figure 9a), nor on the average reduction rate of ΔCO_2 at 3 min (Figure 9b). The Student's t-test showed no significant relationship between the rate of reduction of ΔCO_2 compared to two different speed ranges: 1–20 km/h and 21–40 km/h. It may be due to the flow of the HVAC system, which generates internal drafts so that the inflow of air through the window does not alter the ventilation rates substantially.

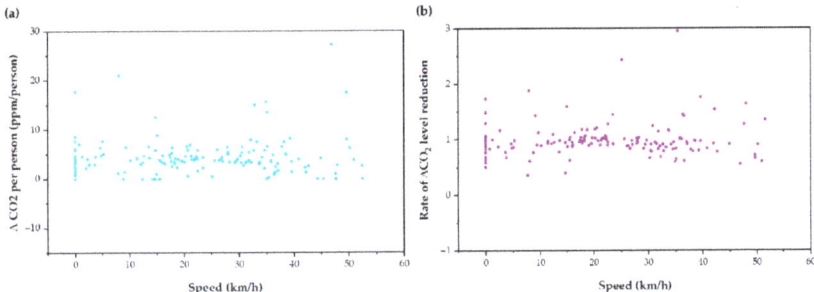

Figure 9. CO_2 measurements depending on Tram speed. (**a**) ΔCO_2 per person ratio, and (**b**) average reduction rate of ΔCO_2 depending on the Tram speed.

3.6. The Filtration System Is Not Efficient against Submicron Matter

The tests have been carried out with the filter usually installed on the Tram (Coarse 75% Filter Media). However, the Coarse 75% filter specially implemented due to the current COVID-19 pandemic has been characterized in the laboratory. The Air Changes per Hour (ACH) of the Zaragoza Tram remained in the unit's regular operation at 25 ACH. As shown in Figure 10, the Coarse 75% filter presented an approximate retention efficiency of 27.9% for 300 nm particles at a flow rate of ~2500 m^3/h. The filtering efficiency decreases up to 2.4 and 2.3% using ~162 and ~622 m^3/h, respectively. The largest particles present more inertia at high flow rates [67,68], resulting in a higher retention rate in the filter medium. Even though the clogging of NaCl particles observed in the head loss tests may have overestimated these results, which could be seen as an increase up to 440 Pascals of pressure drop (Table 4), this flow would be the most representative of the working conditions in the HVAC of the Tram system.

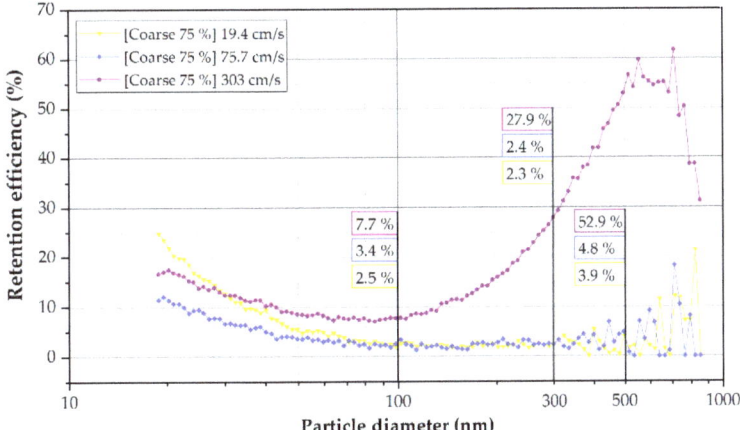

Figure 10. Coarse 75% filter retention efficiency depending on the particle diameter at different speeds (flow rates).

Table 4. Conditions used in the filtration tests and pressure drop determination.

Area	Flow Rate	Velocity in Filter	Pressure Drop
2281.6 cm^2	~161.8 m^3/h	19.4 cm/s	6 Pa
2281.6 cm^2	~621.8 m^3/h	75.7 cm/s	34 Pa
2281.6 cm^2	~2488.8 m^3/h	303.0 cm/s	440 Pa

3.7. Probability of Infection

The probability of infection and the attack rate were calculated following the models proposed by Peng and Jiménez [22] and Aireamos [31]. Based on the average daily CO_2 values collected in Tables S1 and S2, an attack rate of 0.06% was determined in the least favorable case (higher CO_2 values) and an attack rate of 0.04% in the average case (global average CO_2). According to Peng et Jiménez's proposal, the probability of contagion <0.01% is acceptable, so the Tramway did not represent a high risk of contagion under the conditions studied, as shown in Table 5.

Table 5. Determination of the infection probability and attack rate by aerosols in two different scenarios simulates the Tram's ventilation conditions, using Covid Risk Airborne [31] based on the model Wells–Riley [64].

Scenario	Facemask	Occupation	Exposure Time	CO$_2$ Level	Variant	p	Attack Rate
#1 (global average)	Surgical mask	60 pax	10 min	689 ppm (average)/1038 ppm (max)	Omicron	0.01% *	0.04% *
#2 (maximum average)	Surgical mask	60 pax	10 min	810 ppm (average)/1520 ppm (max)	Omicron	0.01% *	0.06% *

* Considering a 78% vaccination with a proportionate immunity of 70%; a cumulative incidence (CI) of 1150 to 14 days/100,000 hab.

4. Discussion

SARS-CoV-2 bioaerosols dissemination in infected individuals' exhalation is widely demonstrated [69–71]. In addition, the virus's presence and persistence in the environmental air have also been extensively studied [10,11,72–78]. Given the apparent predominance of the airborne route of transmission of COVID-19, various strategies have been investigated to mitigate the risk of contagion. Public transport environments represent the second sector with the highest transmission of SARS-CoV-2, only behind the health sector [57]. However, computational studies point to a 1.5–1.6% attack rate [79,80]. Even though numerous works have been aimed at evaluating the behavior of bioaerosols in collective transport by computational fluid dynamics [81–85], extrapolation to actual conditions is an enormous limitation. One of the strategies that allow the indoor ventilation rate to be quantified in situ is the measurement of CO_2, which has positioned itself as a standard for air control [22,86,87].

In this work, CO_2 measurements were collected in 88 round trips, which is equivalent to more than 79,200 records obtained from eight sensors strategically distributed in the Tram. The distribution of CO_2 throughout the vehicle follows a similar trend (RSD 0.09 ± 0.02), so the location of the HVAC systems and natural air intakes seem to favor all points of the Tram equally. The average absolute CO_2 of all the routes studied was 685 ± 59 ppm (572 ± 75 ppm–835 ± 232 ppm). This value suggests that the percentage of air already breathed is <0.7%. Considering the virus emission rates in exhaled breath [71,88], average time spent in the Tram (~7 min), and the mandatory use of facemasks, the interior of the vehicle does not represent a risk space of contagion by aerosols (probability of infection [22], $p = 0.01\%$; attack rate < 0.1%) in the most unfavorable scenario (844 ppm average; 1571 ppm maximum). In this sense, Moreno et al. [78] reported attack rates between 0.00–0.72% in buses depending on the respiratory activity, bus air conditions, and the infected individual without a mask. Thus, the environment of the bus at that time was more dangerous.

Before the pandemic, some reports pointed to metabolic CO_2 concentrations of up to 3700 ppm in buses [58–61]. However, a study on the bus in Barcelona (Spain) points to concentrations close to 1000 ppm that can be easily reduced to <800 ppm by implementing simple ventilation measures (i.e., opening windows) [45]. The operating subways conditions require a reinforcement of artificial ventilation, for which values close to 1000 ppm have been found [62,63].

In this paper, we propose using ppm/person indicator as a measure that allows ΔCO_2 levels comparison on different days and circumstances. A key aspect and an obvious one is the increase in ΔCO_2 as the number of passengers increases. Analyzing the ΔCO_2 data measurements, a gradual increase in CO_2 concentration could be misinterpreted as an accumulation. However, looking at the ppm/person ratio, it can be seen that the increase in ΔCO_2 comes from an increase in capacity.

Trams are typically similar to buses since they circulate outside and substantially favor measures to reinforce natural ventilation. In this work, it was found that the speed of the external wind reduced the ppm/person rates to around 2.3 ± 3.3 ppm. Although it seems a slight benefit, it represents a reduction of between 31 and 44% compared to days with less wind. Closing the air return (total external air intake) favored ventilation, reducing the ΔCO_2 level between 9 and 36%. Tram speed did not affect ventilation rate, at least in two data sets with different speed ranges (2–20 km/h versus 20–40 km/h). However, the data could not be compared with the stopped Tram since the conditions were different at that moment. There are no sources of CO_2 generation (there are no passengers), and the doors open entirely, so the air is wholly recirculated in a few minutes.

Favoring natural ventilation (opening windows), the HVAC system, and the use of masks have been shown to significantly reduce the risk of transmission [30,79,84,89,90]. Masks reduce the bioaerosols emission variably, depending on the type of mask and the aerodynamics of the scattered particles [91–94]. In addition, HVAC systems should consider the filter, but it is also possible to optimize it to maintain adverse thermodynamic conditions for the virus [95,96].

One of the most significant limitations of CO_2 measurement is that its interpretation cannot be generalized but must be individualized. Aerosol generation fluctuates substantially depending on the individual's respiratory event [2,33,97–99]. In addition, environmental conditions directly influence the spread and persistence of the virus [2,100,101]. Therefore, it is not easy to define an effective viral load dependent on CO_2, at least in absolute terms. However, this and other studies demonstrate the effectiveness of CO_2 measurement to implement effective air renewal patterns and reduce the risk of transmission of infectious diseases.

5. Conclusions and Recommendations

This work suggests that the measurement of the ΔCO_2 concentration inside collective transport constitutes a cost-efficiency strategy that can reduce the rates of spread of the respiratory virus by aerosols, as is the case of the SARS-CoV-2 virus. In this work, the interpretation of the exhaled CO_2 levels per person (ppm/person) has made it possible to analyze the behavior of the air inside the Zaragoza Tram. Maintaining the typical parameters of the HVAC units and implementing the partial opening of the windows, the maximum CO_2 level was 1249 ppm. On average, 835 ± 232 ppm have not been exceeded on any of the routes studied, which indicates that air recirculation is adequate for vehicle occupancy. In addition, the absolute CO_2 in all the routes studied was 685 and 690 ± 59 ppm, on average and median, respectively. However, it must be considered that capacity was reduced on the studied days due to the COVID-19 pandemic restrictions. It presents a limitation when extrapolating the data to post-pandemic operating conditions. The passengers' exposure to the Tram air must also be considered since the average route usually lasts around 7 min, and passengers wear a mask and keep their distance when possible. Under the conditions studied, the following recommendations are suggested to reduce the risk of infection by aerosols and/or improve ventilation performance:

- Maximize outside air intake: by opening windows, increasing door openings in stations, and minimizing the rate of return air in HVAC units;
- Completely recirculate the air between outbound and return routes to avoid exposing new passengers to the air breathed by previous passengers;
- Consider implementing efficient filtration systems against particles (0.1–100 μm) instead of coarse-type filters, efficient against pollen or dust. Additionally to filtration systems, other air purification technologies can be beneficial in improving air quality. Even so, its performance needs to be demonstrated under operating conditions and not just in the laboratory or theoretically;
- Limit the respiratory activity of passengers to calm breathing and speech and the use of masks and other personal protection equipment and promote interpersonal distance.

In addition, from experience gathered during the CO_2 measurement experiments in public transport, the following recommendations can be drawn:

- Initially, characterizing the distribution of CO_2 inside the vehicle is essential so that the location of the sensors allows representative measurements of the space to be taken;
- Analyzing the increase in CO_2 instead of absolute CO_2 allows for quantifying only the CO_2 generated by passengers, discriminating external pollution. Additionally, we propose to use the ppm/person ratio as the main indicator to compare the exhaled CO_2 measurements on different scenarios. This ratio can be easily calculated by dividing the increase by the number of people. For example, if the increase in CO_2 is 500 and there are 50 people, the ratio will be 10 ppm/person. In case of studying two separate days, for example with different weather, we can find that one day the ratio is 10 ppm/person and another day it is 30 ppm/person. With this information, we can determine how the change of variables affects independently of the occupation.
- Place the gauges at a sufficient height to avoid the direct exhalation of the passengers. For example, they were placed 2.25 m above ground level for this work. Moreover, locating meters near doors and windows should avoid underestimating CO_2 levels.
- Evaluate weather conditions, especially airspeed, to interpret the measurement results on measurement days correctly. For example, in our study, the weather substantially affected the ventilation ratio inside the Tram. On the days with the greatest wind, ppm/person rates of up to 44% lower were recorded with respect to the days with the least wind.
- Recording occupancy levels (number of passengers) is essential to estimate the ventilation rate and to be able to compare data in different samples.
- Deduct the minimum number of meters to obtain representative measurements of the space. The heterogeneity in vehicle occupancy requires a consistent distribution of meters. For example, a meter was placed for every 35 m^3 of air in this work.
- Considering the respiratory activity of the vehicle occupants is desirable when normalizing the ppm/person rates. In addition, the CO_2 records must be individually interpreted depending on variables such as interpersonal distance, the use of masks or other PPE, and the implemented filtration systems (or other air purification devices).

Under the conditions studied, the Tram does not present itself as a space with a high risk of infection by aerosols (by using Aireamos Covid Risk Airborne tool [31]; see Section 3.7). Air quality monitoring began to gain popularity due to the COVID-19 pandemic. However, once the focus is on the air [2], a post-pandemic scenario presents uncertainty when the windows are completely closed and the capacity increases. Consequently, it will be necessary to implement a standard that allows air quality to be regulated in these post-pandemic conditions. The poor filtration performance against the submicronic matter of the typically implemented filters is a significant limitation. It is necessary to find new air control and purification strategies that reduce the risk of disease transmission in the future.

Supplementary Materials: The following supporting information can be downloaded at: https://www.mdpi.com/article/10.3390/ijerph19116605/s1, Table S1: Weekend journeys data analysis (from Friday evening to Sunday), and Table S2: Weekday journeys data analysis (from Monday to Friday evening).

Author Contributions: Conceptualization, M.B., J.J.A. and A.J.S.; Data curation, M.B.; Formal analysis, M.B., J.J.A. and A.J.S.; Investigation, M.B. and J.J.A.; Methodology, M.B. and A.J.S.; Project administration, J.J.A. and A.J.S.; Resources, J.J.A.; Supervision, A.J.S.; Writing—original draft, M.B., J.J.A. and A.J.S. All authors have read and agreed to the published version of the manuscript.

Funding: This research was funded by the Instituto de Investigación Sanitaria Aragón: Campaña Investiga COVID-19 (CoviBlock).

Acknowledgments: We would like to express our gratitude to "Los Tranvías de Zaragoza S.E.M." and "CAF Spain S.A." for supporting this research and its invaluable collaboration. We also would like to thank "Ayuntamiento de Zaragoza" and "Institute for Health Research Aragón" for the received support.

Conflicts of Interest: The authors declare that they have no known competing financial interests or personal relationships that could have appeared to influence the work reported in this paper.

References

1. Siegel, J.D.; Rhinehart, E.; Jackson, M.; Chiarello, L. Healthcare Infection Control Practices Advisory Committee 2007 Guideline for Isolation Precautions: Preventing Transmission of Infectious Agents in Healthcare Settings (Updated July 2019). *Cent. Diasease Control. Prev.* **2019**, *35*, S65–S164. [CrossRef]
2. Wang, C.C.; Prather, K.A.; Sznitman, J.; Jimenez, J.L.; Lakdawala, S.S.; Tufekci, Z.; Marr, L.C. Airborne Transmission of Respiratory Viruses. *Science* **2021**, *373*, eabd9149. [CrossRef] [PubMed]
3. Beldomenico, P.M. Do Superspreaders Generate New Superspreaders? A Hypothesis to Explain the Propagation Pattern of COVID-19. *Int. J. Infect. Dis.* **2020**, *96*, 19–22. [CrossRef]
4. Lewis, B.D. Why the WHO Took Two Years to Say COVID Is Airborne. *Nature* **2022**, *604*, 26–31. [CrossRef]
5. Greenhalgh, T.; Jimenez, J.L.; Prather, K.A.; Tufekci, Z.; Fisman, D.; Schooley, R. Ten Scientific Reasons in Support of Airborne Transmission of SARS-CoV-2. *Lancet* **2021**, *397*, 1603–1605. [CrossRef]
6. Kim, J.-M.; Chung, Y.-S.; Jo, H.J.; Lee, N.-J.; Kim, M.S.; Woo, S.H.; Park, S.; Kim, J.W.; Kim, H.M.; Han, M.-G. Article History: Identification of Coronavirus Isolated from a Patient in Korea with COVID-19 Osong Public Health and Research Perspectives. *Public Health Res. Perspect.* **2020**, *11*, 3–7. [CrossRef] [PubMed]
7. Park, W.B.; Kwon, N.J.; Choi, S.J.; Kang, C.K.; Choe, P.G.; Kim, J.Y.; Yun, J.; Lee, G.W.; Seong, M.W.; Kim, N.J.; et al. Virus Isolation from the First Patient with SARS-CoV-2 in Korea. *J. Korean Med. Sci.* **2020**, *35*, 10–14. [CrossRef]
8. Wölfel, R.; Corman, V.M.; Guggemos, W.; Seilmaier, M.; Zange, S.; Müller, M.A.; Niemeyer, D.; Jones, T.C.; Vollmar, P.; Rothe, C.; et al. Virological Assessment of Hospitalized Patients with COVID-2019. *Nature* **2020**, *581*, 465–469. [CrossRef]
9. Lee, B.U. Minimum Sizes of Respiratory Particles Carrying SARS-CoV-2 and the Possibility of Aerosol Generation. *Int. J. Environ. Res. Public Health* **2020**, *17*, 6960. [CrossRef]
10. Liu, Y.; Ning, Z.; Chen, Y.; Guo, M.; Liu, Y.; Gali, N.K.; Sun, L.; Duan, Y.; Cai, J.; Westerdahl, D.; et al. Aerodynamic Analysis of SARS-CoV-2 in Two Wuhan Hospitals. *Nature* **2020**, *582*, 557–560. [CrossRef]
11. Chia, P.Y.; Coleman, K.K.; Tan, Y.K.; Ong, S.W.X.; Gum, M.; Lau, S.K.; Lim, X.F.; Lim, A.S.; Sutjipto, S.; Lee, P.H.; et al. Detection of Air and Surface Contamination by SARS-CoV-2 in Hospital Rooms of Infected Patients. *Nat. Commun.* **2020**, *11*, 2800. [CrossRef] [PubMed]
12. Kenarkoohi, A.; Noorimotlagh, Z.; Falahi, S.; Amarloei, A.; Abbas, S. Hospital Indoor Air Quality Monitoring for the Detection of SARS-CoV-2 (COVID-19) Virus. *Sci. Total Environ.* **2020**, *748*, 141324. [CrossRef] [PubMed]
13. Stern, R.A.; Koutrakis, P.; Martins, M.A.G.; Lemos, B.; Dowd, S.E.; Sunderland, E.M.; Garshick, E. Characterization of Hospital Airborne SARS-CoV-2. *Respir. Res.* **2021**, *22*, 73. [CrossRef] [PubMed]
14. Kutter, J.S.; de Meulder, D.; Bestebroer, T.M.; Lexmond, P.; Mulders, A.; Richard, M.; Fouchier, R.A.M.; Herfst, S. SARS-CoV and SARS-CoV-2 Are Transmitted through the Air between Ferrets over More than One Meter Distance. *Nat. Commun.* **2021**, *12*, 1653. [CrossRef]
15. Shi, J.; Wen, Z.; Zhong, G.; Yang, H.; Wang, C.; Huang, B.; Liu, R.; He, X.; Shuai, L.; Sun, Z.; et al. Susceptibility of Ferrets, Cats, Dogs and Other Domesticated Animals to SARS-Coronavirus 2. *Science* **2020**, *368*, 1016–1020. [CrossRef] [PubMed]
16. Lewis, B.D. The Superspreading Problem. *Nature* **2021**, *950*, 544–548. [CrossRef] [PubMed]
17. Eichler, N.; Thornley, C.; Swadi, T.; Devine, T.; McElnay, C.; Sherwood, J.; Brunton, C.; Williamson, F.; Freeman, J.; Berger, S.; et al. Transmission of Severe Acute Respiratory Syndrome Coronavirus 2 during Border Quarantine and Air Travel, New Zealand (Aotearoa). *Emerg. Infect. Dis.* **2021**, *27*, 1274–1278. [CrossRef]

18. Johansson, M.A.; Quandelacy, T.M.; Kada, S.; Prasad, P.V.; Steele, M.; Brooks, J.T.; Slayton, R.B.; Biggerstaff, M.; Butler, J.C. SARS-CoV-2 Transmission from People without COVID-19 Symptoms. *JAMA Netw. Open* **2021**, *4*, e2035057. [CrossRef]
19. Bulfone, T.C.; Malekinejad, M.; Rutherford, G.W.; Razani, N. Outdoor Transmission of SARS-CoV-2 and Other Respiratory Viruses: A Systematic Review. *J. Infect. Dis.* **2021**, *223*, 550–561. [CrossRef]
20. Shen, Y.; Li, C.; Dong, H.; Wang, Z.; Martinez, L.; Sun, Z.; Handel, A.; Chen, Z.; Chen, E.; Ebell, M.H.; et al. Community Outbreak Investigation of SARS-CoV-2 Transmission among Bus Riders in Eastern China. *JAMA Intern. Med.* **2020**, *180*, 1665–1671. [CrossRef]
21. He, X.; Lau, E.H.Y.; Wu, P.; Deng, X.; Wang, J.; Hao, X.; Lau, Y.C.; Wong, J.Y.; Guan, Y.; Tan, X.; et al. Temporal Dynamics in Viral Shedding and Transmissibility of COVID-19. *Nat. Med.* **2020**, *26*, 672–675. [CrossRef] [PubMed]
22. Peng, Z.; Jimenez, J.L. Exhaled CO_2 as a COVID-19 Infection Risk Proxy for Different Indoor Environments and Activities. *Environ. Sci. Technol. Lett.* **2021**, *8*, 392–397. [CrossRef]
23. De Chaumont, F. On the Theory of Ventilation: An Attempt to Establish a Positive Basis for the Calculation of the Amount of Fresh Air Required for an Inhabited Air-Space. *Proc. R. Soc. Lond.* **1875**, *23*, 187–201.
24. Schibuola, L.; Scarpa, M.; Tambani, C. Natural Ventilation Level Assessment in a School Building by CO_2 Concentration Measures. *Energy Procedia* **2016**, *101*, 257–264. [CrossRef]
25. Milton, D.K. Risk of Sick Leave Associated with Outdoor Air Supply Rate, Humidification and Occupant Complaints. *Indoor Air* **2000**, *10*, 212–221. [CrossRef]
26. Zemitis, J.; Bogdanovics, R.; Bogdanovica, S. The Study of CO_2 Concentration in A Classroom during the Covid-19 Safety Measures. *E3S Web Conf.* **2021**, *246*, 01004. [CrossRef]
27. Trilles, S.; Juan, P.; Chaudhuri, S.; Fortea, A.B.V. Data on CO_2, Temperature and Air Humidity Records in Spanish Classrooms during the Reopening of Schools in the COVID-19 Pandemic. *Data Br.* **2021**, *39*, 107489. [CrossRef]
28. Kappelt, N.; Russell, H.S.; Kwiatkowski, S.; Afshari, A.; Johnson, M.S. Correlation of Respiratory Aerosols and Metabolic Carbon Dioxide. *Sustainability* **2021**, *13*, 12203. [CrossRef]
29. Baselga, M.; Güemes, A.; Alba, J.J.; Schuhmacher, A.J. SARS-CoV-2 Droplet and Airborne Transmission Heterogeneity. *J. Clin. Med.* **2022**, *11*, 2607. [CrossRef]
30. Schade, W.; Reimer, V.; Seipenbusch, M.; Willer, U. Experimental Investigation of Aerosol and CO_2 Dispersion for Evaluation of Covid-19 Infection Risk in a Concert Hall. *Int. J. Environ. Res. Public Health* **2021**, *18*, 3037. [CrossRef]
31. Aireamos Covid Risk Airborne. Available online: https://www.aireamos.org/herramienta/ (accessed on 26 May 2022).
32. Liu, L.J.S.; Krahmer, M.; Fox, A.; Feigley, C.E.; Featherstone, A.; Saraf, A.; Larsson, L. Investigation of the Concentration of Bacteria and Their Cell Envelope Components in Indoor Air in Two Elementary Schools. *J. Air Waste Manag. Assoc.* **2000**, *50*, 1957–1967. [CrossRef] [PubMed]
33. Johnson, G.R.; Morawska, L.; Ristovski, Z.D.; Hargreaves, M.; Mengersen, K.; Chao, C.Y.H.; Wan, M.P.; Li, Y.; Xie, X.; Katoshevski, D.; et al. Modality of Human Expired Aerosol Size Distributions. *J. Aerosol Sci.* **2011**, *42*, 839–851. [CrossRef]
34. Shim, E.; Tariq, A.; Choi, W.; Lee, Y.; Chowell, G. Transmission Potential and Severity of COVID-19 in South Korea. *Int. J. Infect. Dis.* **2020**, *93*, 339–344. [CrossRef] [PubMed]
35. Zauzmer, J. Washington-Post 'Take It Very Seriously': Pastor at Arkansas Church Where 34 People Came down with Coronavirus Sends a Warning. Available online: https://www.washingtonpost.com/religion/2020/03/24/pastor-arkansas-church-coronavirus-warning-greers-ferry (accessed on 26 May 2022).
36. Mackie, R. The Guardian. Did Singing Together Spread Coronavirus to Four Choirs? Available online: https://www.theguardian.com/world/2020/may/17/did-singing-together-spread-coronavirus-to-four-choirs (accessed on 26 May 2022).
37. Dashboard of the COVID-19 Virus Outbreak in Singapore. Available online: https://covid19.who.int/region/wpro/country/sg (accessed on 26 May 2022).
38. Adam, D.C.; Wu, P.; Wong, J.Y.; Lau, E.H.Y.; Tsang, T.K.; Cauchemez, S.; Leung, G.M.; Cowling, B.J. Clustering and Superspreading Potential of SARS-CoV-2 Infections in Hong Kong. *Nat. Med.* **2020**, *26*, 1714–1719. [CrossRef] [PubMed]
39. DW. Coronavirus: German Slaughterhouse Outbreak Crosses. Available online: https://www.dw.com/en/coronavirus-german-slaughterhouse-outbreak-crosses-1000/a-53883372 (accessed on 26 May 2022).
40. Cannon, A. Spike in COVID-19 Cases in Iowa Packing Plants a Big Part of 389 New Cases, State's Largest Single-Day Increase. Available online: https://eu.desmoinesregister.com/story/news/2020/04/19/coronavirus-iowa-largest-single-day-increase-iowa-covid-19-cases-tied-meatpacking-plants/5162127002/ (accessed on 26 May 2022).
41. GOV.UK. All Schools to Receive Carbon Dioxide Monitors. Available online: https://www.gov.uk/government/news/all-schools-to-receive-carbon-dioxide-monitors (accessed on 26 May 2022).
42. The White House. Biden Administration Launches Effort to Improve Ventilation and Reduce the Spread of COVID-19 in Buildings. Available online: https://www.whitehouse.gov/briefing-room/statements-releases/2022/03/17/fact-sheet-biden-administration-launches-effort-to-improve-ventilation-and-reduce-the-spread-of-covid-19-in-buildings/#:~{}:text=Today%20the%20Administration%20is%20launching,their%20buildings%20and%20reduce%20the (accessed on 26 May 2022).
43. Ryukyu, A.; Haebaru, H.; Ono, K. Providing Visualized Information on "Safety and Security" Installation of CO_2 Concentration Monitors for Customers at Aeon Stores. 2021; pp. 1–3. Available online: https://www.aeondelight.co.jp/english/news/20210901_installation-of-co2-concentration-monitors-for-customers-at-aeon-stores.pdf (accessed on 26 May 2022).

44. Salthammer, T.; Fauck, C.; Omelan, A.; Wientzek, S.; Uhde, E. Time and Spatially Resolved Tracking of the Air Quality in Local Public Transport. *Sci. Rep.* **2022**, *12*, 3262. [CrossRef]
45. Querol, X.; Alastuey, A.; Moreno, N.; Minguillón, M.C.; Moreno, T.; Karanasiou, A.; Jimenez, J.L.; Li, Y.; Morguí, J.A.; Felisi, J.M. How Can Ventilation Be Improved on Public Transportation Buses? Insights from CO_2 Measurements. *Environ. Res.* **2022**, *205*, 112451. [CrossRef]
46. Woodward, H.; Fan, S.; Bhagat, R.K.; Dadonau, M.; Wykes, M.D.; Martin, E.; Hama, S.; Tiwari, A.; Dalziel, S.B.; Jones, R.L.; et al. Air Flow Experiments on a Train Carriage—Towards Understanding the Risk of Airborne Transmission. *Atmosphere* **2021**, *12*, 1267. [CrossRef]
47. Bazant, M.Z.; Kodio, O.; Cohen, A.E.; Khan, K.; Gu, Z.; Bush, J.W.M. Monitoring Carbon Dioxide to Quantify the Risk of Indoor Airborne Transmission of COVID-19. *Flow* **2021**, *1*, 1–18. [CrossRef]
48. Chillon, S.A.; Millan, M.; Aramendia, I.; Fernandez-Gamiz, U.; Zulueta, E.; Mendaza-Sagastizabal, X. Natural Ventilation Characterization in a Classroom under Different Scenarios. *Int. J. Environ. Res. Public Health* **2021**, *18*, 5425. [CrossRef]
49. Zhang, D.; Ding, E.; Bluyssen, P.M. Guidance to Assess Ventilation Performance of a Classroom Based on CO_2 Monitoring. *Indoor Built Environ.* **2022**, *31*, 1107–1126. [CrossRef]
50. McNeill, V.F.; Corsi, R.; Huffman, J.A.; King, C.; Klein, R.; Lamore, M.; Maeng, D.Y.; Miller, S.L.; Lee Ng, N.; Olsiewski, P.; et al. Room-Level Ventilation in Schools and Universities. *Atmos. Environ. X* **2022**, *13*, 100152. [CrossRef] [PubMed]
51. Avella, F.; Gupta, A.; Peretti, C.; Fulici, G.; Verdi, L.; Belleri, A.; Babich, F. Low-Invasive CO_2-Based Visual Alerting Systems to Manage Natural Ventilation and Improve IAQ in Historic School Buildings. *Heritage* **2021**, *4*, 3442–3468. [CrossRef]
52. Zivelonghi, A.; Lai, M. Mitigating Aerosol Infection Risk in School Buildings: The Role of Natural Ventilation, Volume, Occupancy and CO_2 Monitoring. *Build. Environ.* **2021**, *204*, 108139. [CrossRef]
53. Jones, G.; Parodi, E.; Heinrich, M. Italian Study Shows Ventilation Can Cut School COVID Cases by 82%. *Reuters*. Available online: https://www.reuters.com/world/europe/italian-study-shows-ventilation-can-cut-school-covid-cases-by-82-2022-03-22/ (accessed on 26 May 2022).
54. Ingenieros Industriales de Aragón y la Rioja. *Guía de Referencia Covid*; Ingenieros Industriales de Aragón y la Rioja: Zaragoza, Spain, 2021; Available online: http://www.zaragoza.es/contenidos/coronavirus/guia-referencia-covid.pdf (accessed on 26 May 2022).
55. Cheng, S.Y.; Wang, C.J.; Shen, A.C.T.; Chang, S.C. How to Safely Reopen Colleges and Universities during COVID-19: Experiences from Taiwan. *Ann. Intern. Med.* **2020**, *173*, 638–641. [CrossRef]
56. Verma, A.; Raturi, V.; Kanimozhee, S. Urban Transit Technology Selection for Many-to-Many Travel Demand Using Social Welfare Optimization Approach. *J. Urban Plan. Dev.* **2018**, *144*, 04017021. [CrossRef]
57. Lan, I.; Wei, C.; Id, Y.H.; Christiani, D.C. Work-Related COVID-19 Transmission in Six Asian Countries Areas: A Follow-up Study. *PLoS ONE* **2020**, *15*, e0233588. [CrossRef]
58. Chan, M.Y. Commuters' Exposure to Carbon Monoxide and Carbon Dioxide in Air-Conditioned Buses in Hong Kong. *Indoor Built Environ.* **2005**, *14*, 397–403. [CrossRef]
59. Huang, H.L.; Hsu, D.J. Exposure Levels of Particulate Matter in Long-Distance Buses in Taiwan. *Indoor Air* **2009**, *19*, 234–242. [CrossRef]
60. Hsu, D.J.; Huang, H.L. Concentrations of Volatile Organic Compounds, Carbon Monoxide, Carbon Dioxide and Particulate Matter in Buses on Highways in Taiwan. *Atmos. Environ.* **2009**, *43*, 5723–5730. [CrossRef]
61. Chiu, C.F.; Chen, M.H.; Chang, F.H. Carbon Dioxide Concentrations and Temperatures within Tour Buses under Real-Time Traffic Conditions. *PLoS ONE* **2015**, *10*, e0125117. [CrossRef] [PubMed]
62. Barmparesos, N.; Assimakopoulos, V.D.; Assimakopoulos, M.N.; Tsairidi, E. Particulate Matter Levels and Comfort Conditions in the Trains and Platforms of the Athens Underground Metro. *AIMS Environ. Sci.* **2016**, *3*, 199–219. [CrossRef]
63. Bascompta Massanés, M.; Sanmiquel Pera, L.; Oliva Moncunill, J. Ventilation Management System for Underground Environments. *Tunn. Undergr. Space Technol.* **2015**, *50*, 516–522. [CrossRef]
64. Riley, C.E.; Murphy, G.; Riley, R.L. Copyright O 1978 by The Johns Hopkins University School of Hygiene and Public Health. *Am. J. Epidemiol.* **1978**, *107*, 421–432. [CrossRef]
65. Rudnick, S.; Milton, D. Risk of Indoor Airborne Infection Transmission Estimated from Carbon Dioxide Concentration. *Indoor Air* **2003**, *13*, 237–245. [CrossRef]
66. Anonymous. RWiki in Proyecto R UCA. Available online: http://knuth.uca.es/R/doku.php?id=r_wiki (accessed on 26 May 2022).
67. Yeh, H.; Liu, B. Aerosol Filtraton by Fibrous Filters. I: Theoretical. *J. Aerosol Sci.* **1974**, *5*, 191–204. [CrossRef]
68. Yeh, H.; Liu, B. Aerosol Filtraton by Fibrous Filters. II: Experimental. *J. Aerosol Sci.* **1974**, *5*, 205–217. [CrossRef]
69. Ma, J.; Qi, X.; Chen, H.; Li, X.; Zhang, Z.; Wang, H.; Sun, L.; Zhang, L.; Guo, J.; Morawska, L.; et al. Exhaled Breath Is a Significant Source of SARS-CoV-2 Emission. *medRxiv* **2020**, 1–8. [CrossRef]
70. Malik, M.; Kunze, A.; Bahmer, T.; Herget-rosenthal, S.; Kunze, T. SARS-CoV-2: Viral Loads of Exhaled Breath and Oronasopharyngeal Specimens in Hospitalized Patients with COVID-19. *Int. J. Infect. Dis.* **2021**, *110*, 105–110. [CrossRef]
71. Viklund, E.; Kokelj, S.; Larsson, P.; Nordén, R.; Andersson, M.; Beck, O.; Westin, J.; Olin, A.C. Severe Acute Respiratory Syndrome Coronavirus 2 Can Be Detected in Exhaled Aerosol Sampled during a Few Minutes of Breathing or Coughing. *Influenza Other Respi. Viruses* **2022**, *16*, 402–410. [CrossRef]

72. Chen, G.M.; Ji, J.J.; Jiang, S.; Xiao, Y.Q.; Zhang, R.L.; Huang, D.N.; Liu, H.; Yu, S.Y. Detecting Environmental Contamination of Acute Respiratory Syndrome Coronavirus 2 (SARS-CoV-2) in Isolation Wards and Fever Clinics. *Biomed. Environ. Sci.* **2020**, *33*, 943–947. [CrossRef] [PubMed]
73. Santarpia, J.L.; Rivera, D.N.; Herrera, V.L.; Morwitzer, M.J.; Creager, H.M.; Santarpia, G.W.; Crown, K.K.; Brett-Major, D.M.; Schnaubelt, E.R.; Broadhurst, M.J.; et al. Aerosol and Surface Contamination of SARS-CoV-2 Observed in Quarantine and Isolation Care. *Sci. Rep.* **2020**, *10*, 12732. [CrossRef] [PubMed]
74. Zhou, A.J.; Otter, J.A.; Price, J.R.; Cimpeanu, C.; Garcia, M.; Kinross, J.; Boshier, P.R.; Mason, S.; Bolt, F.; Alison, H.; et al. Investigating SARS-CoV-2 Surface and Air Contamination in an Acute Healthcare 2 Setting during the Peak of the COVID-19 Pandemic in London. *medRxiv Prepr.* **2020**, *73*, e1870–e1877.
75. Moore, G.; Rickard, H.; Stevenson, D.; Aranega-Bou, P.; Pitman, J.; Crook, A.; Davies, K.; Spencer, A.; Burton, C.; Easterbrook, L.; et al. Detection of SARS-CoV-2 within the Healthcare Environment: A Multi-Centre Study Conducted during the First Wave of the COVID-19 Outbreak in England. *J. Hosp. Infect.* **2021**, *108*, 189–196. [CrossRef] [PubMed]
76. Dumont-Leblond, N.; Veillette, M.; Mubareka, S.; Yip, L.; Longtin, Y.; Jouvet, P.; Paquet Bolduc, B.; Godbout, S.; Kobinger, G.; McGeer, A.; et al. Low Incidence of Airborne SARS-CoV-2 in Acute Care Hospital Rooms with Optimized Ventilation. *Emerg. Microbes Infect.* **2020**, *9*, 2597–2605. [CrossRef] [PubMed]
77. Song, Z.G.; Chen, Y.M.; Wu, F.; Xu, L.; Wang, B.F.; Shi, L.; Chen, X.; Dai, F.H.; She, J.L.; Chen, J.M.; et al. Identifying the Risk of SARS-CoV-2 Infection and Environmental Monitoring in Airborne Infectious Isolation Rooms (AIIRs). *Virol. Sin.* **2020**, *35*, 785–792. [CrossRef]
78. Moreno, T.; Pintó, R.M.; Bosch, A.; Moreno, N.; Alastuey, A.; Minguillón, M.C.; Anfruns-Estrada, E.; Guix, S.; Fuentes, C.; Buonanno, G.; et al. Tracing Surface and Airborne SARS-CoV-2 RNA inside Public Buses and Subway Trains. *Environ. Int.* **2021**, *147*, 106326. [CrossRef]
79. Lelieveld, J.; Helleis, F.; Borrmann, S.; Cheng, Y.; Drewnick, F.; Haug, G.; Klimach, T.; Sciare, J.; Su, H.; Pöschl, U. Model Calculations of Aerosol Transmission and Infection Risk of COVID-19 in Indoor Environments. *Int. J. Environ. Res. Public Health* **2020**, *17*, 8114. [CrossRef]
80. Park, J.; Kim, G. Risk of Covid-19 Infection in Public Transportation: The Development of a Model. *Int. J. Environ. Res. Public Health* **2021**, *18*, 12790. [CrossRef]
81. Yang, X.; Ou, C.; Yang, H.; Liu, L.; Song, T.; Kang, M.; Lin, H.; Hang, J. Transmission of Pathogen-Laden Expiratory Droplets in a Coach Bus. *J. Hazard. Mater.* **2020**, *397*, 122609. [CrossRef]
82. Zhang, Z.; Han, T.; Yoo, K.H.; Capecelatro, J.; Boehman, A.L.; Maki, K. Disease Transmission through Expiratory Aerosols on an Urban Bus. *Phys. Fluids* **2021**, *33*, 015116. [CrossRef] [PubMed]
83. Li, F.; Lee, E.S.; Zhou, B.; Liu, J.; Zhu, Y. Effects of the Window Openings on the Micro-Environmental Condition in a School Bus. *Atmos. Environ.* **2017**, *167*, 434–443. [CrossRef]
84. Edwards, N.J.; Widrick, R.; Wilmes, J.; Breisch, B.; Gerschefske, M.; Sullivan, J.; Potember, R.; Espinoza-Calvio, A. Reducing COVID-19 Airborne Transmission Risks on Public Transportation Buses: An Empirical Study on Aerosol Dispersion and Control. *Aerosol Sci. Technol.* **2021**, *55*, 1378–1397. [CrossRef]
85. Hartmann, A.; Kriegel, M. Risk Assessment of Aerosols Loaded with Virus Based on CO_2 Concentration. Hermann Rietschel Inst. (Fachgebiet Gebäude-Energie-Systeme), 2020. Available online: https://d-nb.info/1214708838/34 (accessed on 26 May 2022).
86. Kriegel, M.; Hartmann, A.; Buchholz, U.; Seifried, J.; Baumgarte, S.; Gastmeier, P. Sars-Cov-2 Aerosol Transmission Indoors: A Closer Look at Viral Load, Infectivity, the Effectiveness of Preventive Measures and a Simple Approach for Practical Recommendations. *Int. J. Environ. Res. Public Health* **2022**, *19*, 220. [CrossRef] [PubMed]
87. Pang, Z.; Hu, P.; Lu, X.; Wang, Q.; Neill, Z.O. A Smart CO_2-Based Ventilation Control Framework to Minimize the Infection Risk of COVID-19 in Public Buildings. 2021. Available online: https://www.researchgate.net/publication/349121056_A_Smart_CO2-Based_Ventilation_Control_Framework_to_Minimize_the_Infection_Risk_of_COVID-19_In_Public_Buildings (accessed on 26 May 2022).
88. Hawks, S.A.; Prussin, A.J.; Kuchinsky, S.C.; Pan, J.; Marr, L.C.; Duggal, N.K. Infectious SARS-CoV-2 Is Emitted in Aerosol Particles. *bioRxiv* **2021**, *12*, e02527-21. [CrossRef] [PubMed]
89. Ku, D.; Yeon, C.; Lee, S.; Lee, K.; Hwang, K.; Li, Y.C.; Wong, S.C. Safe Traveling in Public Transport amid COVID-19. *Sci. Adv.* **2021**, *7*, eabg3691. [CrossRef] [PubMed]
90. Hussein, T.; Löndahl, J.; Thuresson, S.; Alsved, M.; Al-Hunaiti, A.; Saksela, K.; Aqel, H.; Junninen, H.; Mahura, A.; Kulmala, M. Indoor Model Simulation for Covid-19 Transport and Exposure. *Int. J. Environ. Res. Public Health* **2021**, *18*, 2972. [CrossRef]
91. Bar-On, Y.M.; Flamholz, A.; Phillips, R.; Milo, R. SARS-CoV-2 (COVID-19) by the Numbers. *Elife* **2020**, *9*, e57309. [CrossRef]
92. Li, Y.; Guo, Y.P.; Wong, K.C.T.; Chung, W.Y.J.; Gohel, M.D.I.; Leung, H.M.P. Transmission of Communicable Respiratory Infections and Facemasks. *J. Multidiscip. Healthc.* **2008**, *1*, 17–27. [CrossRef]
93. Sharma, A.; Omidvarborna, H.; Kumar, P. Efficacy of Facemasks in Mitigating Respiratory Exposure to Submicron Aerosols. *J. Hazard. Mater.* **2022**, *422*, 126783. [CrossRef]
94. Williams, C.M.; Pan, D.; Decker, J.; Wisniewska, A.; Fletcher, E.; Sze, S.; Assadi, S.; Haigh, R.; Abdulwhhab, M.; Bird, P.; et al. Exhaled SARS-CoV-2 Quantified by Face-Mask Sampling in Hospitalised Patients with COVID-19. *J. Infect.* **2021**, *82*, 253–259. [CrossRef] [PubMed]

95. Spena, A.; Palombi, L.; Corcione, M.; Carestia, M.; Spena, V.A. On the Optimal Indoor Air Conditions for Sars-Cov-2 Inactivation. An Enthalpy-Based Approach. *Int. J. Environ. Res. Public Health* **2020**, *17*, 6083. [CrossRef] [PubMed]
96. Drag, M. Model-Based Fiber Diameter Determination Approach to Fine Particulate Matter Fraction (Pm2.5) Removal in Hvac Systems. *Appl. Sci.* **2021**, *11*, 1014. [CrossRef]
97. Chao, C.Y.H.; Wan, M.P.; Morawska, L.; Johnson, G.R.; Ristovski, Z.D.; Hargreaves, M.; Mengersen, K.; Corbett, S.; Li, Y.; Xie, X.; et al. Characterization of Expiration Air Jets and Droplet Size Distributions Immediately at the Mouth Opening. *J. Aerosol Sci.* **2009**, *40*, 122–133. [CrossRef]
98. Shao, S.; Zhou, D.; He, R.; Li, J.; Zou, S.; Mallery, K.; Kumar, S.; Yang, S.; Hong, J. Risk Assessment of Airborne Transmission of COVID-19 by Asymptomatic Individuals under Different Practical Settings. *J. Aerosol Sci.* **2021**, *151*, 105661. [CrossRef]
99. Fabian, P.; Brain, J.; Houseman, E.; Gern, J.; Milton, D. Origin of Exhaled Breath Particles from Healthy and Human Rhinovirus-Infected Subjects. *J. Aerosol Med. Pulm. Drug Deliv.* **2011**, *24*, 137–147. [CrossRef]
100. Hinds, W. *Aerosol Technology: Properties, Behavior, and Measurement of Airborne Particles*; John Wiley & Sons, Inc.: Hoboken, NJ, USA, 1999.
101. Van Doremalen, N.; Bushmaker, T.; Morris, D.; Holbrook, M.; Gamble, A.; Williamson, B.; Munster, V. Aerosol and Surface Stability of SARS-CoV-2 as Compared with SARS-CoV-1. *N. Engl. J. Med.* **2020**, *382*, 1177–1179. [CrossRef]

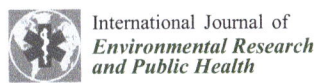

International Journal of *Environmental Research and Public Health*

Article

Environmental Effects of the COVID-19 Pandemic: The Experience of Bogotá, 2020

Jeadran Malagón-Rojas [1,2,*], Daniela Mendez-Molano [1], Julia Almentero [1], Yesith G. Toloza-Pérez [1], Eliana L. Parra-Barrera [1] and Claudia P. Gómez-Rendón [2]

1 Instituto Nacional de Salud, Bogotá 111321, Colombia; damemo27@gmail.com (D.M.-M.); jalmentero@ins.gov.co (J.A.); ytoloza@ins.gov.co (Y.G.T.-P.); elipabarrera@yahoo.es (E.L.P.-B.)
2 Doctorado en Salud Pública, El Bosque University, Bogotá 110121, Colombia; gomezclaudiap@unbosque.edu.co
* Correspondence: jnmalagon@unbosque.edu.co; Tel.: +57-1-2207700

Abstract: During the novel coronavirus disease (COVID-19) pandemic, several environmental factors have influenced activities and protection policy measures in cities. This has had a major effect on climate change and global environmental catastrophe. In many countries, the strategy of closing various activities such as tourism and industrial production stopped normal life, transportation, etc. This closure has a positive impact on the environment. However, the massive use of masks and personal protection could significantly increase pollution worldwide. The impact on the environment needs to be calculated to have information for public health actions. In this study, we present a first overview of the potential impacts of COVID-19 on some environmental matrices in Bogotá, Colombia.

Keywords: COVID-19; SARS-CoV-2; global environment; solid waste; air quality; transport

Citation: Malagón-Rojas, J.; Mendez-Molano, D.; Almentero, J.; Toloza-Pérez, Y.G.; Parra-Barrera, E.L.; Gómez-Rendón, C.P. Environmental Effects of the COVID-19 Pandemic: The Experience of Bogotá, 2020. *Int. J. Environ. Res. Public Health* **2022**, *19*, 6350. https://doi.org/10.3390/ijerph19106350

Academic Editors: Sachiko Kodera and Essam A. Rashed

Received: 24 March 2022
Accepted: 4 May 2022
Published: 23 May 2022

Publisher's Note: MDPI stays neutral with regard to jurisdictional claims in published maps and institutional affiliations.

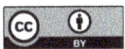

Copyright: © 2022 by the authors. Licensee MDPI, Basel, Switzerland. This article is an open access article distributed under the terms and conditions of the Creative Commons Attribution (CC BY) license (https://creativecommons.org/licenses/by/4.0/).

1. Introduction

The worldwide spread of severe acute respiratory syndrome (SARS-CoV-2) has had a relevant impact on economies, societies, road traffic, tourism, and human interaction [1]. Since COVID-19 was declared a pandemic disease by the WHO on 11 March 2020, strategies have been focused on individual lifestyles protection, suggesting individual isolation, confinement, and introducing behavioral practices such as regular hand washing, and the use of a face mask to help prevent viral transmission, particularly in public spaces [2].

The adoption of measures for preventing COVID-19 transmission has impacted the environment in many ways. Some authors have postulated that the COVID-19 pandemic is an opportunity to "reset" the current practices that are putting in check the planetary sustainability [3–5]. In this vein, a better understanding of pro-environmental behaviors and practices that took part during the global lockdown may contribute to improving health globally [6].

In addition, it seems that the imposed restrictions on mobility have drastically modified patterns and personal behaviors toward energy consumption [7–9]. Additionally, the COVID-19 pandemic decimated tourism and business travel, as well as labor migration [10], and modified the patterns of city mobility, increasing the usage of individual transport modes and behaviors toward bike and car usage [11–13]. In addition, pandemic restrictions have positively impacted indicators of air and water quality and noise pollution [14], and environmental noise has been reduced by 75%. This may be associated with a notable decrease in vehicle traffic, social mobility, international trips, and the temporary closure of factories [15]. In addition, some authors have stated that countries in which a social confinement strategy was applied to stop the spread of coronavirus infection showed a notable decrease in pollution and the emission of greenhouse gases [16–18]. This coincides with reports of a significant reduction in carbon emissions in highly industrialized countries [19]. Nevertheless, other authors have claimed that the potential benefits of the quarantine period have been eclipsed by lifestyles based on the increase in the use of single-use products, such as personal protective equipment, thwarting efforts toward reducing plastic pollution [20–22].

Some reports have indicated that the production of solid waste has increased four times [14,23]. Nevertheless, there is still not enough evidence of the effects on the generation of solid waste and the generation of environmental and air pollutants during the current pandemic. It is necessary to consider the negative impacts of the pandemic in terms of global warming and hospital and general waste to formulate policies regarding waste management and environmental pollution [24]. Understanding how the lockdown and social distancing measures have impacted the environment may inspire ideas supporting the goals of achieving more sustainable cities and communities in 2030 [25]. Therefore, this study is intended to expose and evaluate the environmental impact of the COVID-19 pandemic in 2020 in Bogotá, Colombia.

2. Materials and Methods

2.1. Study Area

Bogotá, the capital of Colombia, was selected as the study area. By May 2021, the city had more than 800 thousand infections since the beginning of the pandemic [26]. Bogotá has approximately 7.2 million inhabitants. The city is located at an average of 2625 m above sea level and is in the center of Colombia. It has a length of 33 km from south to north and 16 km from east to west (Figure 1). The economy is mainly based on the service sector, commerce, manufacturing, and construction. Additionally, it is one of the most polluted cities in Latin America. Pollution is mainly derived from diesel fuel, natural gas, industrial pollution, and the destruction of forests [27]. By 2019, 2.4 million vehicles were circulating in Bogotá, among which 50% were automobiles, 20% were motorcycles, 14% were vans, and 5% were public transport vehicles [28].

During the first year of the pandemic, Colombia reported almost 1.6 million confirmed cases and roughly 42,000 deaths related to COVID-19 [29]. The national lockdown was established between 25 March and 15 April, followed by a slow increase in mobility until August 2020 [29]. Since September 2020, COVID-19 mitigation strategies were fundamentally based on promoting remote work, the usage of personal protective equipment, and preventing social contacts, such as closing schools and universities. Additionally, the Ministry of health's guidance included social distancing, case isolation, and shielding to limit community-level transmission of SARS-CoV-2 and protect vulnerable groups.

In the specific case of Bogotá, community mobility was restricted based on the rates of occupancy of intensive care units (ICUs), through the strategy *"pico y cédula"*, which allowed mobility in the city and access to banks, supermarkets, and public transport based on the ending number of ID cards [30].

Similar to what has been observed in other scenarios, the SARS-CoV-2 epidemic in Colombia and Bogotá has been highly heterogeneous spatially. While some municipalities experienced explosive early spikes, followed by periods of very low transmission despite the near absence of NPI, many others experienced several moderate spikes interspersed with plateaus of sustained transmission [29,31].

2.2. Study Design

A retrospective ecological study was designed. The observed period was January 2019 to June 2021. To select the sources of information, we considered a matrix of environmental factors that may be affected by human activities [32]. In Supplementary Table S1, the environmental factors included in the study are listed, which were considered based on the availability and quality of the data and the relevance and strategic importance of the provided information.

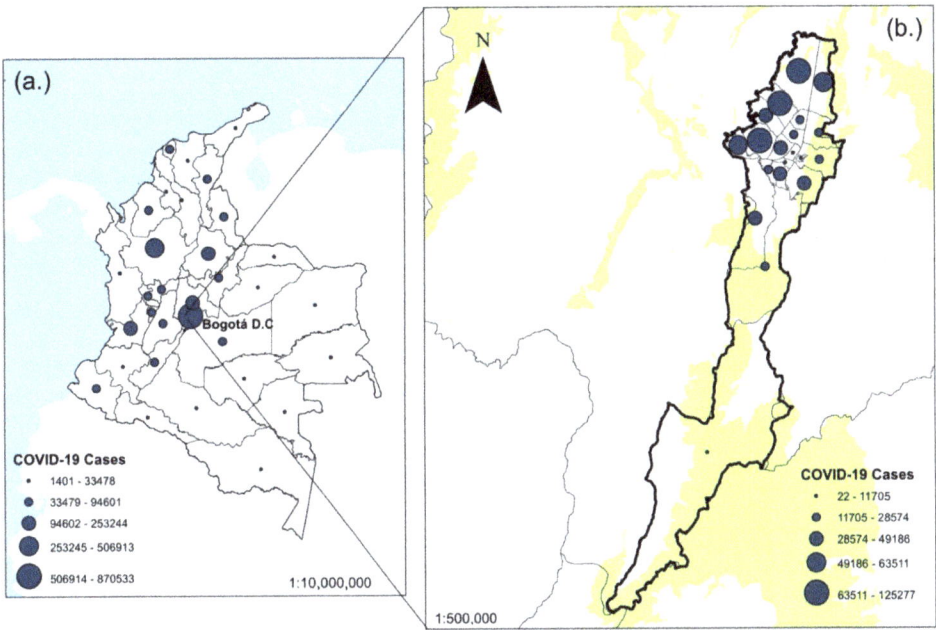

Figure 1. (a) SARS-CoV-2 cases in Colombia from 6 March 2020 until 18 May 2021; (b) study area, showing COVID-19 cases in Bogotá until 18 May 2021. The size of the circles is directly related to the number of infections since the first day of reporting. The geographical information system ArcGIS 10.5 for Desktop version 10.5.0.6491 was used to generate Figure 1. The Colombian administrative divisions and other geographic layers were downloaded from https://www.datos.gov.co/browse?sortBy=newest&utf8=%E2%9C%93 (accessed on 15 March 2022). COVID-19 data were obtained from Health Minister in Colombia, from 6 March 2020 to 18 May 2021.

2.3. Solid Waste Data Analysis

To analyze changes in the generation of solid waste in Bogotá, two sets of data were analyzed. The first set corresponds to the solid waste disposed of in the capital's sanitary landfill. For this analysis, a time series was made comparing its generation in 2019 with that in 2020. For the second dataset, the hospital waste in the biosanitary category obtained from the Special Administrative Unit of Public Services (UAESPs) was analyzed. In this study, the generation of solid waste in kg/month by large producers (LPs), medium producers (MPs), small producers (PPs), and micro-producers type A (MA), type B (MB), and type C (MC) was determined. We included information from all companies (n = 12) who are in charge of solid waste collection in the city (Supplementary Table S2).

2.4. Air Quality

Secondary data from the Bogotá Air Quality Monitoring Network (RMCAB) were used to analyze changes in the concentration of criteria pollutants during the pandemic period. Additionally, a time-series analysis was performed for criteria pollutants carbon monoxide (CO), nitrogen dioxide (NO_2), and particulate matter less than 10 microns in diameter (PM_{10}) and less than 2.5 microns in diameter ($PM_{2.5}$). Information from 11 stations operating during the 2 years was used.

Additionally, we included data from the Air Contamination And Health Effects in Microenvironments in Bogotá (ITHACA) study related to questions regarding the perception of air quality of people on their way to work or study and the personal protective elements they use to travel [33,34]. In this study, we used the data from 1821 citizens (more details are provided in Supplementary Table S3). The data were collected between February 2019 and June 2021.

2.5. Water Resources

Information on physical and chemical profiles of water for human consumption reported by Bogotá Aqueduct Company was included. Values are reported for turbidity in UNT, the concentration of manganese, organic matter, ammonium, dissolved oxygen in mg/L, and conductivity in µS/cm. The values are averages and maximums recorded for 2019 and 2020.

2.6. Transport

To analyze changes in transportation dynamics, the survey conducted in the ITHACA project was used. The survey records participants' answers to questions associated with their transportation and air quality during the COVID-19 pandemic (n = 1821).

In addition, information on the number of trips in the city's BRT system (Transmilenio S.A.) was collected. These values report the number of entries in three modes of transport that are part of the system. The first refers to BRT buses that run on the main lines of the city, the second mode of transport is zonal buses that run in mixed lanes, and the third mode is dual buses.

2.7. Statistical Analysis

For quantitative variables, averages and standard deviations were estimated. For categorical variables, frequencies were obtained. Location measures, such as quartiles, were used for some variables.

A time-series visual analysis was performed for air quality and transport (urban trips and air trips) by month and year. To establish differences between months and years, a bivariate analysis was performed using a t-test or Mann–Whitney U test for continuous variables and Chi^2 test for discrete variables, where $p > 0.05$ indicated a significant difference. In addition, the data from 2020 were divided into four phases: (1) baseline (1 February 2019 to 24 March 2020); (2) strict national lockdown (25 March to 26 April); (3) first relaxation (27 April to 31 May); and (4) gradual economic opening (from 1 June onwards) (Supplementary Figures).

The analysis was performed using R version 4.1 (Vienna, Austria) and Wolfram Mathematica version 12.0 (Champaign, IL, USA).

3. Results

3.1. Solid Waste

A decrease (33%) in disposed waste was observed in April 2020, compared with that in 2019. Nevertheless, after performing a temporal series analysis, it was observed that disposal quantities returned to their recurrent trend after the first measures of the pandemic strategy were removed (Supplementary Figure S1).

It was found that large producers of biosanitary waste and micro-producers A and B significantly increased their waste generation (Figure 2), with large producers presenting an increase from 67,000 kg in March to 89,000 kg in August 2020 and micro-producers A and B presenting a 100% increase in solid waste from March to July 2020.

For LPs, an increase in biosanitary waste generation was observed between April and August 2020. For MPs and PPs, a small increase was also observed, but this coincided with the economic reopening of the sites where these types of waste are produced, which presented the largest figures for 2019. Concerning MA, MB, and MC generators, increases were observed between April and August 2020, corresponding to normalization in the generation of biosanitary waste.

The Mann–Whitney U test showed significant differences between total waste production in 2019 and 2020 (p-value < 0.05). Nevertheless, the median amounts of biosanitary waste in 2019 and 2020 were not different (*p*-value > 0.05) (Supplementary Table S4). When comparing only the LPs, large differences were found (*p* value < 0.05).

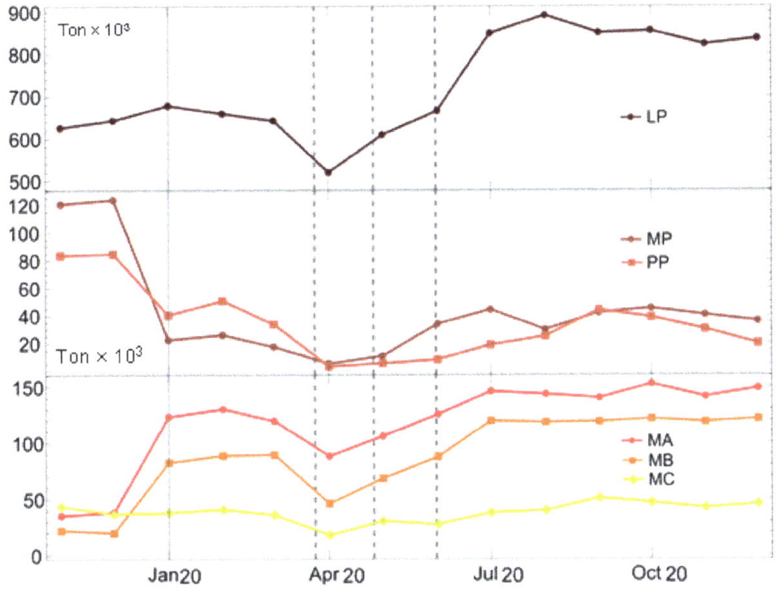

Figure 2. Bio-sanitary waste disposal series at the Bogotá sanitary landfill. The first panel shows biosanitary residues for the year 2020 for large producers (LPs), the second panel shows medium producers (MPs) and small producers (PPs), and the third panel shows micro-producers A, B, and C in red, orange and yellow, respectively.

3.2. Air Quality and Citizens' Perception

Regarding the data provided by the Bogotá Air Quality Monitoring Network, there was a decrease in criteria pollutants, such as carbon monoxide (CO), nitrogen oxides (NO_2), particulate matter less than 10 microns in diameter (PM_{10}), and fine particulate matter ($PM_{2.5}$). For the strict quarantine stage, there was an average reduction of ~51% for CO and ~61% for NO_2 (Figure 3a,b). These reductions were due to the decrease in transportation and halt of activities that produce fixed emissions.

Regarding particulate matter concentrations, there was a reduction of ~36% for PM_{10} and ~19% for $PM_{2.5}$ (Figure 3c,d). It is important to highlight that the strict lockdown began at a time when the city presented critical air pollution conditions due to the atmospheric conditions of the capital. Between February and March, there are usually air pollution alerts that exceed the maximum values allowed by the WHO, as shown in the timeline for 2019.

The *t*-test and Mann–Whitney U test showed significant differences in CO, NO_2, and PM_{10} concentrations between 2019 and 2020 (*p*-value < 0.05) (Supplementary Table S5).

In addition, it was found that the perception of air quality improved significantly during the pandemic period compared with 2019 (Chi^2 = 25.73; *p* = 0.00001) (Supplementary Figure S2). Air quality perceptions are related to the intention to use personal protective equipment (PPE) (*p*-value = <0.001, X-squared = 20.0). This relationship is evident only in surveys conducted during the pandemic. We found that before the pandemic, the use of PPE was not significant. The pandemic modified this trend and promoted the use of PPE, leading to the emergence of similar trends in the perception of the relationship between air quality and health effects (Supplementary Figure S2).

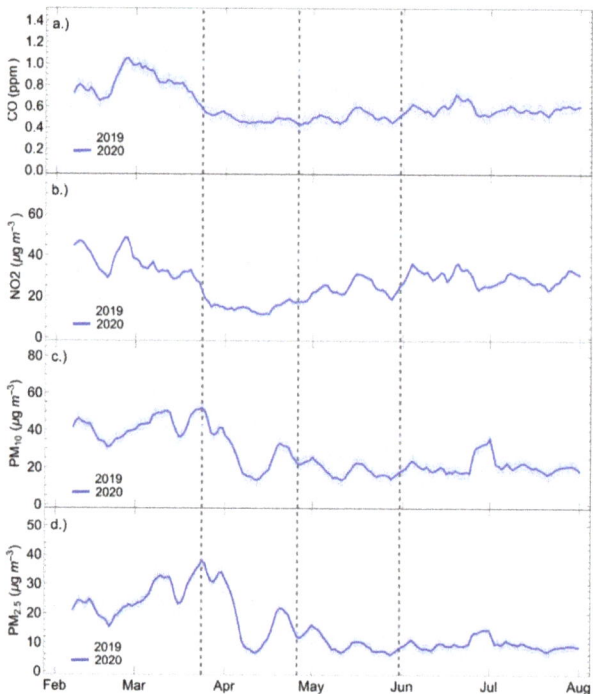

Figure 3. Air quality timeline: (**a**) daily average concentrations of carbon monoxide (CO); (**b**) nitrogen dioxide (NO_2) concentrations; (**c**) the first panel corresponds to concentrations of particulate matter below 10 microns (PM_{10}); (**d**) particulate matter below 2.5 microns ($PM_{2.5}$). The light blue series shows moving concentrations in 2019 and the dark blue series shows concentrations in 2020.

3.3. Transport

From the time-series analysis of the data provided by Transmilenio S.A., declines of 70–80% in revenues to the city's BRT system were observed between April and June, compared with the data of 2019 (Supplementary Figure S3). This decline had not returned to habitual levels by December 2020, showing 37% fewer revenues than the previous year. The figures show the effect of the strict quarantine and are consistent with the reduction in air pollutant emissions.

From the responses obtained from the participants of the ITHACA survey, changes in the choice of a preferred mode of transportation were found (Figure 4). There was a tendency to decrease the use of public transport, such as BRT and conventional buses, along with eight-point and one-point increases in the choice of private transportation by car and by motorcycle, respectively. There was also an increase in the use of active transport modes, reaching almost four points for walking and approximately five points for biking.

3.4. Water Resources

When analyzing water quality according to the reports generated by the Bogotá Water and Sewerage Company, significant reductions were observed in the different pollutants analyzed. In the case of organic matter, a reduction of approximately 7 mg/L was observed in 2020 compared with 2019. Additionally, ammonium was reduced by 38%, manganese was reduced by 75.8%, turbidity was reduced by 46%, and conductivity was reduced by 49%. These values refer to the maximum concentrations observed for the two years of analysis and represent a significant decrease and, thus, favorable conditions in the city for

2020. This effect may be associated with the decrease in discharges from industries located upstream of the plant's catchment point, i.e., in the upper basin (Supplementary Figure S4).

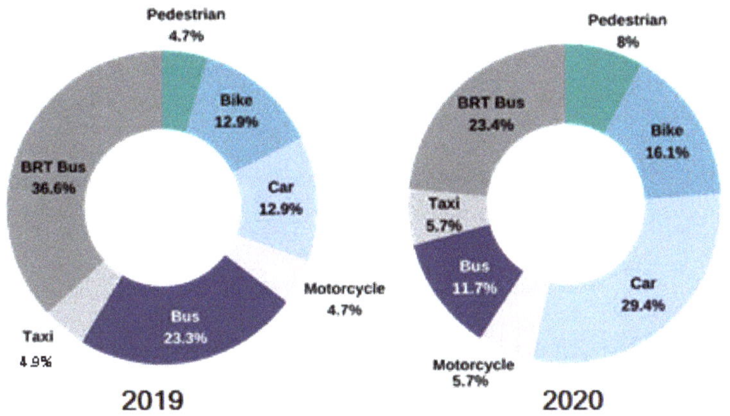

Figure 4. Transport modes in 2019 compared to 2020 or pandemic times according to the ITHACA perception survey.

4. Discussion

To our knowledge, this is the first study carried out about a city in Latin America exploring the effects of the COVID-19 on environmental matrices, including effects on water, air quality, mobility patterns, and waste production. Some studies explored descriptively the effects of the pandemic on air quality in Argentina, Chile, Colombia, and Mexico [35–38], while others reported the effects of deforestation patterns in Brazil and Peru [39]. Nevertheless, information related to solid waste production and water quality is scarce.

The restrictions established by the government generated a change in the dynamics of the city. The strict quarantine led to the closure of many places with economic activities that produce waste, atmospheric emissions, and water pollution and to an increase in solid biosanitary waste. The decrease in different environmental effects was reflected in several scenarios, generally having positive effects on the environment.

First, there was a 32% reduction in solid waste in comparison with the normal amount produced in the most critical month. However, this reduction was evident only until the gradual economic opening, at which time the tons of solid waste arriving at the landfill corresponded to the average values of previous years. In addition, there was a significant increase in the generation of biosanitary waste from large producers, from 600,000 tons per month to almost 900,000 tons/year. Some authors consider that waste production has risen as a result of COVID-19, although these changes do not follow the same pattern in different areas [40]. The increase in waste production is explained in two ways: first, disease prevention or treatment activities (hospital and lab PPE) [41] and, second, the effects of the pandemic on lifestyles, such as increased in-home cooking and online shopping. Additionally, as a result of the massive usage of PPE, this waste category substantially increased, between 18% and 425% [42,43].

On the other hand, atmospheric pollution greatly benefited from the city's mobility restrictions. The Colombian capital tends to present atmospheric conditions that are not characterized exclusively by local emissions, as the influence of regional pollution has been demonstrated [44]. Despite this influence, mobility and industrial activities that are usually critical for the city slowed down for months. Authors have reported similar results in different regions. A study carried out in 10 countries in North America, Europe, and Asia (n = 9394) observed that a reduction in pollutant concentration was perceived, although to different extents, by all populations [45]. According to the authors, except for participants from China and Norway, participants from all countries perceived a drop in the air pollution concentration during the quarantine period. However, the large decline observed in much of the world is projected to be exceeded again by the end of 2021 [46]. The "rebound effect" of the pandemic is estimated to produce an increase of 36.4 billion tons of carbon emissions from burning fossil fuels, an increase of 4.9% in 2021 compared with the previous year, reaffirming the continued reliance of the planet on carbon-based technologies.

Air quality is directly reflected in the third matrix evaluated, which refers to transportation. Clear decreases were observed in the use of the city's BRT system, and the transition of transport modes must be evaluated. A notable proportion of people shifted from public to private transport, which is logical given the exposure to COVID-19 in mass transit modes. These findings are similar to those reported in a study carried out in Pakistan [47]. Travelers seem to prefer not to use public transport during the pandemic situation. Survey participants stated that they feared being infected with the virus while traveling on public transport, as there are chances of interacting with a person who is a carrier of the COVID-19 virus. Another study carried out in more than 15 countries in Asia, Europe, and North America found that most commuters have changed their trip habits. Shopping became the primary purpose for travel during COVID-19 [48].

This change might not be very beneficial if the percentage of people who start using vehicles or motorcycles increases to the extent that the vehicle fleet starts to have a greater impact on air pollution [49]. This situation may be prevented by the increase in the choice of active modes of transport, which generate enormous benefits given sustainable mobility.

We similarly observed an improvement in sewage water quality parameters. Reports from different regions around the world likewise show a reduction in water pollutants during the quarantine period [24]. This may be explained by the decrease in industrial water consumption. Although the report analyzed in this paper refers to the conditions in only one period of the two years of study, the decrease in parameters such as organic matter and turbidity represents a great relief for the city's water bodies and their treatment logistics.

This study has many limitations. The first concerns the design of the study. Ecological studies look for associations between the occurrence of disease and exposure to known or suspected causes. However, because it is not possible to control different variables, biases can interfere with the analysis regarding the association between exposure and outcomes. Second, we did not include variables related to the effect of the pandemic on biodiversity due to the lack of data. Third, the data on changes in transport modes and perception of air quality are not representative of all cities. Finally, data were not available in the same format for all variables, i.e., the frequency of collection differed depending on the environmental matrix and source of the query, so data between matrices could not be compared to more accurately estimate the interrelationships among matrices.

5. Conclusions

This study showed the COVID-19 pandemic impact on the environment, offering an overview of changes in pollutants during 2019 and 2020 in Bogotá. The COVID-19 pandemic was a unique chance to analyze environmental impacts due to the fact that activities in large cities, such as Bogotá, were stopped over lockdown. The effects were both positive and negative. During the pandemic, Bogotá, like most cities around the world, adopted a strict lockdown to contain the spread of the virus. The months of strict restrictions generated significant changes associated with environmental and ecological conditions. The main air pollutants decreased markedly, attributed to travel restrictions by private cars or public transport.

This is relevant, considering that there is a long-term—potentially permanent—downward impact on the levels of environmental pressure, with stronger effects for pressure related to capital-intensive economic activities [50]. The promotion of telework as a result of lessons learned from the pandemic may positively impact some environmental matrices. Social experiments such as "a day without a car" have been undertaken in cities such as Paris, Berlin, Bogotá, and Toledo [51–53]. These experiences offer interesting results for improving mobility and air quality. More detailed studies are urged to understand and apply the lessons learned from the COVID-19 pandemic and its effects on the environment.

Supplementary Materials: The following supporting information can be downloaded at: https://www.mdpi.com/article/10.3390/ijerph19106350/s1, Table S1: Variables to be analyzed and information sources; Table S2: Types of generators according to their production in kilograms per day and the frequency of waste collection; Table S3: Sociodemographic characteristics of the survey participants ITHACA; Table S4: U-Mann Whitney test to total solid waste and biosanitary waste; Table S5: U-Mann Whitney and t-test to Air Quality data; Figure S1: Solid waste disposal series at the Bogota sanitary landfill. The gray line with circular markers indicates the tons per month for 2019, the blue line with square markers indicates the tons disposed of in 2020, the year of the pandemic; Figure S2: Air quality perception: (a) the air quality on house from job. (b) Only pandemic answers about the existence of a relationship between air quality and usage of personal protection; Figure S3: BRT system admissions timeline. The light blue series shows moving concentrations in 2019 and the dark blue series shows concentrations in 2020; Figure S4: Water Quality reported Bogota Water and Sewer Service 2019–2020.

Author Contributions: Conceptualization, J.M.-R. and C.P.G.-R.; methodology, J.M.-R., D.M.-M. and Y.G.T.-P.; software, Y.G.T.-P. and D.M.-M.; formal analysis, D.M.-M., Y.G.T.-P., J.A. and E.L.P.-B.; investigation, D.M.-M., Y.G.T.-P., J.A. and E.L.P.-B.; data curation, D.M.-M., Y.G.T.-P. and J.A., writing—original draft preparation D.M.-M., Y.G.T.-P., J.A. and E.L.P.-B.; writing—review and editing, J.M.-R., J.A., E.L.P.-B. and C.P.G.-R. All authors have read and agreed to the published version of the manuscript.

Funding: The project was partially funded by MinCiencias Colombia, Project Number 2010484467564 (call number 844 of 2019).

Institutional Review Board Statement: The study was conducted in accordance with the Declaration of Helsinki and approved by the Research Ethics and Methodologies Committee (CEMIN) at the National Institute of Health of Colombia (Protocol Code 014/2019, March 2019 for studies involving humans.

Informed Consent Statement: Informed consent was obtained from all subjects involved in the study.

Data Availability Statement: Not applicable.

Acknowledgments: The authors want to thank Hugo Saenz and Sergio Salazar-Sánchez from Secretaria Distrital de Ambiente de Bogotá for their collaboration in providing the public data on air quality and water. Additionally, the authors want to thank the Special Administrative Unit of Public Services in Bogotá for providing us with the data on solid waste. Finally, J.M.R. would like to express his sincere gratitude to Fernando Gutierrez at El Bosque University, for their recommendations in the final version of the manuscript.

Conflicts of Interest: The authors declare no conflict of interest. The funders had no role in the design of the study; in the collection, analyses, or interpretation of data; in the writing of the manuscript; or in the decision to publish the results.

References

1. Saadat, S.; Rawtani, D.; Hussain, C.M. Environmental Perspective of COVID-19. *Sci. Total Environ.* **2020**, *728*, 138870. [CrossRef] [PubMed]
2. Park, J.-H.; Lee, S.-G.; Ahn, S.; Kim, J.Y.; Song, J.; Moon, S.; Cho, H. Strategies to Prevent COVID-19 Transmission in the Emergency Department of a Regional Base Hospital in Korea: From Index Patient until Pandemic Declaration. *Am. J. Emerg. Med.* **2021**, *46*, 247–253. [CrossRef] [PubMed]
3. Kumar, A.; Malla, M.A.; Dubey, A. With Corona Outbreak: Nature Started Hitting the Reset Button Globally. *Front. Public Health* **2020**, *8*, 569353. [CrossRef] [PubMed]
4. COVID-19: The 4 Building Blocks of the Great Reset. Available online: https://www.weforum.org/agenda/2020/08/building-blocks-of-the-great-reset/ (accessed on 25 April 2022).
5. Hawkes, C. Five Steps towards a Global Reset: Lessons from COVID-19. *Glob. Sustain.* **2020**, *3*, e30. [CrossRef]
6. Ramkissoon, H. COVID-19 Place Confinement, Pro-Social, Pro-Environmental Behaviors, and Residents' Wellbeing: A New Conceptual Framework. *Front. Psychol.* **2020**, *11*, 02248. [CrossRef] [PubMed]

7. Buechler, E.; Powell, S.; Sun, T.; Astier, N.; Zanocco, C.; Bolorinos, J.; Flora, J.; Boudet, H.; Rajagopal, R. Global Changes in Electricity Consumption during COVID-19. *iScience* **2022**, *25*, 103568. [CrossRef] [PubMed]
8. Jiang, P.; Fan, Y.V.; Klemeš, J.J. Impacts of COVID-19 on Energy Demand and Consumption: Challenges, Lessons and Emerging Opportunities. *Appl. Energy* **2021**, *285*, 116441. [CrossRef]
9. Kang, H.; An, J.; Kim, H.; Ji, C.; Hong, T.; Lee, S. Changes in Energy Consumption According to Building Use Type under COVID-19 Pandemic in South Korea. *Renew. Sustain. Energy Rev.* **2021**, *148*, 111294. [CrossRef]
10. Benton, M.; Batalova, J.; Davidoff-Gore, S.; Schmidt, T. *COVID-19 and the State of Global Mobility in 2020*; International Organization for Migration: Grand-Saconnex, Switzerland, 2020.
11. IEA Changes in Transport Behaviour during the COVID-19 Crisis–Analysis. Available online: https://www.iea.org/articles/changes-in-transport-behaviour-during-the-COVID-19-crisis (accessed on 25 April 2022).
12. Echaniz, E.; Rodríguez, A.; Cordera, R.; Benavente, J.; Alonso, B.; Sañudo, R. Behavioural Changes in Transport and Future Repercussions of the COVID-19 Outbreak in Spain. *Transp. Policy* **2021**, *111*, 38–52. [CrossRef]
13. Habib, M.A.; Anik, M.A.H. Impacts of COVID-19 on Transport Modes and Mobility Behavior: Analysis of Public Discourse in Twitter. *Transp. Res. Rec.* **2021**. [CrossRef]
14. Mostafa, M.K.; Gamal, G.; Wafiq, A. The Impact of COVID 19 on Air Pollution Levels and Other Environmental Indicators—A Case Study of Egypt. *J. Environ. Manag.* **2021**, *277*, 111496. [CrossRef] [PubMed]
15. Rodríguez-Urrego, D.; Rodríguez-Urrego, L. Air Quality during the COVID-19: PM2.5 Analysis in the 50 Most Polluted Capital Cities in the World. *Environ. Pollut.* **2020**, *266*, 115042. [CrossRef] [PubMed]
16. Khan, I.; Shah, D.; Shah, S.S. COVID-19 Pandemic and Its Positive Impacts on Environment: An Updated Review. *Int. J. Environ. Sci. Technol.* **2021**, *18*, 521–530. [CrossRef] [PubMed]
17. Le Quéré, C.; Jackson, R.B.; Jones, M.W.; Smith, A.J.P.; Abernethy, S.; Andrew, R.M.; De-Gol, A.J.; Willis, D.R.; Shan, Y.; Canadell, J.G.; et al. Temporary Reduction in Daily Global CO2 Emissions during the COVID-19 Forced Confinement. *Nat. Clim. Chang.* **2020**, *10*, 647–653. [CrossRef]
18. Muhammad, S.; Long, X.; Salman, M. COVID-19 Pandemic and Environmental Pollution: A Blessing in Disguise? *Sci. Total Environ.* **2020**, *728*, 138820. [CrossRef]
19. Tollefson, J. COVID Curbed Carbon Emissions in 2020—But Not by Much. *Nature* **2021**, *589*, 343. [CrossRef]
20. Benson, N.U.; Fred-Ahmadu, O.H.; Bassey, D.E.; Atayero, A.A. COVID-19 Pandemic and Emerging Plastic-Based Personal Protective Equipment Waste Pollution and Management in Africa. *J. Environ. Chem. Eng.* **2021**, *9*, 105222. [CrossRef]
21. Sarkodie, S.A.; Owusu, P.A. Impact of COVID-19 Pandemic on Waste Management. *Environ. Dev. Sustain.* **2021**, *23*, 7951–7960. [CrossRef]
22. Zhang, R.; Zhang, Y.; Lin, H.; Feng, X.; Fu, T.-M.; Wang, Y. NOx Emission Reduction and Recovery during COVID-19 in East China. *Atmosphere* **2020**, *11*, 433. [CrossRef]
23. Kumar, A.; Agrawal, A. Recent Trends in Solid Waste Management Status, Challenges, and Potential for the Future Indian Cities—A Review. *Curr. Res. Environ. Sustain.* **2020**, *2*, 100011. [CrossRef]
24. Cheval, S.; Mihai Adamescu, C.; Georgiadis, T.; Herrnegger, M.; Piticar, A.; Legates, D.R. Observed and Potential Impacts of the COVID-19 Pandemic on the Environment. *Int. J. Environ. Res. Public Health* **2020**, *17*, 4140. [CrossRef]
25. Shulla, K.; Voigt, B.-F.; Cibian, S.; Scandone, G.; Martinez, E.; Nelkovski, F.; Salehi, P. Effects of COVID-19 on the Sustainable Development Goals (SDGs). *Discov. Sustain.* **2021**, *2*, 15. [CrossRef] [PubMed]
26. Instituto Nacional de Salud COVID-19 En Colombia. Available online: https://www.ins.gov.co/Noticias/paginas/coronavirus.aspx (accessed on 4 March 2022).
27. Vargas, F.A.; Rojas, N.Y.; Pachon, J.E.; Russell, A.G. PM10 Characterization and Source Apportionment at Two Residential Areas in Bogota. *Atmos. Pollut. Res.* **2012**, *3*, 72–80. [CrossRef]
28. Oróstegui, O. Lo que necesita Bogotá en este 2019. Bogotá Cómo Vamos. 2018. Available online: https://bogotacomovamos.org/que-necesita-bogota-para-el-2019/ (accessed on 30 January 2022).
29. Mercado-Reyes, M.; Malagón-Rojas, J.; Rodríguez-Barraquer, I.; Zapata-Bedoya, S.; Wiesner, M.; Cucunubá, Z.; Toloza-Pérez, Y.G.; Hernández-Ortiz, J.P.; Acosta-Reyes, J.; Parra-Barrera, E.; et al. Seroprevalence of Anti-SARS-CoV-2 Antibodies in Colombia, 2020: A Population-Based Study. *Lancet Reg. Health Am.* **2022**, *9*, 100195. [CrossRef] [PubMed]
30. ¿Pico y Cédula, y Ahora Toque de Queda?: Experiencia del Departamento del Atlántico en las Medidas de Contención Frente al COVID-19-Departamento Economía-Uninorte. Available online: https://www.uninorte.edu.co/web/deptoeconomia/home/-/blogs/-pico-y-cedula-y-ahora-toque-de-queda-experiencia-del-departamento-del-atlantico-en-las-medidas-de-contencion-frente-al-COVID-19 (accessed on 25 April 2022).
31. Malagón-Rojas, J.N.; Mercado-Reyes, M.; Toloza-Pérez, Y.G.; Parra Barrera, E.L.; Palma, M.; Muñoz, E.; López, R.; Almentero, J.; Rubio, V.V.; Ibáñez, E.; et al. Seroprevalence of the SARS-CoV-2 Antibody in Healthcare Workers: A Multicentre Cross-Sectional Study in 10 Colombian Cities. *Occup. Environ. Med.* **2021**. [CrossRef] [PubMed]
32. Oyague, E.; Yaja, A.; Franco, P. Efectos Ambientales Del Confinamiento Debido a La Pandemia de COVID-19. *Cienc. Desarro.* **2020**, *26*, 2–19. [CrossRef]
33. Malagon-Rojas, J.; Pinzón-Silva, D.C.; Parra, E.L.; Lagos, L.; Toloza-Perez, Y.G.; Hernández Florez, L.J.; Morales, R.; Romero Díaz, S.A.; Ríos Cabra, A.P.; Sarmiento, O.L. Assessment of Personal Exposure to Particulate Air Pollution in Different Microenviron-

ments and Traveling by Several Modes of Transportation in Bogotá, Colombia: Protocol for a Mixed-Methods Study. (Preprint). *JMIR Res. Protoc.* **2020**, *11*, e25690. [CrossRef]
34. Malagon-Rojas, J.; Parra-Barrera, E.L.; Toloza-Pérez, Y.G.; Soto, H.; Lagos, L.F.; Méndez, D.; Rico, A.; Almentero, J.E.; Quintana-Cortés, M.A.; Pinzón-Silva, D.C.; et al. Assessment of Factors Influencing Personal Exposure to Air Pollution on Main Roads in Bogota: A Mixed-Method Study. *Preprints* **2022**. [CrossRef]
35. Blackman, A.; Bonilla, J.; Villalobos, L. Quantifying COVID-19's Silver Lining: Avoided Deaths from Air Quality Improvements in Bogotá | Publications. Available online: https://publications.iadb.org/publications/english/document/Quantifying-COVID-19s-Silver-Lining-Avoided-Deaths-from-Air-Quality-Improvements-in-Bogota.pdf (accessed on 25 April 2022).
36. Morales-Solís, K.; Ahumada, H.; Rojas, J.P.; Urdanivia, F.R.; Catalán, F.; Claramunt, T.; Toro, R.A.; Manzano, C.A.; Leiva-Guzmán, M.A. The Effect of COVID-19 Lockdowns on the Air Pollution of Urban Areas of Central and Southern Chile. *Aerosol Air Qual. Res.* **2021**, *21*, 200677. [CrossRef]
37. Arregocés, H.A.; Rojano, R.; Restrepo, G. Effects of Lockdown due to the COVID-19 Pandemic on Air Quality at Latin America's Largest Open-Pit Coal Mine. *Aerosol Air Qual. Res.* **2021**, *21*, 200664. [CrossRef]
38. Sanap, S.D. Global and Regional Variations in Aerosol Loading during COVID-19 Imposed Lockdown. *Atmos. Environ.* **2021**, *246*, 118132. [CrossRef] [PubMed]
39. López-Feldman, A.; Chávez, C.; Vélez, M.A.; Bejarano, H.; Chimeli, A.B.; Féres, J.; Robalino, J.; Salcedo, R.; Viteri, C. Environmental Impacts and Policy Responses to COVID-19: A View from Latin America. *Environ. Resour. Econ.* **2020**, *76*, 447–517. [CrossRef]
40. Yousefi, M.; Oskoei, V.; Jonidi Jafari, A.; Farzadkia, M.; Hasham Firooz, M.; Abdollahinejad, B.; Torkashvand, J. Municipal Solid Waste Management during COVID-19 Pandemic: Effects and Repercussions. *Environ. Sci. Pollut. Res.* **2021**, *28*, 32200–32209. [CrossRef] [PubMed]
41. Zambrano-Monserrate, M.A.; Ruano, M.A.; Sanchez-Alcalde, L. Indirect Effects of COVID-19 on the Environment. *Sci. Total Environ.* **2020**, *728*, 138813. [CrossRef] [PubMed]
42. Liang, Y.; Song, Q.; Wu, N.; Li, J.; Zhong, Y.; Zeng, W. Repercussions of COVID-19 Pandemic on Solid Waste Generation and Management Strategies. *Front. Environ. Sci. Eng.* **2021**, *15*, 115. [CrossRef]
43. Zand, A.D.; Heir, A.V. Environmental Impacts of New Coronavirus Outbreak in Iran with an Emphasis on Waste Management Sector. *J. Mater. Cycles Waste Manag.* **2021**, *23*, 240–247. [CrossRef]
44. Franco, J.F.; Pacheco, J.; Behrentz, E.; Belalcázar, L.C. Characterization and Source Identification of VOC Species in Bogotá, Colombia. *Atmósfera* **2015**, *28*, 1–11. [CrossRef]
45. Lou, B.; Barbieri, D.M.; Passavanti, M.; Hui, C.; Gupta, A.; Hoff, I.; Lessa, D.A.; Sikka, G.; Chang, K.; Fang, K.; et al. Air Pollution Perception in Ten Countries during the COVID-19 Pandemic. *Ambio* **2021**, *51*, 531–545. [CrossRef]
46. Tollefson, J. Carbon Emissions Rapidly Rebounded Following COVID Pandemic Dip. *Nature* **2021**. [CrossRef]
47. Ashraf Javid, M.; Abdullah, M.; Ali, N.; Dias, C. Structural Equation Modeling of Public Transport Use with COVID-19 Precautions: An Extension of the Norm Activation Model. *Transp. Res. Interdiscip. Perspect.* **2021**, *12*, 100474. [CrossRef]
48. Abdullah, M.; Dias, C.; Muley, D.; Shahin, M. Exploring the Impacts of COVID-19 on Travel Behavior and Mode Preferences. *Transp. Res. Interdiscip. Perspect.* **2020**, *8*, 100255. [CrossRef] [PubMed]
49. Rume, T.; Islam, S.M.D.-U. Environmental Effects of COVID-19 Pandemic and Potential Strategies of Sustainability. *Heliyon* **2020**, *6*, e04965. [CrossRef] [PubMed]
50. OECD The Long-Term Environmental Implications of COVID-19. Available online: https://www.oecd.org/coronavirus/policy-responses/the-long-term-environmental-implications-of-COVID-19-4b7a9937/ (accessed on 11 November 2021).
51. Berlin Takes Part in 'Car-Free Day.' Berl. Spect. 2021. Available online: https://berlinspectator.com/2021/09/22/political-correctness-berlin-takes-part-in-car-free-day-2/ (accessed on 30 January 2022).
52. Noticias de Día Sin Carro 2021 en Bogotá | Bogota.gov.co. Available online: https://bogota.gov.co/tag/dia-sin-carro-2021 (accessed on 12 November 2021).
53. Convention and Visitors Bureau Car-Free Day in Paris-Celebration-Paris Tourist Office. Available online: https://en.parisinfo.com/paris-show-exhibition/170120/third-car-free-day-in-paris (accessed on 11 November 2021).

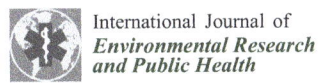

Article

Ethnopharmacology for Skin Diseases and Cosmetics during the COVID-19 Pandemic in Lithuania

Zivile Praskuniene [1,2,*], Rugile Grisiute [2], Andrius Pranskunas [3] and Jurga Bernatoniene [1,2]

1. Department of Drug Technology and Social Pharmacy, Lithuanian University of Health Sciences, LT-50162 Kaunas, Lithuania; jurga.bernatoniene@lsmuni.lt
2. Institute of Pharmaceutical Technologies, Lithuanian University of Health Sciences, LT-50162 Kaunas, Lithuania; rugile.grisiute@stud.lsmu.lt
3. Department of Intensive Care Medicine, Lithuanian University of Health Sciences, LT-50161 Kaunas, Lithuania; andrius.pranskunas@lsmuni.lt
* Correspondence: zivile.pranskuniene@lsmuni.lt

Citation: Pranskuniene, Z.; Grisiute, R.; Pranskunas, A.; Bernatoniene, J. Ethnopharmacology for Skin Diseases and Cosmetics during the COVID-19 Pandemic in Lithuania. *Int. J. Environ. Res. Public Health* **2022**, *19*, 4054. https://doi.org/10.3390/ijerph19074054

Academic Editors: Sachiko Kodera and Essam A. Rashed

Received: 12 February 2022
Accepted: 25 March 2022
Published: 29 March 2022

Publisher's Note: MDPI stays neutral with regard to jurisdictional claims in published maps and institutional affiliations.

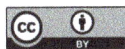

Copyright: © 2022 by the authors. Licensee MDPI, Basel, Switzerland. This article is an open access article distributed under the terms and conditions of the Creative Commons Attribution (CC BY) license (https://creativecommons.org/licenses/by/4.0/).

Abstract: The documentation of ethnopharmaceutical knowledge has always been important for the preservation of countries' cultural, social, and economic identity. The COVID-19 pandemic with the collapse of healthcare, which has left the individual health to self-care, has also forced us to look back at ethnopharmacology from a practical point of view. This is the first study in Lithuania, dedicated entirely to ethnopharmaceuticals used for skin diseases and cosmetics, and the first study to analyse ethnopharmacology as a Lithuanian phenomenon during the ongoing COVID-19 pandemic. The main purpose of this study was to collect and evaluate ethnopharmaceutical knowledge regarding skin diseases and cosmetics in Šiauliai District, Lithuania during the COVID-19 pandemic from July 2020 to October 2021. This study surveyed 50 respondents; the survey was conducted using the deep interview method. The respondents mentioned 67 species of medicinal plants from 37 different families used for skin diseases (64.18%), cosmetics (13.44%) and cosmeceuticals (22.38%). Of the 67 plant species, 43 (64%) were not included in the European Medicines Agency monographs and only 14 species (21%) of all included species were used with European Medicines Agency approved medical indications for skin diseases. In terms of public health, the safety of "self-treatment" and recovery rituals for skin diseases are no less important than ethnopharmacological knowledge and its application, this being especially relevant during the COVID-19 pandemic.

Keywords: ethnopharmacology; skin diseases; cosmetics; COVID-19; Lithuania

1. Introduction

Lithuanian scientists first viewed ethnopharmacology as a cultural phenomenon. It was analyzed in historical, ethnocultural and geographical contexts. Traditional folk medicine is an area of folk culture which includes medicinal knowledge, beliefs, and treatments that existed in traditional rural communities [1]. It is necessary to document traditional knowledge since many communities are losing their cultural, social, and economic characteristics [2].

Lithuanian medics, interested in ethnopharmacology, are viewing it not only as a part of the Lithuanian history of medicine, but also as a significant opportunity for medical science and practice. The use of ethnopharmaceuticals, analyzed from both ethnological and ethnomedical aspects, has forced us to view ethnopharmacology as a whole entity. An opinion that ethnopharmacology is not only a way of treatment but also the means of health care and disease prevention has formed [3,4].

Currently, the interest in ethnopharmacological research is not only noticeable in developing countries but in the developed world as well. The COVID-19 pandemic with the collapse of healthcare, which has left the health of individuals to self-care, has forced us to look back at ethnopharmacology from a practical point of view [5].

The World Health Organization has estimated that more than 6 billion people depend on plant-based and animal-based medicine. Various populations have natural, widely used pharmacopoeia, where animal and plant derived ingredients are used in the preparation of modern medicines, herbal, and traditional medicines [6]. In the 21st century, medicinal plants have not lost their significance in human lives. Their application value for prophylactic and treatment purposes keeps increasing. The inhabitants of various countries actively make use of local and imported plants and their parts. As many as 80% of the world's medicinal products are made from medicinal plants, consequently the research of plants is still relevant. Today, as in the past, there are still specialists in phytotherapy since the knowledge and analysis of plants to this day remains a relevant issue.

One of the areas of research and application of ethnopharmacology is dedicated to very important human organ, the skin. The European Medicines Agency, as well as the World Health Organization and the European Scientific Cooperative on Phytotherapy, have confirmed that one of the most frequent indications for which many medicinal plants are used in the European Community and in the rest of the world, is the treatment of skin disorders and minor wounds [7]. Researchers around the world are researching plants and looking for natural means to treat skin diseases and create cosmetics [8–11].

Skin care and preventative treatments have a strong impact on the condition of skin, consequently scientists pay a lot of attention to cosmetics and cosmeceuticals (the active and science-based cosmetics). Natural agents are gaining popularity nowadays as most women prefer natural products for their personal care. These products supply the body with nutrients and enhance health and at the same time are free from synthetic chemicals and have relatively less side-effects compared to synthetic cosmetics. Following this tendency, more medicinal plants are used for the development of new drugs, cosmeceuticals, and pharmaceutical applications [12]. The investment in ethnobotanical studies can minimize the loss of knowledge and, with specialized analytics and more complex in vitro skin models, can develop and help better understand the effects that plants have on human skin [7]. In addition, preventative cosmetic procedures can reduce psychological disorders that may increase in patients during the COVID-19 pandemic situation [13].

Studies have shown that during the COVID-19 pandemic, patients were concerned with their appearance and continued to undergo cosmetic procedures and pay attention to their skincare [14]. The emotional health and well-being of a person heavily depends on aesthetic appearance, therefore the disrupted availability of cosmetology services due to the pandemic was a stressful occurrence in Lithuania as well. This is the first study in Lithuania dedicated entirely to skin diseases and cosmetic ethnopharmaceuticals, and the first study to analyze ethnopharmacology as a phenomenon in Lithuania during the ongoing COVID-19 pandemic. The main purpose of this study was to collect and evaluate ethnopharmaceutical knowledge regarding skin diseases and cosmetics in the Šiauliai District during the COVID-19 pandemic in Lithuania.

2. Materials and Methods

2.1. Study Area

The climate of Lithuania is transitional between the continental type in the East and the oceanic type of Western Europe. Therefore, here predominate air masses influenced by the Atlantic alternating with continental Eurasian or Arctic air masses. The coldest month in Lithuania is January with an average temperature of -5 °C; the warmest month is July with an average temperature of 17 °C. The average annual rainfall is about 800 mm [15]. Climate change also affects Lithuanian vegetation, which inhabits several different regions. The maritime region is dominated by pine forests, the sand dunes by shrubby plants, spruce dominate in the hilly eastern part, oaks in the central part, birches, black alder, aspen in the north, while pine forests are prevalent in the south. About 1/3 of the vegetation consists of forests, 1/5 is meadows, and a small part is wetlands. Dzūkija is the most forested ethnographic area in Lithuania, while the least forested is Suvalkija. Coniferous trees make up 56% of Lithuania's forests, while deciduous trees make up 39% and hardwoods 4%. The average age of forests in Lithuania is from 50 to 69 years [16].

The regions in Lithuania that have formed throughout the course of history are called ethnographic regions. Their boundaries roughly coincide with the boundaries of Lithuanian dialects. The regions differ in their internal structure, cultural traditions, architecture, dialects, and activities [17]. Samogitia is a unique ethnographic region of Lithuania, first mentioned in the Volhynian Chronicle in 1219. It stands out from other homesteads in terms of planning, landscaping, work tools, household utensils, landscape, traditions, and dialect. The traditional dishes of Samogitia are cibulynė, or blood sausage with groats, and boiled potatoes with hemp. Samogitians have a reputation for being very stubborn, sincere, unhurried, and hospitable people. Samogitia is characterized by these craftsmen: carpenters, shoemakers, tailors, weavers, wheelers, and blacksmiths. Pottery is especially popular. Samogitia used to be famous for its wooden chapels, chapel columns, crosses, and figurines of saints [18].

Šiauliai district is in the Northwest of Lithuania, located directly on the border between Aukštaitija and Samogitia, although it is considered a part of Samogitia. The district covers 1807 square kilometres, consists of 11 elderships, with a population density of 26 people/sq. km. The district has 1 city, 7 towns and 521 villages within its territory. The highest point is Grinikai hill (183.4 m). Šiauliai district is in the middle plain of the Venta river, in the lowland of the Mūša Nemunėlis and in the Eastern Samogitian plateau. Forests cover 34.8% of the district's territory. Spruce and birch forests are predominant. The most important extractable minerals in the district are gravel and sand [17,18]. Most of the respondents lived closer to the border of Samogitia (Kuršėnai, Daugėliai, Kužiai, Gruzdžiai, Lukšiai, etc.) (Figure 1). Although the Samogitian dialect is quite prevalent in Samogitia, people who can speak the dialect usually use it only with people they are close to with, in a private environment and less often in public. Although the respondents were mostly from the Samogitian side of the border, they did not use the dialect during the interviews.

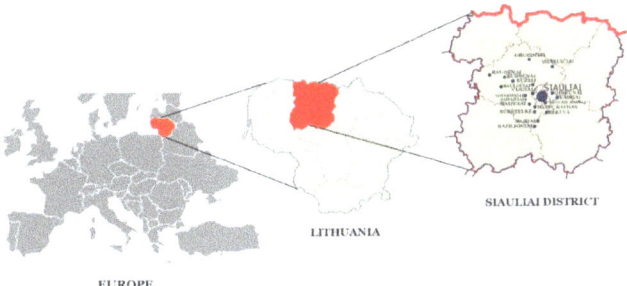

Figure 1. Study area.

2.2. Methods

The study was conducted from July 2020 to October 2021 in Šiauliai district, in the territory of the Samogitia ethnographic region (Figure 1). The purpose of this study was explained to each interviewee and an informed consent form was signed prior to the study. The study was conducted in accordance with the Code of Ethics of the International Society of Ethnobiology [19]. The research was approved by the Bioethics Centre of the Lithuanian University of Health Sciences (No. BEC-FF-30). The study surveyed 50 respondents, 9 men (18%) and 41 women (82%). The respondents were mostly farmers, housewives and even medical professionals, practically all of whom were interested in the use of medicinal plants for medicinal purposes (herbalists). Permission to conduct the study was obtained from local community leaders. A study guide identified the members of the target group as respondents who used ethnopharmacology for skin diseases and cosmetics. The study group formation employed the "snowball" technique. All safety measures were taken according to requirements of the pandemic situation (i.e., wearing face masks and gloves and maintaining a safe distance).

The research method was a structured interview. It was carried out in two stages. During the first stage, using the prepared questionnaire File S1 (Supplementary Materials), the researcher wrote down the respondent's answers. The prepared questionnaire consisted of 17 questions. The first stage started with the main questions for demographic data and closed questions to assess the source of ethnopharmaceutical information and to evaluate how many respondents chose to consult a healthcare professional (pharmacist or doctor) as a qualified consultant regarding ethnopharmacology for skin diseases and cosmetics. Much attention was paid to the sources of ethnobotanical knowledge obtained by the respondents. The aim of the second stage was to gather as much information as possible about products of natural origin, to identify medicinal raw materials used for medicinal and cosmetic purposes, their preparation methods, indications for use, doses, duration of use, and storage conditions (Figure 2). This information was obtained in the form of a free interview, and informants were allowed to speak spontaneously and without pressure. Interviews were voice recorded with permission from the respondents, and field notes were also taken and encoded. It was attempted to capture information about collected medicinal substances: where they were collected and how and under what conditions they were dried and stored. Respondents were visited a second time to supplement information if needed. The indications for skin diseases identified in the study were compared with the European Union herbal monographs by the Committee on Herbal Medicinal Products published by the European Medicines Agency (EMA) [20]. In this way, an attempt was made to determine the extent to which the indications for use in this study matched the indications approved in the EMA studies.

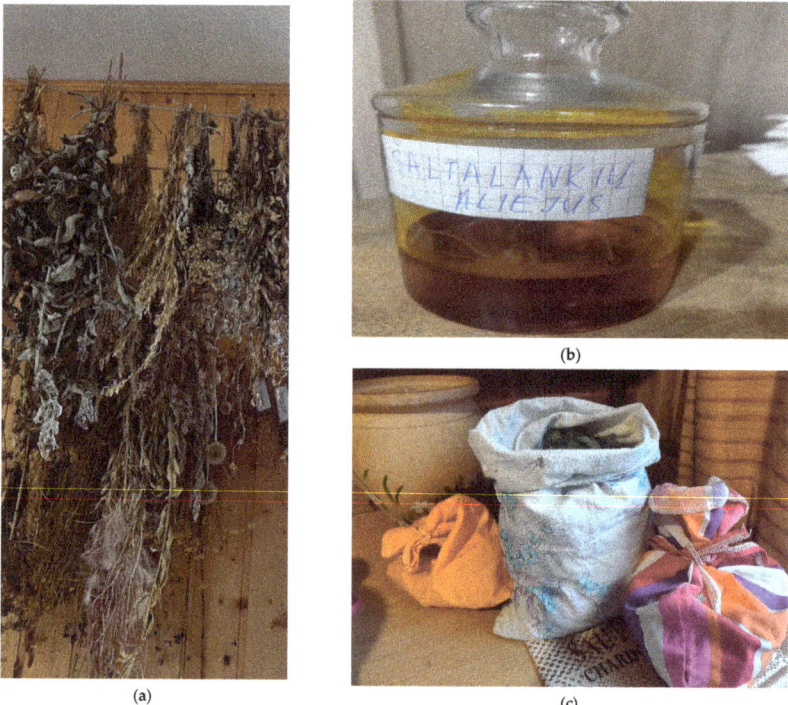

Figure 2. Preparation and storage conditions of medicinal raw materials used for skin diseases and/or cosmetics: (**a**) drying of various herbs; (**b**) prepared Sea buckthorn oil; (**c**) storage of dried plants in canvas bags.

Taxonomic identification, botanical nomenclature and plant family assignment were performed based on validated databases, namely World Flora Online [21] and the Angiosperm Phylogeny Group IV [22]. Plant species were identified using writings on traditional Lithuanian flora [23–25].

The research data is stored in the Lithuanian Museum of the History of Medicine and Pharmacy of the Lithuanian University of Health Sciences.

3. Results and Discussion

3.1. Characteristics of Informants and Sources of Ethnopharmaceutical Knowledge

50 respondents were interviewed: 9 men (18%) and 41 (82%) women. The age of the respondents ranged from 23 to 94 years. 30% of the respondents were over the age of 65. When interviewing the respondents, it was important to determine whether the respondents were permanent residents of Šiauliai district and to determine if they were born there. Four respondents have changed their place of residence (moved to another district), but all of them named Šiauliai district as their place of residence. Therefore, we can assume that part of the ethnopharmaceutical knowledge collected in the study area is of local use. Respondents from 18 different residential areas of Šiauliai district were interviewed in this study. Most respondents lived in villages-Kužiai 15%, Voveriškiai 13%, Gruzdžiai 11% (Figure 1).

The respondents' education was also an important indicator in the survey. The oldest respondents in the survey, who were over 80 years old, had primary education 7 respondens (14%), secondary education 4 respondents (8%), vocational education 8 respondents (16%), higher education 7 (14%), and university education 24 (48%) respondents. This shows that in the first decades of the 21st century, 22% of the respondents did not have a profession and were primarily agricultural workers. A total of 20 (40%) respondents with vocational, higher and university education were engaged in agricultural activities. The other 19 (38%) respondents were not involved with agricultural work (studying or working in the city).

Knowledge about the use of ethnopharmaceuticals for the treatment of skin diseases and for cosmetic purposes was obtained mainly from parents, grandparents, and relatives 45 (90%) of all respondents. Other sources of information were neighbors 27 (54%), the internet and television 26 (52%), doctors 9 (18%), pharmacists 25 (50%), and books 13 (26%). Every second respondent consulted a pharmacist on the use of ethnopharmaceuticals, which is a high percentage, considering that in our previous studies in Lithuania this percentage was incredibly low—0% [3], 8% [26] and 28% [27] of all respondents. A study on the attitude of the Lithuanian population towards phytotherapy revealed that only 1% of patients in all age groups turned to a pharmacist as a source of information on herbal medicine [28]. The reasons for not referring to a pharmacist were mainly distrust of pharmacists and their lack of knowledge about ethnopharmacology, and sometimes even the pharmacist's ridicule of the patient for using such measures. In this study, due to the increase in the number of patients turning to a pharmacist for information on ethnopharmacology, the COVID-19 pandemic can be identified as the cause, due to it causing difficulties in reaching a physician or cosmetologist, leaving pharmacists as the most widely available healthcare professionals. On the other hand, the question arises as to whether the consultation and the knowledge of the pharmacist were sufficient and met the expectations of patients.

3.2. Skin Diseases and Ethnopharmacology

We documented 67 species of medicinal plants from 37 families used for skin diseases and cosmetics. All of the collected data are summarized in Table S1 (Supplementary Materials). According to our results, the most common indication of skin diseases were wounds (39%) (Figure 3).

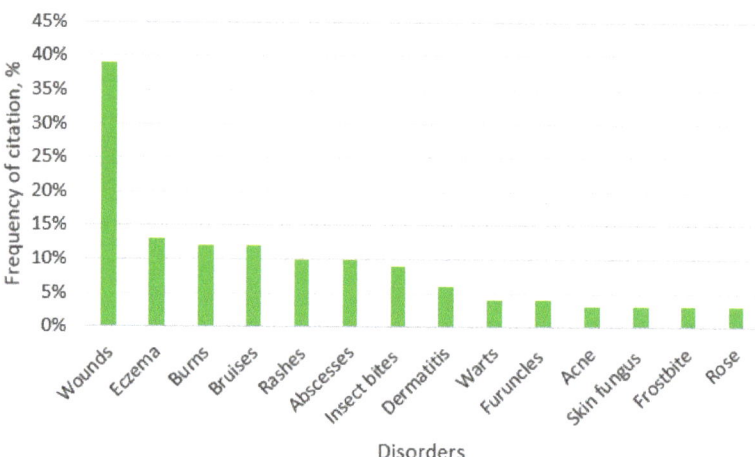

Figure 3. Ethnopharmaceutical preparations for skin disorders.

According to studies by other researchers, this is the most common indication of all skin diseases for which ethnobotanical measures are used [7]. For thousands of years, medicinal plants have represented the only remedy for wound care, and they still maintain an important therapeutic role. Of course, the main properties of plants used for wound care are antimicrobial and anti-inflammatory activities [29]. Although homemade herbal products in general are less expensive than modern treatments, they can lead to unexpected allergic reactions and side effects [30]. This is especially true when applied to the affected area of skin (excluding wounds, the main indications were eczema, burns, abscesses). In this study, all ethnopharmaceuticals were used externally, mostly as decoction, compress, juice, and oil applications (Figure 4).

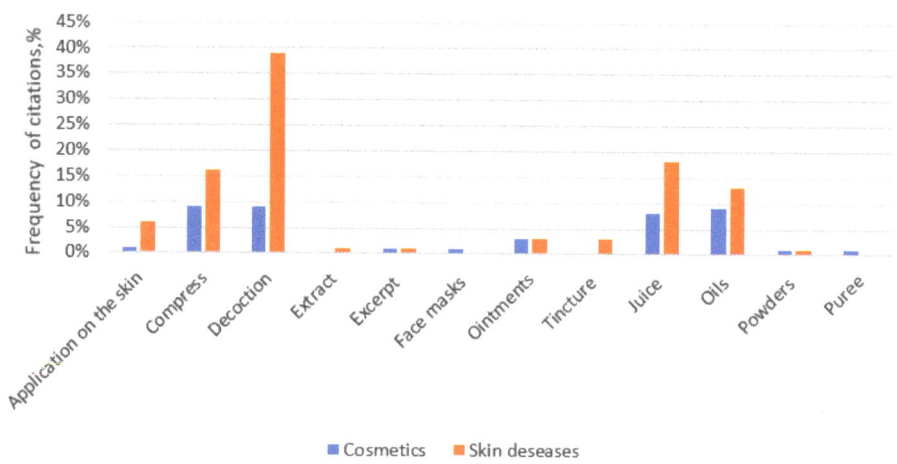

Figure 4. Methods of ethnopharmaceutical preparation for the treatment of skin diseases and cosmetics.

Although the most common method of administration is decoction usually used internally, in this case a decoction is prepared from plant-based raw materials and placed externally on the area affected by skin diseases. Only two types of plant raw materials were used internally, namely the decoction of *Viola tricolor* L. aerial parts for the treatment of furuncles, eczema, and rashes, the other internally used substance being a decoction made with roots of *Elytrigia repens* L., used to treat skin lesions, furuncles, and rashes. Decoction was the most common method of preparation in this study, using a soft above-ground part of the plant, so it is not surprising that the most used parts of the plant were aerial parts, leaves and flowers (Figure 5). The hard parts of plants (i.e., the seeds, stem, bark, and the fruits) were used less often, and less common preparation methods were used to prepare them, such as extraction with oil and tinctures.

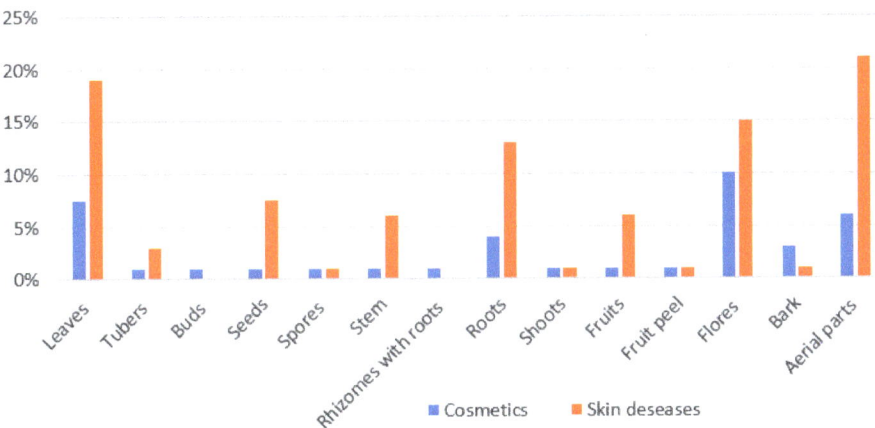

Figure 5. Parts of the plants used for ethnopharmaceutical preparations for skin diseases and cosmetics.

Jarič S and colleagues in their study on traditional wound-healing plants used in the Balkan region (Southeast Europe) [31] mentioned that the applications used for wound healing were external, in the form of infusions, decoctions, tinctures, syrups, oils, ointments, and balms, and were applied directly onto the skin, with *Plantago major* L. being the most popular medicinal plant.

In our study, the most cited plants for the care of skin diseases were *Plantago major* L. (80%) and *Chelidonium majus* L. (70%). *Plantago major* L. leaves have been used to treat wounds and traumas for centuries in almost all parts of the Europe [7,32]. According to our study, it was usually applied directly onto the skin. *Chelidonium majus* L. (70%) is a well-known plant in Lithuania, frequently the fresh juice of this plant is used to destroy warts. The plant accumulates alkaloids, so ingestion without medical supervision can be dangerous. In our study, the plant was used only externally to treat warts or psoriasis. *Chelidonium majus* L. has traditionally been used for the treatment of various inflammatory diseases and recently there were studies conducted on its use for atopic dermatitis [33] and antibacterial wound dressing applications [34].

In our study not only the frequency of use was identified, but also a comparative safety analysis with EMA monographs was carried out (Table S1). Modern pharmacological investigations have shown that many medicinal plants used in ethnobotanical traditions worldwide are being currently used in a very rational way, mainly synthesizing new and old information. Most clinical uses of medicinal plants have been similar to their traditional uses. However, there are some plants which have clinical uses that differ from traditional uses [7,35]. Despite their clinical effectiveness, a guarantee of the safety and quality of medicinal plants in developed countries is challenging as people increasingly return to herbal remedies refusing chemical drugs [27]. According to our study, respondents in Šiauliai district mentioned 67 species of medicinal plants from 37 different families used for the treatment of skin diseases and/or production of cosmetics. Only 24 species are described in the official herbal monographs of the European Medicines Agency (EMA) [20]. Sile I and colleagues from Latvia [36] have analyzed archives and found out that one of the most common health conditions were skin disorders. Analysis of EMA monographs showed that only 59 out of 211 taxa mentioned in this study are included in the official herbal monographs. EMA herbal monographs provide scientific information on safety and efficacy and deserve further exploration as traditional herbal medicines. In our study, 43 of 67 plant species were not included in the EMA monographs and only 14 species (21%) of all included species were used with EMA approved medical indications for the treatment of skin diseases. Other medicinal plants were used without EMA approved medical indications and were based solely on folk knowledge and experience in medicine.

In the treatment of skin diseases, phytotherapy plays an important role, and other materials are also used as main or additional remedy bases. In our previous study regarding historical uses of the bee products, according to archival sources, honey and propolis were used to treat wounds and abscesses [37]. In this study, honey was used as an excipient (for example by preparing a home-made ointment, which is made by mixing pine shoots and honey) to treat psoriasis. For acne-prone skin, a facial mask is made by mixing a tablespoon of honey with 10 mL of almond oil and one egg yolk. To treat burns, 10 g of birch tar is mixed with 0.5 kg of honey and then the mixture is spread on the skin area affected by burns. Lard is often used as a base for the ointment. Melted hare fat is a popular remedy for treating splinters, and it is used as a poultice on the opposite side of where the splinter is. Cases where the whole animal is used instead of its products are usually only isolated occurrences (for example, the treatment of cold sores by rubbing a small frog's abdomen on the affected area).

3.3. Ethnopharmacology and Cosmetics

Data on ethnopharmaceutical applications for cosmetic use made up 13.44% of our research (Table S1). Ethnobotanical studies combined with modern analyses of plants have a potential to enrich modern cosmetic products. Plants with cosmetic uses have often been neglected in ethnobotanical surveys which focus mainly on plants with medicinal and culinary uses [38–40]. Often, the target of researchers is the measures for treatment of skin conditions, but during the course of the study, it has been revealed that many of the plant preparations for therapeutic purposes were also used for cosmetic purposes, and making a clear distinction among the recorded preparations between cosmetics, cosmeceuticals and pharmaceuticals for the treatment of skin diseases is very problematic [41–43]. Although it may seem that the treatment of skin diseases is more important than skin care for cleanliness, prevention and restoration, beautification has also played an important role in rural communities. Studies show that the need for beauty treatments, including natural ones, has not diminished during the COVID-19 pandemic [44]. In our study during the COVID-19 pandemic in Lithuania, the main cosmetic uses were skin (20% of reports) and hair hydration (17%) and sweat reduction (17%) (Figure 6).

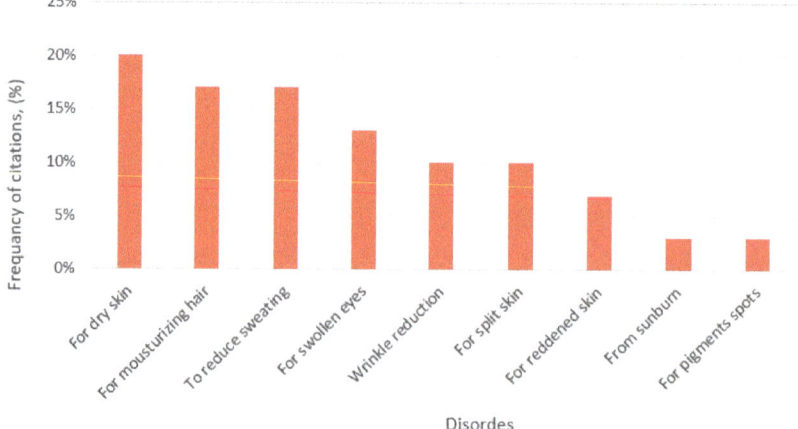

Figure 6. Ethnopharmaceutical usage for cosmetics.

According to our knowledge, there are only some ethnobotanical studies in the world that research the medicinal properties of plants and their use for cosmetic purposes. Xenia J and colleagues [39] have conducted an ethnobotanical survey of cosmetic plants used in the Marquesas Islands (French Polynesia). The most referred application areas were the skin, the hair, and the genitalia, whereas the main cosmetic uses were perfume, hydration, medicinal care, and healing. In our study the most common areas of application were the face (40% of reports), the body (38%), the feet (16%), and the hair (7%). 15.5% of facial treatments were used to reduce eye swelling.

If in Marquesas Islands the perfumed coconut oil, also known as monoi, was the main Marquesan cosmetic preparation used on skin and hair, in our study the main cosmetic preparation of *Aloe vera* L. (70%) juice was also used on skin and hair (Table S1). Our previous study on plants cultivated in Lithuania and the archival sources have revealed that *Aloe vera* L., usually called "the plant of elders", was very popular to grow at home and was "always at hand when needed" [26,45]. Due to its special composition of amino acids, lectin, lipids, minerals, lactates, phenols, etc. and its soothing and cooling properties, aloe was not only used to improve the condition of the skin but also to treat it. It reduces itching and swelling, treats light cuts, bruises, eczema, has antibacterial, antifungal properties, and improves blood flow in the affected areas [46]. In our study, several cosmetic recipes are presented. For example, for acne, one tablespoon of crushed aloe mixed with three tablespoons of calendula oil. The mixture is applied on the face and left there for 20 min; an aloe mask used for application under the eyes, is made with 1 tablespoon of aloe juice, 1 tablespoon almond oil and half a grated cucumber, everything is mixed and applied under the eyes. The mixture is left there for 15–20 min. Burns are treated by applying the flesh of a peeled aloe leaf to the affected area. This plant is popular in today's cosmetic products [47] and the modern consumer is usually aware of its beneficial properties for skin and hair.

As in treatment of skin diseases, honey, pig fat, eggs, and buttermilk represented the most reported ingredients of animal origin in cosmetic applications. The face was washed with whey to remove freckles so that the skin was "clear". The acid of ants was also used to remove freckles. This acid was acquired by throwing a scarf on an anthill, and when it dampened, the freckles were rubbed with it. Decoction, juice, and tincture with oil were most popular ways of preparation (Figure 4). As pointed out by Svanberg I [10], birch sap was the second most valuable product after wood to be found in the forest. It is renowned for antioxidative nutrients and high content of minerals. In northern Europe, birch sap has long been used not only as a food source but also for healing and cosmetics. The cosmetic use of birch sap was widespread in Estonia, where in the 19th century it was believed that washing the face with the first drops of birch sap will get rid of freckles and that the face will stay clear all summer. It was also used to treat skin diseases. In Lithuania, it was popular to rinse hair with birch sap. In this study, birch sap was also used to remove freckles and treat acne, blackheads, dry skin etc. Among the respondents, it was mentioned that the juice is frozen to ice and used to treat swollen eyes and to smoothen small wrinkles. To treat an oily scalp, two tablespoons of honey are mixed with four tablespoons of juice and a pinch of heated salt. The mixture is then diluted in half a glass of vodka, and it is then kept in a dark place for 10 days. The mixture is then rubbed into the oily scalp before washing.

The data from our study shows that the same plants are often used for cosmetic purposes and for the treatment of skin diseases. This distinguishes a separate group of cosmeceuticals. The term "cosmeceuticals" was first used by Raymond Reed in 1961 and the word and concept were further popularized by Dr Albert Kligman in the late 1970s [12]. Cosmeceuticals are both cosmetic and pharmaceutical preparations, intended to enhance health and beauty through ingredients that influence the skin's biological function. These are cosmetic products that are not just used for beautification but also for different skin ailments, from acne-control and anti-wrinkle effects to sun protection. Medicinal plants as ingredients act not only as cosmetics, but also as pharmaceuticals [12]. In this study we highlighted medicinal plants used for cosmetics and for the treatment of skin diseases (Table S1). According to the results of our study, medicinal plants used for the treatment of medical disorders and for cosmetic purposes can be singled out as potential cosmeceuticals (Figure 7).

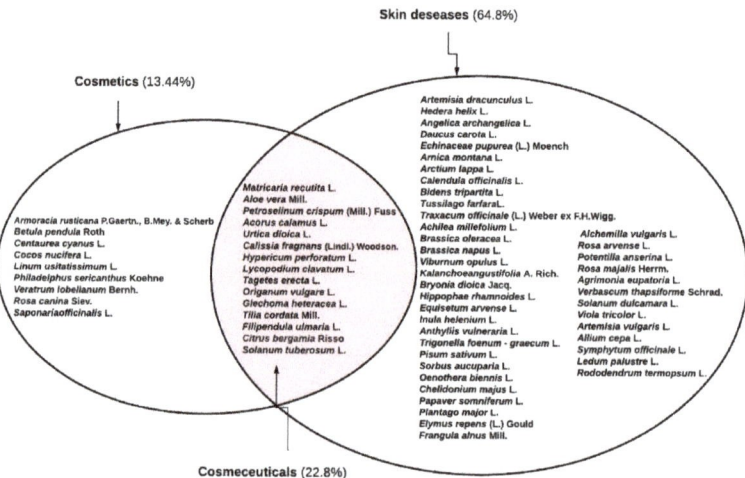

Figure 7. Use categories of medicinal plants.

4. Conclusions

The documentation of ethnopharmacological knowledge is important for the preservation of country's cultural, social, and economic identity. Also, the application of modern methods of analysis enables the development of pharmaceutical and cosmetic products acceptable to the modern consumer. In terms of public health, not only ethnopharmaceutical knowledge and its application are relevant, but also the safety of "self-treatment" and recovery rituals for the treatment of skin diseases (which is especially relevant during the COVID-19 pandemic). Our study showed that only 21% of the indications for the use of ethnopharmaceuticals for the treatment of skin diseases coincide with the EMA assessment. The use of natural cosmetics and cosmeceuticals during the COVID-19 pandemic was popular in Lithuania. Improper use of ethnopharmaceuticals for cosmetic purposes and in the treatment of skin diseases can cause not only aesthetic but also health problems, and therefore ethnopharmacological knowledge must be critically assessed and based on scientific research. The ethnopharmacological knowledge of healthcare professionals (especially pharmacists) must be sufficient for the patient consultation and an adequate care.

Supplementary Materials: The following supporting information can be downloaded at: https://www.mdpi.com/article/10.3390/ijerph19074054/s1, File S1: Questionnaire, Table S1: Ethnopharmaceuticals for skin diseases and cosmetics in Siauliai district, Lithuania.

Author Contributions: Data curation, A.P.; formal analysis, R.G.; investigation, Z.P. and R.G.; methodology, Z.P., A.P. and J.B.; supervision, Z.P. and J.B.; writing—original draft, Z.P.; writing—review and editing, A.P. and J.B. All authors have read and agreed to the published version of the manuscript.

Funding: This research received no external funding.

Institutional Review Board Statement: The study was conducted according to the guidelines of the Declaration of Helsinki, and approved by the Bioethics Center of the LITHUANIAN UNIVERSITY OF HEALTH SCIENCES (No. BEC-FF-30, data of approval 16 June 2020).

Informed Consent Statement: Informed consent was obtained from all subjects involved in the study.

Data Availability Statement: The data generated for this study are available from the authors upon request.

Acknowledgments: We thank all the local people who kindly shared their knowledge and lifestyle.

Conflicts of Interest: The authors declare no conflict of interest.

References

1. Savoniakaite, V. Rethinking history of Lithuanian ethnology. *Lituanistica* **2008**, *2008*, 59–66. Available online: https://explore.openaire.eu/search/publication?articleId=od_____2712::04ef88cbbc929408aad4e6bc8468bbbf (accessed on 26 September 2021).
2. Alves, R.R.N.; Rosa, I.L. Why Study the Use of Animal Products in Traditional Medicines. *J. Ethnobiol. Ethnomed.* **2005**, *1*, 5. [CrossRef] [PubMed]
3. Pranskuniene, Z.; Dauliute, R.; Pranskunas, A.; Bernatoniene, J. Ethnopharmaceutical knowledge in Samogitia region of Lithuania: Where old traditions overlap with modern medicine. *J. Ethnobiol. Ethnomed.* **2018**, *14*, 1–26. [CrossRef]
4. Tilvikas, J. Lietuvininkų Liaudies Medicina Nuo XX A.Vidurio Iki XXI A. Pradžios. 2017. Available online: http://www.ekgt.lt/media/dokumentai/veikla/Tyrimai/2017tyrimai/Tilvikas_tyrimas.pdf (accessed on 20 September 2021).
5. Pieroni, A.; Vandebroek, I.; Prakofjewa, J.; Bussmann, R.W.; Paniagua-Zambrana, N.Y.; Maroyi, A.; Torri, L.; Zocchi, D.M.; Dam, A.T.K.; Khan, S.M.; et al. Taming the pandemic? The importance of homemade plant-based foods and beverages as community responses to COVID-19. *J. Ethnobiol. Ethnomed.* **2020**, *16*, 75–79. [CrossRef]
6. Dugani, S.; Wasan, K.M.; Kissoon, N. World Health Organization and Essential Medicines. *J. Pharm. Sci.* **2018**, *107*, 1261–1262. [CrossRef] [PubMed]
7. Tsioutsiou, E.E.; Miraldi, E.; Governa, P.; Biagi, M.; Giordani, P.; Cornara, L. Skin Wound Healing: From Mediterranean Ethnobotany to Evidence based Phytotherapy. *Athens. J. Sci.* **2017**, *4*, 199–212. [CrossRef]
8. Koskovac, M.; Cupara, S.; Kipic, M.; Barjaktarevic, A.; Milovanovic, O.; Kojicic, K.; Markovic, M. Sea Buckthorn Oil—A Valuable Source for Cosmeceuticals. *Cosmetics* **2017**, *4*, 40. Available online: https://search.proquest.com/docview/2124637370 (accessed on 12 January 2022). [CrossRef]
9. Vaughn, A.R.; Clark, A.K.; Sivamani, R.K.; Shi, V.Y. Dermatology—Clinical Dermatology; Reports from University of Arizona Highlight Recent Findings in Clinical Dermatology (Natural Oils for Skin-Barrier Repair: Ancient Compounds Now Backed by Modern Science). *Health Med. Week.* **2018**, *19*, 103–117. Available online: https://search.proquest.com/docview/2007625668 (accessed on 10 January 2022).
10. Svanberg, I.; Sõukand, R.; Łuczaj, Ł.; Kalle, R.; Zyryanova, O.; Dénes, A.; Papp, N.; Nedelcheva, A.; Šeškauskaitė, D.; Kołodziejska-Degórska, I.; et al. Uses of tree saps in northern and eastern parts of Europe. *Acta Soc. Bot. Pol.* **2012**, *81*, 343–357. Available online: https://search.proquest.com/docview/1962285827 (accessed on 9 January 2022). [CrossRef]
11. Germanò, M.P.; Cacciola, F.; Donato, P.; Dugo, P.; Certo, G.; D'Angelo, V.; Mondello, L.; Rapisarda, A. Betula pendula leaves: Polyphenolic characterization and potential innovative use in skin whitening products. *Fitoterapia* **2012**, *83*, 877–882. [CrossRef]
12. Palle, A.J.; Ratnamala, K.V. An Overview on Herbal Cosmetics and Cosmeceuticals. *Int. J. Pharm. Sci. Rev. Res.* **2021**, *71*, 75–82. [CrossRef]
13. Türsen, Ü.; Türsen, B.; Lotti, T. Aesthetic dermatology procedures in coronavirus days. *J. Cosmet. Dermatol.* **2020**, *19*, 1822–1825. Available online: https://onlinelibrary.wiley.com/doi/abs/10.1111/jocd.13509 (accessed on 20 December 2021). [CrossRef] [PubMed]
14. Pikoos, T.D.; Buzwell, S.; Sharp, G.; Rossell, S.L. The COVID-19 pandemic: Psychological and behavioral responses to the shutdown of the beauty industry. *Int. J. Eat. Disord.* **2020**, *53*, 1993–2002. Available online: https://onlinelibrary.wiley.com/doi/abs/10.1002/eat.23385 (accessed on 10 December 2021). [CrossRef]
15. Lietuvos Hidrometeorologijos Tarnyba. Available online: http://www.meteo.lt/lt/klimatorajonavimas (accessed on 12 October 2021).
16. Ivavičiūtė, G. The change of forests and their area in Lithuania. *Rural. Environ. Eng. Archit.* **2018**, *1*, 174–180. [CrossRef]
17. Alma Ragauskaite Etnokulturinio Regionavimo Samprata. *Geogr. Metrast.* **2012**, *45*, 78. Available online: https://search.proquest.com/docview/1469669231 (accessed on 12 October 2021).
18. Ramonienė, M. Regional Dialects in the Lithuanian Urban Space: Skills, Practices and Attitudes. In *Multilingualism in the Baltic States*; Palgrave Macmillan: London, UK, 2018; pp. 123–152.
19. International Society of Ethnobiology (2006). International Society of Ethnobiology Code of Ethics (with 2008 Additions). Available online: http://ethnobiology.net/code-of-ethics/ (accessed on 12 September 2021).
20. European Medicines Agency. Guideline on the Assessment of Clinical Safety and Efficacy in the Preparation of Community Herbal Monographs for Well-Established and of Community Herbal Monographs/Entries to the Community List for Traditional Herbal Medicinal Products/Substances/Preparations. 2017. Available online: https://www.ema.europa.eu/en/documents/scientific-guideline/guideline-assessment-clinical-safety-efficacypreparation-eu-herbal-monographs-well-established_en.pdf (accessed on 22 December 2021).
21. WFO. 2021: World Flora Online. Available online: http://www.worldfloraonline.org (accessed on 15 January 2022).
22. Stevens, P.F. Angiosperm Phylogeny Website, Version 13. 2012. Available online: http://www.mobot.org/MOBOT/research/APweb/ (accessed on 15 January 2022).

23. Jankevičienė, R. *Botanikos Vardų Žodynas*; Botanikos Instituto Leidykla: Vilnius, Lithuania, 1998.
24. Vilkonis, K.K. *Lietuvos Žaliasis Rūbas*; Lutute: Kaunas, Lithuania, 2008.
25. Ragažinskienė, O.; Rimkienė, S.; Sasnauskas, V. *Vaistinių Augalų Enciklopedija*; Lutute: Kaunas, Lithuania, 2005.
26. Pranskuniene, Z.; Bajoraite, R.; Simaitiene, Z.; Bernatoniene, J. Home Gardens as a Source of Medicinal, Herbal and Food Preparations: Modern and Historical Approaches in Lithuania. *Appl. Sci.* **2021**, *11*, 9988. Available online: https://doaj.org/article/72979498046c4a8580485ca360755f09 (accessed on 15 January 2022). [CrossRef]
27. Pranskuniene, Z.; Ratkeviciute, K.; Simaitiene, Z.; Pranskunas, A.; Bernatoniene, J. Ethnobotanical Study of Cultivated Plants in Kaisiadorys District, Lithuania: Possible Trends for New Herbal Based Medicines. *Evid.-Based Complement. Altern. Med.* **2019**, *2019*, 3940397. [CrossRef]
28. Gukauskiene, L.; Juknyte, K. Lithuanian population attitude to herbal medicine. *Int. J. Pharm. Chem. Biol. Sci.* **2019**, *9*, 146–150.
29. Dorai, A.A. Wound care with traditional, complementary and alternative medicine. *Indian J. Plast. Surg.* **2012**, *45*, 418–424. [CrossRef]
30. Pereira, R.F.; Bártolo, P.J. Traditional Therapies for Skin Wound Healing. *Adv. Wound Care* **2016**, *5*, 28–229. Available online: https://www.liebertpub.com/doi/abs/10.1089/wound.2013.0506 (accessed on 15 December 2021). [CrossRef]
31. Jarić, S.; Kostić, O.; Mataruga, Z.; Pavlović, D.; Pavlović, M.; Mitrović, M.; Pavlović, P. Traditional wound-healing plants used in the Balkan region (Southeast Europe). *J. Ethnopharmacol.* **2018**, *211*, 311–328. [CrossRef]
32. Bottoni, M.; Milani, F.; Colombo, L.; Nallio, K.; Colombo, P.S.; Giuliani, C.; Bruschi, P.; Fico, G. Using Medicinal Plants in Valmalenco (Italian Alps): From Tradition to Scientific Approaches. *Molecules* **2020**, *25*, 4144. Available online: https://www.ncbi.nlm.nih.gov/pubmed/32927742 (accessed on 16 November 2021). [CrossRef] [PubMed]
33. Yang, G.; Lee, K.; Lee, M.; Kim, S.; Ham, I.; Choi, H. Inhibitory effects of *Chelidonium majus* extract on atopic dermatitis-like skin lesions in NC/Nga mice. *J. Ethnopharmacol.* **2011**, *138*, 398–403. [CrossRef] [PubMed]
34. Mouro, C.; Gomes, A.P.; Ahonen, M.; Fangueiro, R.; Gouveia, I.C. *Chelidoniummajus* L. Incorporated Emulsion Electrospun PCL/PVA_PEC Nanofibrous Meshes for Antibacterial Wound Dressing Applications. *Nanomaterials* **2021**, *11*, 1785. Available online: https://search.proquest.com/docview/2554781609 (accessed on 10 January 2022). [CrossRef]
35. Alan, Z.; Özgüldü, H.; Erdal, M.S.; Bucak, A.Y.; Üresin, A.Y.; Akalın, E. Evaluation of clinical trials of the plants, which have ethnobotanical uses for skin disorders in Turkey: A review. *Clin. Phytosci.* **2021**, *7*, 1–29. Available online: https://link.springer.com/article/10.1186/s40816-021-00316-x (accessed on 12 January 2022). [CrossRef]
36. Sile, I.; Romane, E.; Reinsone, S.; Maurina, B.; Tirzite, D.; Dambrova, M. Medicinal plants and their uses recorded in the Archives of Latvian Folklore from the 19th century. *J. Ethnopharmacol.* **2020**, *249*, 112378. [CrossRef]
37. Pranskuniene, Z.; Bernatoniene, J.; Simaitiene, Z.; Pranskunas, A.; Mekas, T. Ethnomedicinal Uses of Honeybee Products in Lithuania: The First Analysis of Archival Sources. *Evid.-Based Complement. Altern. Med.* **2016**, *2016*, 9272635. [CrossRef] [PubMed]
38. Faccio, G. Plant Complexity and Cosmetic Innovation. *iScience* **2020**, *23*, 101358. [CrossRef] [PubMed]
39. Jost, X.; Ansel, J.; Lecellier, G.; Raharivelomanana, P.; Butaud, J. Ethnobotanical survey of cosmetic plants used in Marquesas Islands (French Polynesia). *J. Ethnobiol. Ethnomed.* **2016**, *12*, 1–22. Available online: https://www.ncbi.nlm.nih.gov/pubmed/27899137 (accessed on 17 November 2021). [CrossRef]
40. Gilca, M.; Tiplica, G.S.; Salavastru, C.M. Traditional and ethnobotanical dermatology practices in Romania and other Eastern European countries. *Clin. Dermatol.* **2018**, *36*, 338–352. Available online: https://www.clinicalkey.es/playcontent/1-s2.0-S0738081X18300440 (accessed on 17 November 2021). [CrossRef]
41. Saikia, A.P.; Ryakala, V.K.; Sharma, P.; Goswami, P.; Bora, U. Ethnobotany of medicinal plants used by Assamese people for various skin ailments and cosmetics. *J. Ethnopharmacol.* **2006**, *106*, 149–157. [CrossRef] [PubMed]
42. Pieroni, A.; Quave, C.L.; Villanelli, M.L.; Mangino, P.; Sabbatini, G.; Santini, L.; Boccetti, T.; Profili, M.; Ciccioli, T.; Rampa, L.G.; et al. Ethnopharmacognostic survey on the natural ingredients used in folk cosmetics, cosmeceuticals and remedies for healing skin diseases in the inland Marches, Central-Eastern Italy. *J. Ethnopharmacol.* **2004**, *91*, 331–344. [CrossRef] [PubMed]
43. Setshego, M.V.; Aremu, A.O.; Mooki, O.; Otang-Mbeng, W. Natural resources used as folk cosmeceuticals among rural communities in Vhembe district municipality, Limpopo province, South Africa. *BMC Complement. Med. Ther.* **2020**, *20*, 81. Available online: https://www.ncbi.nlm.nih.gov/pubmed/32164701 (accessed on 17 November 2021). [CrossRef] [PubMed]
44. Aslan Kayıran, M.; Kara Polat, A.; Alyamaç, G.; Demirseren, D.D.; Taş, B.; Kalkan, G.; Özkök Akbulut, T.; Kaya Özden, H.; Koska, M.C.; Emre, S. Has the COVID-19 pandemic changed attitudes and behaviors concerning cosmetic care and procedures among patients presenting to the dermatology outpatient clinic? A multicenter study with 1437 participants. *J. Cosmet. Dermatol.* **2021**, *20*, 3121–3127. Available online: https://onlinelibrary.wiley.com/doi/abs/10.1111/jocd.14420 (accessed on 15 January 2022). [CrossRef] [PubMed]
45. Žumbakienė, G. *Senieji Lietuvos Gėlių Darželiai*; Lietuvos Liaudies Buities Muziejus: Rumšiškės, Lithuania, 2016.
46. Watson, R.R.; Zibadi, S. *Bioactive Dietary Factors and Plant Extracts in Dermatology*, 1st ed.; Humana Press: Totowa, NJ, USA, 2013.
47. Dal'Belo, S.E.; Gaspar, L.R.; Maia Campos, P.M. Moisturizing effect of cosmetic formulations containing *Aloe vera* extract in different concentrations assessed by skin bioengineering techniques. *Ski. Res. Technol.* **2006**, *12*, 241–246. Available online: https://api.istex.fr/ark:/67375/WNG-44D5QHS6-6/fulltext.pdf (accessed on 18 January 2022). [CrossRef] [PubMed]

Article

COVID-19 Pandemic Lockdown: An Excellent Opportunity to Study the Effects of Trawling Disturbance on Macrobenthic Fauna in the Shallow Waters of the Gulf of Gabès (Tunisia, Central Mediterranean Sea)

Nawfel Mosbahi [1,*], Jean-Philippe Pezy [2], Jean-Claude Dauvin [2] and Lassad Neifar [1]

1 Laboratoire de Biodiversité Marine et Environnement, Faculté des Sciences de Sfax, Université de Sfax, BP 1171, Sfax 3038, Tunisia; lassad.naifar@fss.rnu.tn
2 Laboratoire Morphodynamique Continentale et Côtière, Normandie University, UNICAEN, CNRS, UMR 6143 M2C, 24 Rue des Tilleuls, 14000 Caen, France; jean-philippe.pezy@unicaen.fr (J.-P.P.); jean-claude.dauvin@unicaen.fr (J.-C.D.)
* Correspondence: nawfelmosbahi@hotmail.fr or nawfel.mosbahi.etud@fss.usf.tn

Abstract: This study describes for the first time in the central Mediterranean Sea the effects of bottom trawling on macrobenthic fauna in tidal channels of the Kneiss Islands in the Gulf of Gabès, Tunisia. Following a BACI protocol, two control stations (protected by artificial reefs) and two trawled stations (impacted stations) were sampled during a period with the absence of bottom trawling activity (the COVID-19 pandemic lockdown period from March to May 2020) and during a trawled period. Although bottom trawling had no impact on sediment composition, this anthropogenic activity reduced the concentration of dissolved oxygen and had a noticeable effect on water column turbidity. The absence of trawling led to a significant increase in biomass, number of species, and abundance of total macrofauna. This illustrated the negative effect of trawling activity in shallow waters and the high resilience of macrobenthic communities of the tidal ecosystem of the Kneiss Islands. In the future, it would be very important to control the use of this destructive fishing gear due to its negative impact on the marine habitat and macrofauna, which represents essential prey for fishes and birds living in this protected area.

Keywords: bottom trawling; COVID-19 pandemic lockdown; environmental impacts; macrobenthic fauna; tidal channels; central Mediterranean Sea

1. Introduction

Bottom trawling is one of the most harmful anthropogenic activities on both shallow and deep marine ecosystems [1–3]. It is a relatively non-selective fishing method with global negative impacts on benthic communities and habitats [4–6]. Bottom trawling provokes sediment re-suspension; decreases macrofaunal bioturbation processes; and removes, injures, or kills a wide range of sedentary organisms. It also induces changes in the population demography and can have dire consequences on ecosystem structures and functions [7–10].

The Gulf of Gabès, located in the central part of the Mediterranean, covers the second-widest continental shelf area (35,900 km²) and is characterized by unique geomorphological, climatic, and oceanographic conditions. This gulf has an extensive network of tidal channels and very gentle slopes [11]. The tidal channel environments are of major ecological importance, being considered among the main pathways of passage and migration for several commercial marine species (fish and shrimp) and providing important habitats for the juveniles of many inshore fish species [12,13]. Therefore, the Gulf of Gabès is an important nursery for several fish species and represents one of the main target areas for fishing activities in Tunisia; moreover, it is among the most highly productive zones in the

Mediterranean Sea [14]. The favourable geomorphologic and climatic conditions are combined to support one of the most productive ecosystems around the small tidal channels in the Gulf of Gabès [14,15]. These tidal features are very attractive for many kinds of fishing activity, especially bottom trawling [16]. Around the Kneiss Islands, tidal channels are visible only at low tide; this unique system in the Mediterranean Sea represents the highest energy environment of the Gulf of Gabès and is sensitive to anthropogenic activities and climate change [17,18]. These conditions favour the circulation of seawater, sediments, organic matter, and nutrients between terrestrial and coastal marine environments [19]. Due to their diversity of birds, the Kneiss Islands have been designated as a 'Specially Protected Area of Mediterranean Importance' (SPAMI) in 2001, an 'Important Bird Area' (IBA) in 2003, and as a 'RAMSAR site' since 2007. Nevertheless, despite international protection, intensive human activities occur in this Marine Protected Area [20]. In the tidal channels of the Kneiss Islands, fishers use traditional and impacting fishing gear such as the small bottom trawl known locally as "Kiss". The Kiss trawlers usually display all of the characteristics and gears that can be found on regular trawlers: a net with a lead line; a float line; and a cod end, tied on both sides to otter doors that are usually wooden on Kiss trawlers. The main differences between a Kiss trawler and a regular one are the size of the vessel and those of the net. The mesh size of the Kiss nets is much smaller (18 versus more than 28 mm) than on a regular trawler, which makes them less selective and liable to producing large amounts of by-catch. Kiss trawlers are small versions of the regular ones; they rarely reach 10 m in length, are mainly manufactured with wood, and are equipped with a power winch and an iron bar on the stern of the boat to tow the net. Illegal vessels could operate in areas of shallow water (5 m depth or less), destroying sensitive habitats and spawning grounds, by tearing out the seagrass meadows caused by bottom scraping metal panels towed by the trawler [21].

Such gear unfavourably affects the juveniles of fish and shrimps as well as sensitive benthic habitats such as *Posidonia oceanica* meadows [7,22]. In October 2018, a team of inspectors counted the vessels equipped with unauthorized bottom trawls to estimate the total number of illegal trawlers operating over the whole Gulf of Gabès. Between 400 and 500 of such trawlers were identified in the main ports around the Gulf of Gabès [21]. It is very difficult to recognize and separate illegal Kiss trawlers from other trawlers, as most of them do not display their identification numbers or VMS (vessel monitoring system) used to monitor the location and the activities of commercial fishing vessels required under Tunisian legislation, making legal pursuit and law enforcement harder. We estimated that, around the Kneiss Islands, in the central part of the Gulf of Gabès, approximately 100 vessels carry out trawling activities every day in tidal channels. These vessels came from the ports of Khawala, Skhira, and Mahres. They were small vessels (7 to 10 m of length) equipped with mini trawls to catch target species such as the shrimp *Metapenaeus monoceros* (Fabricius, 1798), several fish species, including *Sparus aurata* Linnaeus, 1758; *Diplodus* spp.; *Solea* spp.; cephalopods *Sepia officinalis* Linnaeus, 1758; and recently, the exotic invasive blue crab *Portunis segnis* (Forskål, 1775).

To study anthropogenic pressures and to assess their effects, ecologists and stakeholders have stressed the key role of the macrofauna in establishing the ecological quality status of benthic communities [23,24] and in assessing the biological integrity of marine systems [25,26]. In fact, benthic invertebrates are considered potentially powerful indicators of marine ecosystem health [24]. Due to their life at the sediment–water interface and their short life spans, these organisms can record both accidental and chronic perturbations in marine environments [27–29].

Coronavirus Disease 2019 (COVID-19) is the official name of a respiratory infectious disease caused by a new coronavirus that was first reported in Wuhan, China, and then spread unexpectedly fast across the world on 11 March 2020, when the World Health Organization (WHO) stated the COVID-19 outbreak as a "pandemic public health menace" [30,31] due to its worldwide spread. Since February 2020, affected countries have locked down their cities and industries to restrict the movement of their citizens and to minimize the spread of the virus [30,32]. Despite the negative aspects of coronavirus on human health, this crisis had a positive impact on the natural environment: improvements in air and water quality, and reductions in industrial effluents and in the discharge of other wastes [33,34]. There had also been a decline in the exploitation of natural resources and a strong rise in the successful recruitment of several marine species observed in certain perturbed ecosystems (harbours, industrial coastal zones, etc.), which was attributed to lowered anthropogenic pressures [35,36]. These might be short-term improvements, but they highlighted the severity of anthropogenic impacts worldwide.

In the Gulf of Gabès, a major part of this scientific work was carried out to assess the interaction between fishing with bottom trawling, and vulnerable and protected animals such as sharks, rays, and marine turtles. Data on the impacts of bottom trawling on macrobenthic fauna in the Gulf of Gabès are few and even rare, because a reference period is required to study anthropogenic activities to understand their environmental effects. Many human activities have developed around the Kneiss Islands, including bait digging [20] and clam harvesting [37], and several research protocols have been implemented to study the effects of each activity (see [20,37]).

This work highlights the response of macrobenthic communities when faced with the cessation of destructive fishing activities during the COVID-19 pandemic lockdown period. Therefore, this study was carried out using a BACI (Before After Control Impact) approach, exploiting the COVID-19 pandemic lockdown period to evaluate the impacts of bottom trawling on soft-bottom macrobenthic communities of the tidal channels of the Kneiss Islands in order to set up an effective management plan for artisanal fishing activity in this subtidal ecosystem of the central Mediterranean Sea.

2. Materials and Methods

2.1. Study Area

Located in the northwestern part of the Gulf of Gabès, between latitudes $34°10'$ N and $34°30'$ N and between longitudes $10°E$ and $10°30'$ E, the Kneiss islands are characterized by the highest tidal range in the western Mediterranean Sea; the tide is semi-diurnal with an amplitude varying from 0.8 to 2.3 m [11]. Tidal currents have created shallow channels in the Gulf of Gabès that are extensively developed around the Kneiss islands. In these ecosystems, sediments are mainly composed of sand and coarse sand; the sedimentary filling of the tidal channels shows decreasing grain size from downstream to upstream, indicating that the action of tidal currents is stronger during a flood tide than during an ebb tide [19]. Moreover, sediments in the shallowest waters are mainly characterized by sand, whilst gravel is found at intermediate-depth stations and deeper stations are dominated by fine sediment including silt [16]. Intensive human activities take place in this protected area of the Kneiss Islands [16,20,37].

2.2. Sampling and Laboratory Procedures

2.2.1. Macrobenthic Sampling and Measurement of Physicochemical Variables

Benthic macrofauna sampling was performed between March and June 2020, and carried out in the tidal channels of the Kneiss Islands at two trawled stations (i.e., stations I1 and I2) in zones where the fishers used bottom trawling and at two other control stations (stations C1 and C2: located in a protected zone preserved by artificial reefs since 2014) (Figures 1 and 2). Five sampling campaigns were organized according to a BACI strategy: one during March before the lockdown period, another at the end of the lockdown period (total cessation of trawler fishing activity controlled by the coast guard and the national navy), and three after the lockdown period (Figure 2). Benthic macrofauna sampling was carried out using a Van Veen grab covering an area of about 0.05 m^2, which penetrated approximately 0.1 m into the sediment. The station positions were accurately determined using a GPS (Global Positioning System, WGS84). For each sampling campaign, five replicates were carried out at each station: four for biological analysis covering a total surface-area of 0.2 m^2 and one for sediment analysis. Each biological sample was sieved through a 1 mm mesh, fixed with buffered 10% formaldehyde, and stained with Rose Bengal to facilitate sorting. In the laboratory, prior to identification, the samples were washed and the organisms were hand-sorted into major taxonomic groups, identified to the lowest practical taxonomic level (usually species level), and then counted. Biomass was obtained as ash-free dry weight (g AFDW) after drying (60 °C for 48 h) and calcination (500 °C for 5 h). Species names were checked using the World Register of Marine Species list (http://www.marinespecies.org accessed on 20 November 2021). In addition, several environmental factors were measured in situ such as depth (m), turbidity (measured by Suspended Solids Concentration "SSC"; mg L^{-1}), temperature (T °C), salinity (measured in situ by WTW multi-meter) and dissolved oxygen concentration (by WTW oximeter; mg L^{-1}).

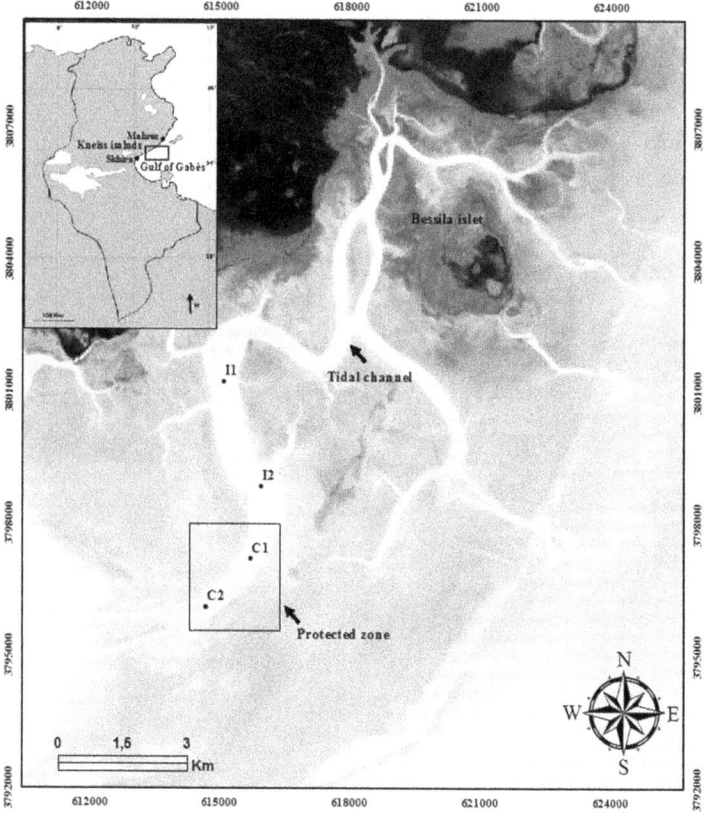

Figure 1. Map of the study area showing the locations of the sampling stations (I1 and I2: trawled zones; C1 and C2: control stations).

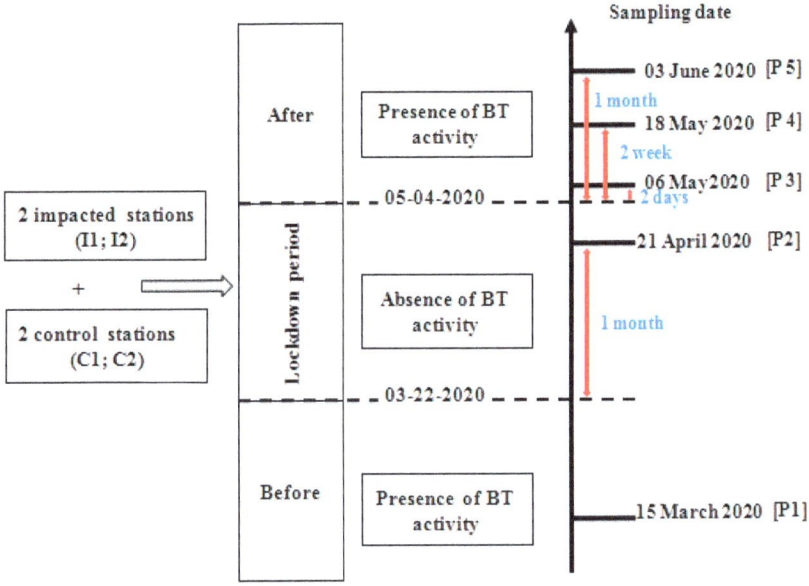

Figure 2. Representation of the sampling strategy used in this study during the five sampling periods, with P1: before lockdown; P2: during lockdown; P3: after two days; P4: after two weeks; P5: one month after the lockdown; and BT: bottom trawling.

2.2.2. Sediment Grain-Size Analysis and Organic Matter Content

The sediment from each sampling period was homogenized and wet-sieved through a 63 μm mesh to separate muddy (including silt and clay), gravely, and sandy fractions (retained on the sieve). After being oven-dried to constant weight at 60 °C, sediment fractions were separated using a mechanical shaker (column of five sieves with mesh sizes of 1000, 500, 250, 125, and 63 μm) for 10 min. All fractions (including <63 μm) were then weighed to determine their percentage relative abundance. For the organic matter content analyses, sediment samples were dried at 60 °C to constant weight and ground to a fine powder. Organic matter content was determined on the powder samples by 'loss on ignition' at 450 °C for 4 h.

2.3. Statistical Analyses

Univariate and multivariate analyses were used to evaluate the changes in the structure and composition of macrobenthic assemblages due to bottom trawling. We considered the number of taxa, abundance, and biomass per station. These biological data were used to calculate, at each station, the abundance (ind. m^{-2}) and the most common biodiversity indices, i.e., taxonomic richness (number of taxa per 0.2 m^2), biomass (g AFDW m^{-2}), Shannon index (H') [38], and Pielou's evenness (J') [39].

A Log (x + 1) transformation was applied to the abundance matrix (data for each station were pooled prior to undertaking further analyses) to minimize the influence of the most dominant taxa, before calculating the Bray–Curtis similarities using the statistical package PRIMER [40]. A dendrogram was created with group averages expressed in the cluster mode. Then, a non-parametric multi-dimensional scaling (n-MDS) ordination was applied to the abundance matrix using the Bray–Curtis similarity measure, with the objective of examining the structure of the macrobenthic assemblages. The SIMilarity PERcentages (SIMPER) routine was applied to establish which species contributed most to the observed differences in the data. Analyses of the data were performed using PRIMER® version 6 (Plymouth Routines in Multivariate Ecological Research) package [40]. Permutational multivariate analysis of variance (PERMANOVA) was also conducted to test the significant differences in macrobenthic fauna composition in response to bottom trawling (one-way analysis) [41].

For the biological parameters, a Shapiro–Wilk normality test and a Bartlett's test for homogeneity of variance were performed prior to each ANOVA to check whether the assumptions of ANOVA were met and if data transformation was necessary. Then, three-way ANOVAs were used to assess the spatiotemporal effect of bottom trawling on taxonomic, abundance, and biomass of macrofauna benthic between sample stations and during each sampling campaign (before lockdown; during lockdown; and after two days, two weeks, and one month of deconfinement). A Tukey Honestly Significant Difference test was employed to determine differences before and after trawling period as well as between the different sediment types. These statistical procedures were performed using the R software vegan package.

3. Results

3.1. Environmental Variables

There were only a very small proportion of fine particles (<63 µm) in the sediment, representing between 2 and 3.4% at stations I2, C1, and C2 and reaching 16% at I1. The sediment was dominated by coarse sand (500–2000 µm) (68 to 82%), except at I1, which was dominated by medium sand (74%). The organic matter content varied between 2.6% (C2) and 4.1% (I1) (Table 1). No significant statistical changes could be identified in sediment type and organic matter content between sampling stations and between dates (in both cases; $p > 0.05$), showing that the sediment variables were stable throughout the BACI study period from March to June 2020.

Table 1. Mean environmental characteristics of the four sampling stations during the five campaigns of the March–June period.

Stations	Coordinates		Depth (m)	OM (%)	Q50 (mm)	Sandy (%)	Silt-Clay (%)	Sediment Type
	Latitude (N)	Longitude (E)						
I1	38.00974	32.614844	5.60	4.1	0.79	83.5 ± 3.62	16.0 ± 5.18	medium sand
I2	37.98597	32.615700	8.30	3.8	1.11	97.3 ± 4.10	2.6 ± 6.22	coarse sand
C1	37.96937	32.615471	7.40	3.6	1.21	96.8 ± 3.12	3.2 ± 4.60	coarse sand
C2	37.95854	32.614429	6.50	2.6	1.14	95.8 ± 2.64	3.4 ± 1.42	coarse sand

Figure 3 showed the variation in physicochemical variables measured during the sampling period. The dissolved oxygen and the turbidity were significantly different (ANOVA; F = 1.38; $p < 0.01$; F = 2.12; $p < 0.01$, respectively) between the control and impacted stations during the five trawling periods (P1, P3, P4, and P5; illustrated in Figure 2), with higher turbidity values in the trawling stations (I1 and I2) and higher dissolved oxygen values at the control stations (C1 and C2). The impacted stations exhibited lower values of dissolved oxygen and higher values of SSC compared with the control stations during the trawling period and particularly at the last date of sampling. Conversely, no significant differences were identified for temperature and salinity between the stations during the five sampling periods for the both environmental variables ($p < 0.05$) (Table 1).

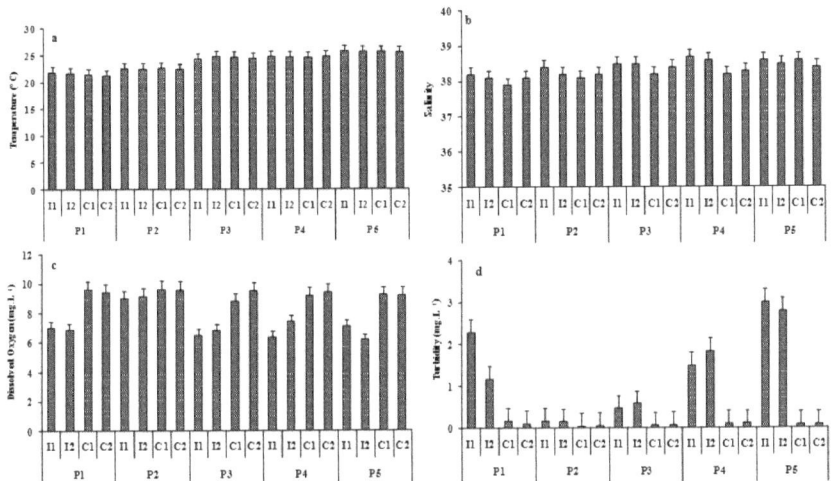

Figure 3. Physicochemical parameters (± SD) during the five sampling periods, with P1: 15 March; P2: 21 April; P3: 6 May; P4: 18 May; and P5: 3 June 2020, were (**a**) temperature (°C), (**b**) salinity, (**c**) dissolved oxygen (mg L^{-1}), and (**d**) turbidity (Suspended solid concentrations; mg L^{-1}).

3.2. General Composition of the Benthic Macrofauna

In total, 4846 macrofaunal individuals were identified belonging to 72 taxa and 6 zoological groups unequally distributed among the sampling stations. Annelid polychaetes were dominant (40% of the total number of taxa), followed by crustaceans (34%), mainly amphipods, decapods, and isopods, along with molluscs (21%), mainly bivalves and gastropods. The other three phyla (echinoderms, cnidarians, and tunicates) accounted for only 5% of the total number of taxa. Similarly, the polychaetes dominate numerically (42% of the total abundance) with the species *Cirratulus cirratus* (O. F. Müller, 1776), *Euclymene lumbricoides* (Quatrefages, 1866), *Amphitritides gracilis* (Grube, 1860), and *Nereis* spp. showing the highest number of individuals.

3.3. Impact of Bottom Trawling on the Macrofauna

Before the lockdown period (15 March 2020), the number of taxa and abundances in the four sampled stations were significantly different, with higher values recorded in the control stations than in the impacted stations (F = 3.9; $p < 0.01$; F = 2.1; $p < 0.01$, respectively). During the lockdown period (21 April 2020), when there were no trawling activities, the number of taxa and abundance increased at both impacted stations. After lockdown, abundances and numbers of taxa at both control stations were higher after two days, two weeks, and one month of the period after confinement compared with the impacted stations (Figure 4; Table 2).

Table 2. Proportion of zoological groups (A: % total abundance; B: % total biomass), the mean taxa number, mean abundance, and mean biomass recorded at the two impacted (I) and two control stations (C) during the five sampling periods: The mean taxa number (number of taxa per 0.2 m^2 ± SD); the mean abundance (number of individuals per m^2 ± SD); the mean biomass (g AFDW per m^2 ± SD); BT: bottom trawling and others groups (echinoderms, cnidarians, and tunicates).

	Presence of BT Activity Before Lockdown				Absence of BT Activity Lockdown				Deconfinement; Presence of BT Activity											
									After Two Days				After Two Weeks				After One Month			
	C		I		C		I		C		I		C		I		C		I	
	A	B	A	B	A	B	A	B	A	B	A	B	A	B	A	B	A	B	A	B
Polychaetes	47	35.1	27.0	14.4	42	34.3	37	24.9	36	35.4	30	21.8	43	31.7	26	16.2	49	31.3	19	13.6

Table 2. Cont.

	Presence of BT Activity Before Lockdown				Absence of BT Activity Lockdown				Deconfinement; Presence of BT Activity											
									After Two Days				After Two Weeks				After One Month			
	C		I		C		I		C		I		C		I		C		I	
	A	B	A	B	A	B	A	B	A	B	A	B	A	B	A	B	A	B	A	B
Crustaceans	27	34.3	44	51.3	33	35.1	35	42.8	38	34.5	39	42.4	31	36.0	42	50.4	26	38.3	42	54.2
Molluscs	22	27.2	27	32.2	21	28.1	25	28.8	24	28.3	30	34.6	23	30.3	32	33.4	22	27.2	39	32.2
Others groups	4	3.4	2	2.1	4	2.4	3	3.5	2	1.8	1	1.2	3	2.0	0	0	3	3.2	0	0
Mean taxa number	35.0 ± 3.0		11.0 ± 2.1		41.5 ± 3.6		33.0 ± 4.2		36.0 ± 2.4		25.5 ± 2.6		36.5 ± 3.2		17.0 ± 1.8		34.5 ± 3.4		9.5 ± 2.2	
Mean abundance	2762 ± 202		1256 ± 112		3187 ± 348		2807 ± 211		2856 ± 262		1923 ± 104		2821 ± 301		1112 ± 96		2634 ± 182		958 ± 62	
Mean biomass	113 ± 20		64 ± 9		186 ± 22		124 ± 12		194 ± 24		102 ± 13		198 ± 14		68 ± 8		211 ± 14		49 ± 6	

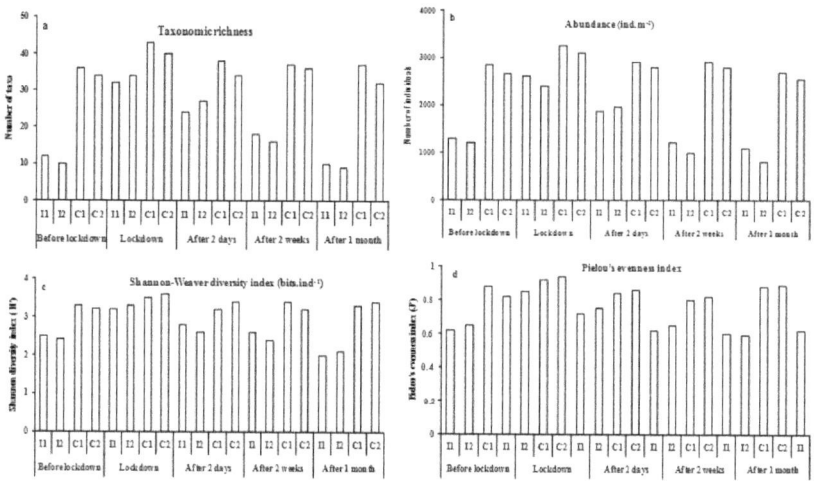

Figure 4. Benthic community parameters: taxonomic richness (**a**), abundance (**b**), Shannon–Wiener index (**c**), and Pielou's evenness (**d**) with standard deviation for all stations sampled before lockdown; during lockdown; and after two days, two weeks, and one month after confinement.

H' and J' varied significantly between stations (F = 2.18; $p < 0.01$; F = 3.11; $p < 0.01$, respectively) (Table 3), with higher values of these indices corresponding to control stations during the lockdown period (H'= 3.6 bits.ind^{-1}; J'= 0.95 in C2) (Figure 4).

Table 3. Results of the ANOVAs with the three factors: time (5 levels; df = 4), trawling (2 levels; df = 1), and site (4 levels; df = 3) for the five biological variables (*: significant variation).

	Factor	F	p
Richness species	Time	3.9	<0.01 *
	Site	1.14	<0.01 *
	Trawling	0.23	0.01 *
Abundance	Time	2.9	<0.01 *
	Site	1.21	<0.01 *
	Trawling	0.84	<0.01 *
Biomass	Time	21.4	0.01 *
	Site	0.86	<0.01 *
	Trawling	12.2	0.01 *
	Time	2.11	<0.01 *

Table 3. Cont.

	Factor	F	p
H'	Site	2.18	<0.01 *
	Trawling	1.14	0.01 *
	Time	2.41	0.01 *
J'	Site	3.11	<0.01 *
	Trawling	1.04	0.01 *

During the lockdown period, the four stations were dominated by polychaetes (~40%), followed by crustaceans and molluscs. During the trawling period, the faunal composition varied between the control and the impacted stations, with lower values in the impacted stations. The abundance of dominant species such as the infaunal polychaetes *Cirratulus cirratus* (O.F. Müller, 1776), *Euclymene oerstedii* (Claparède, 1863), the amphipod *Microdeutopus anomalus* (Rathke, 1843), and the bivalve *Scrobicularia plana* (da Costa, 1778) decreased during the trawling periods at trawled sites compared with the control stations. In contrast, the abundances of the latest species were higher during the lockdown period and even two days after the end of the lockdown in all sampled stations (Figure 5).

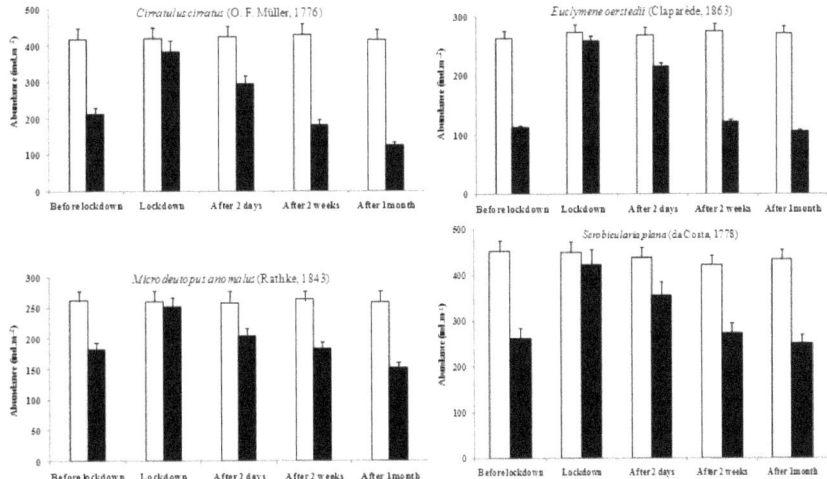

Figure 5. Mean abundance ($\pm$ SD; n = 2) for some representative species at control and impact stations during the five sampling periods (before lockdown; during lockdown; and after two days, two weeks, and one month of deconfinement). White column: control stations; black column: impacted stations.

Several sedentary organisms such as the porifera; echinodermata; cnidaria; and the tubicolous polychaeta (including the Sabellidae *Sabella pavonina* Roule, 1896 and *Branchiomma bombyx* (Dalyell, 1853); the Terebellidae *Terebella lapidaria* Linnaeus, 1767 and *Amphitrite rubra* (Risso, 1826); and the Serpulidae *Serpula vermicularis* Linnaeus, 1767 and *Hydroides dianthus* (Verrill, 1873)) only appeared at trawled stations during the lockdown period and after two days at the end of the lockdown, and then disappeared after two weeks later (18 May 2020). The ANOVA test showed that there were significant difference between biomass recorded during the five sampling periods at all stations (ANOVA; df = 4; F = 21.4; $p < 0.05$) (Table 3). The control stations showed higher biomass compared with both trawled stations during the five sampling campaigns (ANOVA; df = 1; F = 12.2; $p < 0.01$). The biomass of macrobenthic communities was higher at the control stations during the four fishing periods compared with the trawled stations (I1 and I2). During the lockdown period (P2), the biomass increased at the impacted stations simultaneously with the increase in abundance. Equally, the biomass of the main zoological group showed significant variation during the five sampling periods (ANOVA; df = 4; F = 112.4; $p < 0.05$). The biomass of polychaetes recorded at trawled stations gradually decreased with the increase in the number of trawling days (see Table 2).

The dendrogram and n-MDS (Figure 6) showed a remarkable spatial separation between the sampled stations in all three groups. The first group (GI) corresponded to both control stations sampled during the five campaigns plus both impacted stations sampled during the lockdown period. The second group (GII) corresponded to the two impacted stations sampled after only two days of deconfinement (resumption of bottom trawling activity) (I1d and I2d). The last group (GIII) gathered the impacted stations sampled before lockdown, after two weeks and after one month of deconfinement.

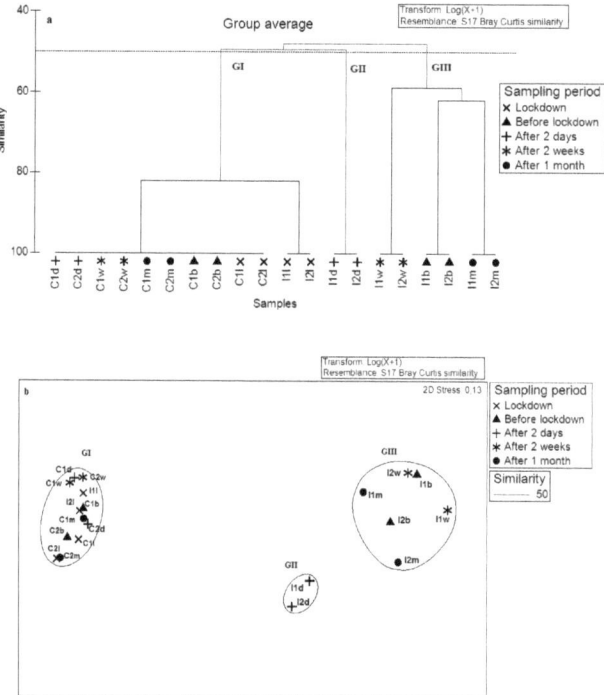

Figure 6. Dendrogram (**a**) and n-MDS ordination plot (**b**) of Bray–Curtis similarities from abundance data (Log (x + 1) transformation) for impacted (I1 and I2) and control (C1 and C2) sampling before lockdown (b); during lockdown (l); and after two days (d), two weeks (w), and one month (m) of deconfinement. Three groups of stations are identified by cluster analysis at a 50% similarity level.

SIMPER was used here to illustrate the biological reasons for the clustering of stations with (before and after lockdown) and without bottom trawling activity (during lockdown period) (Table 4) by showing the group similarity identifying species contributing most to the similarity between groups. The first group (GI; 84.54% contribution to total similarity) was strongly represented by the polychaetes *Cirratulus cirratus*, *Euclymene oerstedii*, *Hediste diversicolor*, *Amphitritides gracilis*, and *Euclymene lumbricoides* and the amphipods *Monocorophium acherusicum* and *Microdeutopus anomalus*. The second group (GII; 59.43%) was represented by the polychaetes *Cirratulus cirratus*, *Hilbigneris gracilis*, and *Perinereis cultrifera*; the molluscs *Cerithium scabridum*, *Scrobicularia plana*, and *Tricolia speciosa*; and the amphipods *Monocorophium insidiosum* and *Dexamine spinosa*. The last group (GIII; 27.82%) corresponded to the impacted stations sampled before lockdown and after two weeks and then one month of deconfinement. This group was represented by the amphipods

Microdeutopus gryllotalpa, *Cymadusa filosa*, and *Dexamine spinosa* and the molluscs *Gibbula ardens*, *Loripes orbiculatus*, and *Calliostoma zizyphinum* (Table 4). The PERMANOVA analysis showed that the three groups are statistically highly separated (PERMANOVA; F = 23.2; $p < 0.01$).

Table 4. Groups formed by n-MDS ordination, with indication of similarities between each group (%) and the most representative species (% of contribution for the similarity within the group) contributing to the similarity within the group, determined with SIMPER analysis.

	GI	GII	GIII
Similarity (%)	64.54	49.43	27.82
Main species	*Cirratulus cirratus*—52.3 *Euclymene oerstedii*—46.0 *Hediste diversicolor*—38.1 *Amphitritides gracilis*—34.2 *Leucothoe incisa*—28.2 *Eulymene lumbricoides*—26.6 *Monocorophium acherusicum*—22.7 *Microdeutopus anomalus*—18.6 *Scrobicularia plana*—11.3 *Melinna palmata*—7.0 *Heteromastus filiformis*—4.2	*Cirratulus cirratus*—48.6 *Hilbigneris gracilis*—44.9 *Perinereis cultrifera*—42.0 *Cerithium scabridum*—37.0 *Euclymene oerstedii*—26.7 *Scrobicularia plana*—21.0 *Melita palmata*—18.2 *Monocorophium insidiosum*—16.1 *Marphysa sanguinea*—10.2 *Tricolia speciosa*—8.6 *Dexamine spinosa*—3.2	*Microdeutopus gryllotalpa*—51.6 *Cymadusa filosa*—48.2 *Dexamine spinosa*—41.0 *Gibbula ardens*—32.2 *Tellina tenius*—28.1 *Tritia cuvierii*—21.4 *Gammarus insensibilis*—20.8 *Euclymene oerstedii*—19.4 *Loripes orbiculatus*—17.3 *Calliostoma zizyphinum*—15.2 *Pinctada (imbricata) radiata*—7.1

4. Discussion

Bottom trawling has global negative impacts on marine biodiversity and habitats and is already considered among the anthropogenic pressures that threaten marine environments [5,6,8,10,42]. This destructive fishing activity is very widespread in the Mediterranean and practiced intensively in the Gulf of Gabès region. In the Mediterranean Sea, many studies have demonstrated the negative environmental impacts of bottom trawling on *Posidonia oceanica* meadows, marine fish productivity, and macroinvertebrate fauna diversity [43–45]. According to different observations in several Mediterranean fisheries, trawling activities have been responsible for the bulk of discards and the decline in fish stocks during the last few decades in the Mediterranean region [5,44].

To study the impacts of bottom trawling on macrobenthic communities in tidal channels of the Kneiss Islands, we use a BACI approach applied before and after the COVID-19 pandemic lockdown in the Gulf of Gabès. In this study, we evaluate for the first time the effects of trawling on the benthic fauna of soft bottom substrates. Many recent studies have indicated that the COVID-19 lockdown had important positive impacts in reducing several human activities and improving environmental quality [35,36]. Similarly, the before/after COVID-19 pandemic lockdown approach is an excellent opportunity used to assess the impacts of trawling on benthic communities in the central part of the Mediterranean Sea.

The macrofauna of the tidal channels of Kneiss Islands is mainly composed of polychaetes belonging to the families *Cirratulidae*, *Maldanidae*, *Nereididae*, and *Lumbrineridae*, followed by the amphipods represented by the *Gammaridae*, *Dexaminidae*, *Corophiidae*, and *Aoridae*. During the five sampling periods (Figure 2), the control stations showed higher diversity indices (taxonomic richness, abundance, and biomass) compared with the trawled stations. The values of abundance and biomass recorded at the control stations in tidal channels of Kneiss islands (3187 ± 348 ind.m^{-2}; 186 ± 22 g AFDW.m^{-2}, respectively) appear to be very high compared with other Mediterranean ecosystems [46], showing that the tidal channels ecosystems form suitable and highly productive habitats for the macrobenthic fauna [16,47].

The seafloor morphologies in the tidal channels are of crucial importance for the functioning of marine ecosystems since they allow for the exchange of water, sediments, nutrients, biota, and pollutants with the open sea [16,48]. The low biodiversity of the macrozoobenthic fauna recorded at trawled stations reflects the strong impact of destructive fishing gear, potentially affecting entire habitats and leading to the damage and/or killing of benthic organisms. As a result, this reduces species taxonomic richness, abundance, and biomass as reported in several other international studies [49–51]. The notable increase in benthic community indices during the COVID-2019 pandemic lockdown period and after two days of deconfinement (5 June 2020) at trawled stations highlights the negative effects of illegal fishing gear on the subtidal benthic soft-bottom communities of the Kneiss Islands. However, in the absence of trawling activities, we observe an increase in the abundance of many species such as the tubicolous polychaetes *Euclymene oerstedii* and *Melinna palmata*; the infaunal polychaetes *Cirratulus cirratus* and *Scolemata impatiens*; the amphipod *Microdeutopus anomalus*; and the bivalves *Scrobicularia plana, Loripes orbiculatus,* and *Pinctada imbricata radiata*. Likewise, other numerous sedentary fauna such as the cnidaria, echinodermata, and tubicolous polychaeta species (e.g., *Sabellidae, Terebellidae,* and *Serpulidae*) appeared only at impacted stations during the lockdown period and after two days of deconfinement. In fact, the continuous fishing disturbance contributes to a decline in the resistance of the macrobenthic assemblages of the Kneiss Islands. The high resilience of these shallow benthic communities during the cessation of fishing activities is indicated by the reappearance of smaller and some sensitive species such as infaunal polychaetes (e.g., tubicolous species) and mobile crustaceans that are unable to withstand environmental changes due to their biological traits (life history, morphology, behaviour of each taxon, inter-specific interactions, and connections between species and their environment); this also proves that the stability of sediment and nutrients of the tidal channels in the absence of bottom trawling promotes the successful recruitment and colonization of several benthic species and increases the trophic availability, which also attracts other mobile organisms from neighbouring ecosystems (intertidal zones). The short-term increase in the number abundance, and biomass of many sensitive and small-sized benthic organisms during the COVID-19 lockdown period in the tidal channels of Kneiss could be explained by the fact that this period coincides with the recruitment period of the majority of the macrobenthic species that generally takes place during the spring and summer season [52]. Previous studies showed that opportunistic species, such as the polychaete families Spionidae and Cirratulidae, are characterized by high growth rates, a short life span, a low reproductive age, and a large reproductive output [53,54]; these are more resistant to change and impose their opportunistic strategy of life to overcome environmental changes caused by anthropogenic pressures including fishing disturbances [45,55].

Trawling stress leads to the selection of species that are adapted to living in soft-bottom habitats. Combined with a strong bottom trawling activity, this implies that the benthic community is able to recolonize this environment rapidly after the cessation of anthropogenic pressures [56]. In fact, mobile species (e.g., amphipods and small species) have the ability to tolerate environmental changes and are able to escape during fishing disturbances [57]. Moreover, the smaller and sensitive macrobenthic organisms are also vulnerable to trawling effects [45,58], often displaying relatively high growth capacity and turnover rates, resulting in shorter recovery times [42,59,60].

The reappearance of some macrobenthic species and the increases in abundance and biomass of macrofauna at the trawled stations during the COVID-19 lockdown suggest that one month without trawling activities is necessary for the restoration of biodiversity and for the recovery of the subtidal ecosystem of the Kneiss Islands. Many authors have shown the strong resilience capacity of benthic communities following the short impacts of fishing disturbances including bottom trawling effects and that the speed and nature of recovery can vary greatly, depending upon the type and duration of impact and upon the physical and life-history characteristics of the species making up the macrobenthic communities [6,60–63].

The depletion in diversity and biomass of macrobenthic communities (especially polychaetes; Cirratulidae, Nereididae, and Maldanidae) observed at trawled stations during the fishing period (almost −70% after a month of fishing) is due to direct and indirect mortality (destruction of tubes, exposure to predators, and habitat destruction) [63–66].

Generally, the diversity and abundance of tubicolous polychaetes decreases after any destructive fishing activity [20,37,65]. Environmental changes caused by destructive fishing gear lead to effects that modify the habitat structure, disrupt food web processes, and eliminate the more vulnerable organisms susceptible to environmental damage. This is because organisms are displaced by the fluidized sediments generated by the pressure wave in front of a moving trawl [67,68]. Usually, macrobenthos respond negatively to fishing pressures, since they are highly vulnerable and can be considerably reduced in diversity and abundance or even eliminated, being extremely fragile and particularly susceptible to damage [45,69]. The increase in macrobenthic fauna biomass at the trawled stations during the COVID-19 lockdown compared with the fishing periods confirms that chronic trawling has a strong negative impact on the biomass and the functional capacity of subtidal benthic macrofaunal communities. These results are in agreement with other previous studies reporting the negative effects of trawling activity on the diversity, size composition, and biomass of benthic communities [50,62]. Equally, biomass is an effective indicator of trawling disturbance. Recently, Sciberras et al. [50] demonstrated that the effects of trawling are most pronounced in long-lived benthic organisms, as these typically take longer to recover after a trawling event. In the tidal channels of the Kneiss Islands, the effects of trawling influence not only the sensitive taxa (infauna polychaetes) but also the larger macrobenthic communities such as the crustacean decapods *Carcinus* spp. and *Metapenaeus Monoceros* (Fabricius, 1798) and the molluscs *Pinctada imbricata radiata* (Leach, 1814) and *Cerastoderma glaucum* (Bruguière, 1789). Evenly, many experimental studies have revealed that large macrofauna are also disproportionately sensitive to trawling disturbance [70–72]. This vulnerability has been linked to a relationship between body size and several key life-history traits [73], whereby larger macrobenthic species tend to grow and reach maturity at a slower rate. Such species have comparatively lower mortality and population growth rates and are therefore more vulnerable to trawling-induced mortality. Repeated and intense trawling would typically result in shifts away from communities dominated by a high biomass of long-lived organisms towards those dominated by highly abundant small macrofauna including opportunistic species [42,71,74]. The frequently trawled tidal channels of the Kneiss islands show increased water turbidity caused by the scraping of the seabed during trawling and the injection of sediments into the water column [75] associated with a decrease in dissolved oxygen concentration [52]. The impact of oxygen deficiency results in various behavioural changes for macrofauna communities. Mobile organisms (i.e., amphipods and decapods) are able to move away from or avoid hypoxic locations, while the behavioural responses of sessile species (i.e., some molluscs, infauna, and tubicolous polychaetes) might express modifications of feeding and bioturbation rates [76]. However, complete faunal depletion is observed at low oxygen concentrations and under anoxic conditions in trawled zones [77]. Generally, various co-varying and interacting factors have been proposed to account for the environmental effects of bottom trawling. These may include the sensitivity of specific marine habitats [7,62], the impact of different gear types [1,78], the magnitude of background human and natural disturbances [52,79], and the capacity of benthic communities to adapt (resistance) to environmental disturbances [62,74]. Either alone or in combination, such factors could obscure the measurable effects of trawling on benthic habitats and organisms and may also explain why indicators sometimes display various different performances [12,80].

5. Conclusions and Future Perspectives

The present study shows the negative effects of bottom trawling on macrobenthic fauna in the tidal channels of the Kneiss Islands. This destructive fishing gear causes a notable reduction in the taxonomic richness, abundance, and biomass of the macrobenthic communities. It is well known that the macrofauna plays a crucial role in the food web either by feeding on detritus or as food for aquatic birds and economically important demersal fish [81]. Thus, it would be very important to ban this illegal destructive fishing activity in the Kneiss Islands, which represents a site of international interest in terms of marine biodiversity (Important Bird Area, SPAMI, and RAMSAR Site). This study shows that just one month of non-fishing is sufficient to allow for the recovery of benthic biodiversity. Finally, this exceptional lockdown period due to the COVID-19 pandemic points to the high resilience of the macrobenthic community after the cessation of trawling disturbances, which affects the interface between the sediment and the bottom layer of the water column and has widespread negative impacts on benthic communities and marine habitat. It could be a significant and important reason to prevent and prohibit the use of this illegal and destructive fishing gear to better protect the marine biodiversity of the tidal channels of Gulf of Gabès.

Several aims might be considered for future work. The first would be to produce an effective management plan integrating stakeholder communities to conserve the fisheries of the Kneiss Islands. Second, it would be interesting to complete an evaluation of the impacts of bottom trawling on macro- and megabenthic fauna in other tidal channels of the Gulf of Gabès (studied recently by Dauvin et al. [16]). Finally, it might be worthwhile carrying out seasonal and annual monitoring at selected stations along these tidal channels to follow the long-term response of macrofauna communities to illegal fishing pressures.

Author Contributions: Conceptualization, N.M. and L.N.; methodology, N.M. and L.N.; software, N.M. and J.-P.P.; writing—original draft preparation, N.M.; writing—review and editing, N.M., J.-P.P.; J.-C.D. and L.N., supervision, J.-C.D. and L.N. All authors have read and agreed to the published version of the manuscript.

Funding: This research received no external funding.

Institutional Review Board Statement: Not applicable.

Informed Consent Statement: Not applicable.

Data Availability Statement: All data used are in the manuscript and are available from the corresponding author.

Acknowledgments: The authors thank the fishers of the Kneiss Islands and General Directorate of Fisheries and Aquaculture of Skhira for their support during the five sampling campaigns, especially during the COVID-19 lockdown period in the Gulf of Gabès (Mach–May 2020), and M. Carpenter for the English revision.

Conflicts of Interest: The authors declare no conflict of interest.

References

1. Eigaard, O.R.; Bastardie, F.; Hintzen, N.; Buhl-Mortensen, L.; Mortensen, P.; Catarino, R.; Dinesen, G.E.; Egekvist, J.; Fock, H.O.; Geitner, K.; et al. The footprint of bottom trawling in European waters: Distribution, intensity, and seabed integrity. *ICES J. Mar. Sci.* **2017**, *74*, 847–865. [CrossRef]
2. Puig, P.; Canals, M.; Company, J.B.; Martin, J.; Amblas, D.; Lastras, G.; Palanques, A.; Calafat, A. Ploughing the deep sea floor. *Nature* **2012**, *489*, 286–289. [CrossRef] [PubMed]
3. Pusceddu, A.; Bianchelli, S.; Martin, J.; Puig, P.; Palanques, A.; Masque, P.; Danovaro, R. Chronic and intensive bottom trawling impairs deep-sea biodiversity and ecosystem functioning. *Proc. Natl. Acad. Sci. USA* **2014**, *111*, 8861–8866. [CrossRef]
4. Kaiser, M.J.; Spencer, B.E. The Effects of Beam-Trawl Disturbance on Infaunal Communities in Different Habitats. *J. Anim. Ecol.* **1996**, *65*, 348. [CrossRef]
5. Smith, C.J.; Papadopoulou, K.N.; DiLiberto, S. Impact of otter trawling on an eastern Mediterranean commercial trawl fishing ground. *ICES J. Mar. Sci.* **2000**, *57*, 1340–1351. [CrossRef]
6. Hall-Spencer, J.M.; Froglia, C.; Atkinson, R.J.A.; Moore, P.G. The impact of Rapido trawling for scallops, *Pecten jacobaeus* (L.), on the benthos of the Gulf of Venice. *ICES J. Mar. Sci.* **1999**, *56*, 111–124. [CrossRef]
7. Ardizzone, G.D.; Tucci, P.; Somaschini, A.; Belluscio, A.; Kaiser, M.J.; de Groot, J. *Is the Bottom Trawling Partly Responsible for the Regression of Posidonia Oceanica Meadows in the Mediterranean Sea? The Effects of Fishing on Non-Target Species and Habitats*; Blackwell Scientific: Oxford, UK, 2000; pp. 37–46.
8. Foden, J.; Rogers, S.; Jones, A. Recovery of UK seabed habitats from benthic fishing and aggregate extraction—Towards a cumulative impact assessment. *Mar. Ecol. Prog. Ser.* **2010**, *411*, 259–270. [CrossRef]
9. Muntadas, O.A. Benthic Communities' Response to Different Trawling Impact Levels: Generalization towards Developing a Mediterranean Model. Ph.D. Thesis, Barcelona University, Barcelona, Spain, 2015; p. 480. Available online: http://hdl.handle.net/10261/126878 (accessed on 4 December 2015).

10. Sciberras, M.; Parker, R.; Powell, C.; Robertson, C.; Kröger, S.; Bolam, S.; Geert Hiddink, J. Impacts of bottom fishing on the sediment infaunal community and biogeochemistry of cohesive and non-cohesive sediments: Trawling impacts on ecosystem processes. *Limnol. Oceanogr.* **2016**, *61*, 2076–2089. [CrossRef]
11. Sammari, C.; Koutitonsky, V.G.; Moussa, M. Sea level variability and tidal resonance in the Gulf of Gabes, Tunisia. *Cont. Shelf Res.* **2006**, *26*, 338–350. [CrossRef]
12. Posey, M.H.; Alphin, T.D.; Cahoon, L.B.; Lindquist, D.G.; Mallin, M.A.; Nevers, M.B. Top-down versus bottom-up limitation in benthic infaunal communities: Direct and indirect effects. *Estuaries* **2002**, *25*, 999–1014. [CrossRef]
13. Mallin, M.A.; Lewitus, A.J. The importance of tidal creek ecosystems. *J. Exp. Mar. Biol. Ecol.* **2004**, *298*, 145–149. [CrossRef]
14. Hattab, T.; Lasram, F.B.R.; Albouy, C.; Romdhane, M.S.; Jarboui, O.; Halouani, G.; Cury, P.; Le Loc'H, F. An ecosystem model of an exploited southern Mediterranean shelf region (Gulf of Gabes, Tunisia) and a comparison with other Mediterranean ecosystem model properties. *J. Mar. Syst.* **2013**, *128*, 159–174. [CrossRef]
15. Halouani, G.; Lasram, B.R.; Shin, Y.-J.; Velez, L.; Verley, P.; Hattab, T.; Oliveros-Ramos, R.; Diaz, F.; Ménard, F.; Baklouti, M.; et al. Modelling food web structure using an end-to-end approach in the coastal ecosystem of the Gulf of Gabes (Tunisia). *Ecol. Model.* **2016**, *339*, 45–57. [CrossRef]
16. Dauvin, J.-C.; Fersi, A.; Pezy, J.-P.; Bakalem, A.; Neifar, L. Macrobenthic communities in the tidal channels around the Gulf of Gabès, Tunisia. *Mar. Pollut. Bull.* **2021**, *162*, 111846. [CrossRef]
17. Hattab, T.; Albouy, C.; Ben Rais Lasram, F.; Somot, S.; Le Loc'h, F.; Leprieur, F. Towards a better understanding of potential impacts of climate change on marine species distribution: A Multiscale modelling approach. *Glob. Ecol. Biog.* **2014**, *23*, 1417–1429. [CrossRef]
18. Mosbahi, N.; Serbaji, M.M.; Pezy, J.-P.; Neifar, L.; Dauvin, J.-C. Response of benthic macrofauna to multiple anthropogenic pressures in the shallow coastal zone south of Sfax (Tunisia, central Mediterranean Sea). *Environ. Pollut.* **2019**, *253*, 474–487. [CrossRef]
19. Bali, M.; Gueddari, M. Les chenaux de marée autour des îles de Kneiss, Tunisie: Sédimentologie et évolution. *Hydrol. Sci. J.* **2011**, *56*, 498–506. [CrossRef]
20. Mosbahi, N.; Pezy, J.-P.; Dauvin, J.-C.; Neifar, L. Short-term impact of bait digging on intertidal macrofauna of tidal mudflats around the Kneiss Islands (Gulf of Gabès, Tunisia). *Aquat. Living Resour.* **2016**, *28*, 111–118. [CrossRef]
21. Zerelli, S. Investigating Illegal Bottom Trawling in the Gulf of Gabès, Tunisia. Rapport Final, Fishact Tunisia 2018. Available online: https://fishact.org/2018/12/investigating-illegal-bottom-trawling-in-the-gulf-of-gabes-tunisia/ (accessed on 2 November 2018).
22. Ben Brahim, M.; Hamza, A.; Hannachi, I.; Rebai, A.; Jarboui, O.; Bouain, A.; Aleya, L. Variability in the structure of epiphytic assemblages of Posidonia oceanica in relation to human interferences in the Gulf of Gabes, Tunisia. *Mar. Environ. Res.* **2010**, *70*, 411–421. [CrossRef]
23. Blanchet, H.; Lavesque, N.; Ruellet, T.; Dauvin, J.; Sauriau, P.-G.; Desroy, N.; Desclaux, C.; Leconte, M.; Bachelet, G.; Janson, A.-L.; et al. Use of biotic indices in semi-enclosed coastal ecosystems and transitional waters habitats—Implications for the implementation of the European Water Framework Directive. *Ecol. Indic.* **2008**, *8*, 360–372. [CrossRef]
24. Hale, S.S.; Heltshe, J.F. Signals from the benthos: Development and evaluation of a benthic index for the nearshore Gulf of Maine. *Ecol. Indic.* **2008**, *8*, 338–350. [CrossRef]
25. Dauvin, J.C.; Alizier, S.; Rolet, C.; Bakalem, A.; Bellan, G.; Gomez Gesteira, J.L.; Grimes, S.; De-La-Ossa-Carretero, J.A.; Del-Pilar-Ruso, Y. Response of the different indices to the diverse human pressures. *Ecol. Ind.* **2012**, *12*, 143–153. [CrossRef]
26. Dauvin, J.; Andrade, H.; De-La-Ossa-Carretero, J.; Del-Pilar-Ruso, Y.; Riera, R. Polychaete/amphipod ratios: An approach to validating simple benthic indicators. *Ecol. Indic.* **2016**, *63*, 89–99. [CrossRef]
27. Reiss, H.; Kröncke, I. Seasonal variability of benthic indices: An approach to test the applicability of different indices for ecosystem quality assessment. *Mar. Pollut. Bull.* **2005**, *50*, 1490–1499. [CrossRef]
28. Dauvin, J.C. Le benthos: Témoin des variations de l'environnement. *Océanis* **1993**, *19*, 25–53.
29. Dauvin, J.-C. Paradox of estuarine quality: Benthic indicators and indices, consensus or debate for the future. *Mar. Pollut. Bull.* **2007**, *55*, 271–281. [CrossRef]
30. Cucinotta, D.; Vanelli, M. WHO declares COVID-19 a pandemic. *Acta Biomed.* **2020**, *91*, 157–160. [CrossRef]
31. McKay, B.; Calfas, J.; Ansari, T.; Coronavirus Declared Pandemic by World Health Organization. Wall St J. Archived from the Original on 11 March 2020. Available online: https://www.wsj.com/articles/u-s-coronavirus-cases-top-1-000-11583917794 (accessed on 12 March 2020).
32. Sheahan, T.P.; Frieman, M.B. The continued epidemic threat of SARS-CoV-2 and implications for the future of global public health. *Curr. Opin. Virol.* **2020**, *40*, 37–40. [CrossRef]
33. Briz-Redón, Á.; Belenguer-Sapiña, C.; Serrano-Aroca, Á. Changes in air pollution during COVID-19 lockdown in Spain: A multi-city study. *J. Environ. Sci.* **2021**, *101*, 16–26. [CrossRef]
34. Nigam, R.; Pandya, K.; Luis, A.J.; Sengupta, R.; Kotha, M. Positive effects of COVID-19 lockdown on air quality of industrial cities (Ankleshwar and Vapi) of Western India. *Sci. Rep.* **2021**, *11*, 4285. [CrossRef]
35. Khan, I.; Shah, D.; Shah, S.S. COVID-19 pandemic and its positive impacts on environment: An updated review. *Int. J. Environ. Sci. Technol.* **2020**, *18*, 521–530. [CrossRef] [PubMed]

36. Bates, A.E.; Primack, R.B.; Moraga, P.; Duarte, C.M. COVID-19 pandemic and associated lockdown as a "Global Human Confinement Experiment" to investigate biodiversity conservation. *Biol. Conserv.* **2020**, *248*, 108665. [CrossRef] [PubMed]
37. Mosbahi, N.; Pezy, J.P.; Dauvin, J.C.; Neifar, L. Immediate Effect of Clam Harvesting on Intertidal Benthic Communities in the Mudflat Zones of Kneiss Islands (Central Mediterranean Sea). *J. Aquac. Res. Dev.* **2016**, *7*, 2155. [CrossRef]
38. Shannon, F.P.; Weaver, W. *The Mathematical Theory of Communication*; University Illinois Press: Champaign, IL, USA, 1963; p. 117.
39. Pielou, E.C. Shannon's Formula as a Measure of Specific Diversity: Its Use and Misuse. *Am. Nat.* **1966**, *100*, 463–465. [CrossRef]
40. Clarke, K.R.; Gorley, R.N. *PRIMER v6: User Manual/Tutorial*; PRIMER-E Ltd.: Plymouth, UK, 2006.
41. Clarke, K.R. Non-parametric multivariate analyses of changes in community structure. *Aust. J. Ecol.* **1993**, *18*, 117–143. [CrossRef]
42. McLaverty, C.; Eigaard, O.R.; Gislason, H.; Bastardie, F.; Brooks, M.E.; Jonsson, P.; Lehmann, A.; Dinesen, G.E. Using large benthic macrofauna to refine and improve ecological indicators of bottom trawling disturbance. *Ecol. Indic.* **2020**, *110*, 105811. [CrossRef]
43. Sánchez-Jerez, P.; Esplá, A.A.R. Detection of environmental impacts by bottom trawling on *Posidonia oceanica* (L.) Delile meadows: Sensitivity of fish and macroinvertebrate communities. *J. Aquat. Ecosyst. Heal.* **1996**, *5*, 239–253. [CrossRef]
44. Sacchi, J. The use of trawling nets in the Mediterranean. Problems and selectivity options. In *The Mediterranean Fisheries Sector. A Reference Publication for The VII Meeting of Ministers of Agriculture and Fisheries of CIHEAM Member Countries (Zaragoza, Spain, 4 February 2008)*; Basurco, B., Ed.; CIHEAM/FAO/GFCM: Zaragoza, Spain, 2008; pp. 87–96, Options Méditerranéennes: Série B. Etudes et Recherches (N 62). Available online: http://om.ciheam.org/article.php?IDPDF=800739 (accessed on 12 March 2020).
45. De Juan, S.; Thrush, S.; Demestre, M. Functional changes as indicators of trawling disturbance on a benthic community located in a fishing ground (NW Mediterranean Sea). *Mar. Ecol. Prog. Ser.* **2007**, *334*, 117–129. [CrossRef]
46. Baldrighi, E.; Lavaleye, M.; Aliani, S.; Conversi, A.; Manini, E. Large Spatial Scale Variability in Bathyal Macrobenthos Abundance, Biomass, α- and β-Diversity along the Mediterranean Continental Margin. *PLoS ONE* **2014**, *9*, e107261. [CrossRef]
47. Fersi, A.; Dauvin, J.C.; Pezy, J.P.; Neifar, L. Amphipods from tidal channels of the Gulf of Gabès (central Mediterranean Sea). *Mediterr. Mar. Sci.* **2018**, *19*, 430–443. [CrossRef]
48. Madricardo, F.; Montereale-Gavazzi, G.; Sigovini, M.; Kruss, A.; Toso, C.; Foglini, F. Seafloor Morphology and Habitats of Tidal Channels in the Venice Lagoon, Italy Tidal Channel Habitats. Available online: https://www.sciencedirect.com/science/article/pii/B9780128149607000099?via%3Dihub (accessed on 12 March 2020).
49. Collie, J.S.; Hall, S.J.; Kaiser, M.J.; Poiner, I.R. A quantitative analysis of fishing impacts on shelf-sea benthos. *J. Anim. Ecol.* **2000**, *69*, 785–798. [CrossRef] [PubMed]
50. Sciberras, M.; Hiddink, J.G.; Jennings, S.; Szostek, C.L.; Hughes, K.M.; Kneafsey, B.; Clarke, L.J.; Ellis, N.; Rijnsdorp, A.D.; McConnaughey, R.A.; et al. Response of benthic fauna to experimental bottom fishing: A global meta-analysis. *Fish Fish.* **2018**, *19*, 698–715. [CrossRef]
51. Mosbahi, N.; Pezy, J.-P.; Dauvin, J.-C.; Neifar, L. Spatial and Temporal Structures of the Macrozoobenthos from the Intertidal Zone of the Kneiss Islands (Central Mediterranean Sea). *Open J. Mar. Sci.* **2016**, *6*, 223–237. [CrossRef]
52. van Denderen, D.; Bolam, S.G.; Friedland, R.; Hiddink, J.G.; Norén, K.; Rijnsdorp, A.D.; Sköld, M.; Törnroos, A.; Virtanen, E.; Valanko, S. Evaluating impacts of bottom trawling and hypoxia on benthic communities at the local, habitat, and regional scale using a modelling approach. *ICES J. Mar. Sci.* **2020**, *77*, 278–289. [CrossRef]
53. Kaiser, M.J. Significance of Bottom-Fishing Disturbance. *Conserv. Biol.* **1998**, *12*, 1230–1235. [CrossRef]
54. Craeymeersch, J.A.; Piet, G.J.; Rijnsdorp, A.D.; Buijs, J. Distribution of macrofauna in relation to the micro distribution of trawling effort. In *The Effects of Fishing on Non-Target Species and Habitats: Biological, Conservation and Socio-Economic Issues*; Kaiser, M.J., de Groot, S.J., Eds.; Blackwell Science: Oxford, UK, 2000; pp. 187–197.
55. Meenakumari, B.; Bhagirathan, U.; Pravin, P. Impact of bottom trawling on benthic communities: A Review. *Fish. Techn.* **2008**, *45*, 1–22.
56. Dauvin, J.; Bakalem, A.; Baffreau, A.; Grimes, S. Benthic ecological status of Algerian harbours. *Mar. Pollut. Bull.* **2017**, *125*, 378–388. [CrossRef]
57. Foveau, A.; Dauvin, J.-C. Surprisingly diversified macrofauna in mobile gravels and pebbles from high-energy hydrodynamic environment of the 'Raz Blanchard' (English Channel). *Reg. Stud. Mar. Sci.* **2017**, *16*, 188–197. [CrossRef]
58. Petović, S.; Marković, O.; Ikica, Z.; Đurović, M.; Joksimović, A. Effects of bottom trawling on the benthic assemblages in the south Adriatic Sea (Montenegro). *Acta Adriat.* **2016**, *57*, 81–92.
59. Jennings, S.; Kaiser, M.J. The Effects of Fishing on Marine Ecosystems. *Adv. Mar. Biol.* **1998**, *34*, 201–352. [CrossRef]
60. McConnaughey, R.A.; Syrjala, S.E. Short-term effects of bottom trawling and a storm event on soft-bottom benthos in the eastern Bering Sea. *ICES J. Mar. Sci.* **2014**, *71*, 2469–2483. [CrossRef]
61. Giovanardi, O.; Pranovi, F.; Franceschini, G. "Rapido" trawl fishing in the Northern Adriatic: Preliminary observations of the effects on macrobenthic communities. *Acta Adriat.* **1998**, *39*, 37–52.
62. Kaiser, M.J.; Hormbrey, S.; Booth, J.R.; Hinz, H.; Hiddink, J.G. Recovery linked to life history of sessile epifauna following exclusion of towed mobile fishing gear. *J. Appl. Ecol.* **2018**, *55*, 1060–1070. [CrossRef]
63. Pranovi, F.; Raicevich, S.; Franceschini, G.; Farrace, M.G.; Giovanardi, O. Rapido trawling in the northern Adriatic Sea: Effects on benthic communities in an experimental area. *ICES J. Mar. Sci.* **2000**, *57*, 517–524. [CrossRef]
64. Cowie, P.R.; Widdicombe, S.; Austen, M.C. Effects of physical disturbance on an estuarine intertidal community: Field and mesocosm results compared. *Mar. Biol.* **2000**, *136*, 485–495. [CrossRef]

65. De Carvalho, A.N.; Vaz, A.S.L.; Sérgio, T.I.B.; Dos Santos, P.J.T. Sustainability of bait fishing harvesting in estuarine ecosystems—Case study in the Local Natural Reserve of Douro Estuary, Portugal. *Rev. Gestão Costeira Integr.* **2013**, *13*, 157–168. [CrossRef]
66. Collie, J.; Hiddink, J.G.; Van Kooten, T.; Rijnsdorp, A.D.; Kaiser, M.J.; Jennings, S.; Hilborn, R. Indirect effects of bottom fishing on the productivity of marine fish. *Fish Fish.* **2016**, *18*, 619–637. [CrossRef]
67. Gilkinson, K.; Paulin, M.; Hurley, S.; Schwinghamer, P. Impacts of trawl door scouring on infaunal bivalves: Results of a physical trawl door model/dense sand interaction. *J. Exp. Mar. Biol. Ecol.* **1998**, *224*, 291–312. [CrossRef]
68. Hermsen, J.; Collie, J.; Valentine, P. Mobile fishing gear reduces benthic megafaunal production on Georges Bank. *Mar. Ecol. Prog. Ser.* **2003**, *260*, 97–108. [CrossRef]
69. Kaiser, M.J.; Spencer, B. Fish scavenging behaviour in recently trawled areas. *Mar. Ecol. Prog. Ser.* **1994**, *112*, 41–49. [CrossRef]
70. De Biasi, A.M. Impact of experimental trawling on the benthic assemblage along the Tuscany coast (north Tyrrhenian Sea, Italy). *ICES J. Mar. Sci.* **2004**, *61*, 1260–1266. [CrossRef]
71. Jennings, S.; Nicholson, M.D.; Dinmore, T.; Lancaster, J. Effects of chronic trawling disturbance on the production of infaunal communities. *Mar. Ecol. Prog. Ser.* **2002**, *243*, 251–260. [CrossRef]
72. Duplisea, D.E.; Jennings, S.; Warr, K.J.; Dinmore, T.A. A size-based model of the impacts of bottom trawling on benthic community structure. *Can. J. Fish. Aquat. Sci.* **2002**, *59*, 1785–1795. [CrossRef]
73. Begon, M.; Harper, J.L.; Townsend, C.R. *Ecology: From Individuals to Ecosystems*, 4th ed.; Blackwell Science: Oxford, UK, 2006.
74. Kaiser, M.J.; Ramsay, K.; Richardson, C.A.; Spence, F.E.; Brand, A.R. Chronic fishing disturbance has changed shelf sea benthic community structure. *J. Anim. Ecol.* **2000**, *69*, 494–503. [CrossRef]
75. Palanques, A.; Puig, P.; Guillén, J.; Demestre, M.; Martin, J. Effects of bottom trawling on the Ebro continental shelf sedimentary system (NW Mediterranean). *Cont. Shelf Res.* **2014**, *72*, 83–98. [CrossRef]
76. Villnäs, A.; Norkko, J.; Lukkari, K.; Hewitt, J.; Norkko, A. Consequences of Increasing Hypoxic Disturbance on Benthic Communities and Ecosystem Functioning. *PLoS ONE* **2012**, *7*, e44920. [CrossRef]
77. Diaz, R.J.; Rosenberg, R. Marine benthic hypoxia: A review of its ecological effects and the behavioural responses of benthic macrofauna. *Oceanogr. Mar. Biology Annu. Rev.* **1995**, *33*, 203–245.
78. Hiddink, J.G.; Jennings, S.; Sciberras, M.; Bolam, S.G.; Cambiè, G.; McConnaughey, R.A.; Mazor, T.; Hilborn, R.; Collie, J.S.; Pitcher, C.R.; et al. Assessing bottom trawling impacts based on the longevity of benthic invertebrates. *J. Appl. Ecol.* **2018**, *56*, 1075–1084. [CrossRef]
79. Diesing, M.; Stephens, D.; Aldridge, J. A proposed method for assessing the extent of the seabed significantly affected by demersal fishing in the Greater North Sea. *ICES J. Mar. Sci.* **2013**, *70*, 1085–1096. [CrossRef]
80. Atkinson, L.; Field, J.; Hutchings, L. Effects of demersal trawling along the west coast of southern Africa: Multivariate analysis of benthic assemblages. *Mar. Ecol. Prog. Ser.* **2011**, *430*, 241–255. [CrossRef]
81. Henniger, T.O.; Forenamen, P.W. Macrofaunal community structure in the littoral zone of a freshwater-deprived, permanently open Eastern Cape estuary. *Afr. Zool.* **2011**, *46*, 263–279. [CrossRef]

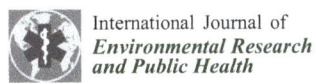

Article

Evidence of Air and Surface Contamination with SARS-CoV-2 in a Major Hospital in Portugal

Priscilla Gomes da Silva [1,2,3], José Gonçalves [4,5], Ariana Isabel Brito Lopes [6], Nury Alves Esteves [6], Gustavo Emanuel Enes Bamba [6], Maria São José Nascimento [7], Pedro T. B. S. Branco [3], Ruben R. G. Soares [8], Sofia I. V. Sousa [3] and João R. Mesquita [1,2,*]

1. ICBAS–School of Medicine and Biomedical Sciences, Porto University, 4050-313 Porto, Portugal; up202002072@edu.icbas.up.pt
2. Epidemiology Research Unit (EPIunit), Institute of Public Health, University of Porto, 4050-600 Porto, Portugal
3. LEPABE–Laboratory for Process Engineering, Environment, Biotechnology and Energy, Faculty of Engineering, University of Porto, 4200-465 Porto, Portugal; up200606911@fe.up.pt (P.T.B.S.B.); sofia.sousa@fe.up.pt (S.I.V.S.)
4. Institute of Sustainable Processes, University of Valladolid, 47011 Valladolid, Spain; zemcg5@gmail.com
5. Department of Chemical Engineering, University of Valladolid, 47011 Valladolid, Spain
6. Unidade Local de Saúde do Alto Minho E.P.E., 4904-858 Viana do Castelo, Portugal; ariana.lopes@ulsam.min-saude.pt (A.I.B.L.); nury.esteves@ulsam.min-saude.pt (N.A.E.); gustavo.bamba@ulsam.min-saude.pt (G.E.E.B.)
7. Faculty of Pharmacy, University of Porto, 4050-313 Porto, Portugal; saojose@ff.up.pt
8. Department of Biochemistry and Biophysics, Science for Life Laboratory, Stockholm University, SE-106 91 Stockholm, Sweden; ruben.soares@scilifelab.se
* Correspondence: jrmesquita@icbas.up.pt

Abstract: As the third wave of the COVID-19 pandemic hit Portugal, it forced the country to reintroduce lockdown measures due to hospitals reaching their full capacities. Under these circumstances, environmental contamination by SARS-CoV-2 in different areas of one of Portugal's major Hospitals was assessed between 21 January and 11 February 2021. Air samples ($n = 44$) were collected from eleven different areas of the Hospital (four COVID-19 and seven non-COVID-19 areas) using Coriolis® µ and Coriolis® Compact cyclone air sampling devices. Surface sampling was also performed ($n = 17$) on four areas (one COVID-19 and three non-COVID-19 areas). RNA extraction followed by a one-step RT-qPCR adapted for quantitative purposes were performed. Of the 44 air samples, two were positive for SARS-CoV-2 RNA (6575 copies/m^3 and 6662.5 copies/m^3, respectively). Of the 17 surface samples, three were positive for SARS-CoV-2 RNA (200.6 copies/cm^2, 179.2 copies/cm^2, and 201.7 copies/cm^2, respectively). SARS-CoV-2 environmental contamination was found both in air and on surfaces in both COVID-19 and non-COVID-19 areas. Moreover, our results suggest that longer collection sessions are needed to detect point contaminations. This reinforces the need to remain cautious at all times, not only when in close contact with infected individuals. Hand hygiene and other standard transmission-prevention guidelines should be continuously followed to avoid nosocomial COVID-19.

Keywords: SARS-CoV-2; environmental contamination; air samples; surface samples

Citation: Silva, P.G.d.; Gonçalves, J.; Lopes, A.I.B.; Esteves, N.A.; Bamba, G.E.E.; Nascimento, M.S.J.; Branco, P.T.B.S.; Soares, R.R.G.; Sousa, S.I.V.; Mesquita, J.R. Evidence of Air and Surface Contamination with SARS-CoV-2 in a Major Hospital in Portugal. *Int. J. Environ. Res. Public Health* **2022**, *19*, 525. https://doi.org/10.3390/ijerph19010525

Academic Editors: Sachiko Kodera and Essam A. Rashed

Received: 3 December 2021
Accepted: 30 December 2021
Published: 4 January 2022

Publisher's Note: MDPI stays neutral with regard to jurisdictional claims in published maps and institutional affiliations.

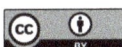

Copyright: © 2022 by the authors. Licensee MDPI, Basel, Switzerland. This article is an open access article distributed under the terms and conditions of the Creative Commons Attribution (CC BY) license (https://creativecommons.org/licenses/by/4.0/).

1. Introduction

SARS-CoV-2 infection causes respiratory illness ranging from mild to severe disease and death, with some infected people being asymptomatic [1]. According to the World Health Organization (WHO), evidence shows that SARS-CoV-2 spreads mainly between people who are standing near one another. In these situations, aerosols or droplets produced by an infected person and which contain the virus are inhaled or come directly into contact with the nose or mouth of a susceptible person, particularly in poorly-ventilated and crowded indoor environments [2].

Respiratory droplets formed from respiratory secretions and saliva are emitted through talking, coughing, sneezing and even breathing, and have a diameter ranging from <1 μm to >100 μm [3]. Respiratory droplets are generally defined as particles that fall to the ground (or any surface) more quickly under the influence of gravity due to their larger size; typically, these are particles > 5–10 μm that fall within 2 m of the source. When these particles settle on surfaces, the contaminated surfaces are then called fomites. Once emitted by humans, these respiratory droplets tend to reduce in size due to evaporation, after which they are termed as droplet nuclei or aerosols, which can be defined as particles that remain suspended due to size and/or environmental conditions; typically, these are particles ≤ 5 μm that stay suspended in air for longer, eventually falling to the ground if the air is motionless for long enough (at least 30 min) [3]. Considering that aerosols are small enough to remain suspended in air, they can accumulate in poorly-ventilated spaces and in turn be inhaled at both short and long ranges by a susceptible person, indicating the importance of improving and ensuring good indoor ventilation in the context of COVID-19 [4]. Moreover, the produced aerosols contain much higher viral loads when compared to viral loads in droplets [5–8]. Hence, proper ventilation can reduce surface contamination by removing virus particles before they can land on surfaces [9].

Despite droplet and fomite transmissions being considered the probable main modes of transmission for SARS-CoV-2, these alone cannot account for superspreading events [10–12], or for differences in transmission between indoor and outdoor environments [8]. SARS-CoV-2 modes of transmission are now distinguished as inhalation of virus, deposition of virus on exposed mucous membranes, and touching mucous membranes with soiled hands contaminated with virus [13]. However, individuals who come into contact with potentially infectious surfaces or aerosols containing viral particles often have close contact with an infected person, making it difficult to distinguish the source of infection as being airborne or through fomites [14], particularly in healthcare institutions where infected individuals continuously excrete high viral loads into the environment, potentially adding to the occupational risk of healthcare professionals [15]. In fact, while the risk of transmission via environmental contamination of SARS-CoV-2 is considered to be generally low [16], a number of factors may increase this risk, particularly considering hospital environments where a high number of symptomatic patients with active infection and increased viral shedding might be present when compared to the situation in the community outside the hospital environment [17].

At the beginning of this study, 21 January 2021, there were 151,226 active cases of COVID-19 in Portugal and 702 people admitted in intensive care units (ICUs) all over the country [18]. To the best of the authors' knowledge, no study on environmental contamination with SARS-CoV-2 in hospital settings has been performed in Portugal; hence, this study aimed to assess air and surface contamination in different areas of a major Hospital in Portugal during the peak of the third wave of COVID-19 in the country (late December 2020 to mid-February 2021). The study also aimed at assessing the performance and suitability of two air samplers (Coriolis® μ and Coriolis® Compact) for SARS-CoV-2 air monitoring. The results may be relevant in establishing interventions to prevent healthcare workers' exposure to SARS-CoV-2 and to optimize and better understand the extent of environmental viral contamination of surfaces in healthcare settings.

2. Materials and Methods

Sampling sites

Environmental sampling took place in a Hospital in Portugal that serves around 2.2% of the Portuguese population, between 21 January and 11 February 2021. Air samples (n = 44) were collected from four COVID-19 and seven non-COVID-19 areas. COVID-19 areas included the COVID-19 ICU, intermediate COVID-19 ICU, COVID-19 nursing area and the COVID-19 testing room. Non-COVID-19 areas included the respiratory diseases observation room, respiratory diseases waiting room, clinical decision unit, non-respiratory diseases patients' waiting room, urgent care (recovery area), the Hospital's outside entrance atrium and the Hospital's staff cafeteria.

Surface sampling ($n = 17$) was performed on four areas, of which three were non-COVID-19 areas (non-respiratory disease waiting room, staff cafeteria, and outside entrance atrium) and one COVID-19 area (the COVID-19 testing room). Further details about each sampling site are summarized in Tables 1 and 2.

Table 1. Air ventilation details about the sampling sites.

	Hospital Area	Type of Ventilation and Pressure	People with Access to This Area
COVID-19 areas	COVID-19 ICU	Mechanic ventilation, negative pressure	Patients and Hospital staff
	Intermediate COVID-19 ICU	Mechanic ventilation, negative pressure	Patients and Hospital staff
	COVID-19 nursing area	Mechanic ventilation, negative pressure	Patients and Hospital staff
	COVID-19 testing room	Mechanic ventilation, negative pressure	Patients and Hospital staff
Non-COVID-19 areas	Respiratory diseases observation room	Natural ventilation, neutral pressure	Patients and Hospital staff
	Respiratory diseases waiting room	Natural ventilation, neutral pressure	Patients, Hospital staff and patients' companions
	Non-respiratory diseases waiting room	Natural ventilation, neutral pressure	Patients, Hospital staff and patients' companions
	Clinical decision unit	Natural ventilation, neutral pressure	Patients and Hospital staff
	Urgency care (recovery area)	Natural ventilation, neutral pressure	Patients and Hospital staff
	Hospital's outside entrance atrium	Natural ventilation, neutral pressure	Open to the general public
	Hospital staff's cafeteria	Natural ventilation, neutral pressure	Hospital staff

Table 2. Details of the air samples' collections for SARS-CoV-2 RNA detection in the Hospital.

Device	Sample ID	Date of Collection	Hospital Area	Sampler Location	Sampling Parameters
Coriolis® Compact	C1	21 January 2021	ICU COVID-19	Air sampler placed approximately 1.3 m above the floor and 2 m from a patient bed, in the center of the room	50 L/min, 60 min
	C2	21 January 2021	ICU intermediate COVID-19	Air sampler placed approximately 1.3 m above the floor and 2 m from a patient bed, in the center of the room	50 L/min, 60 min

Table 2. Cont.

Device	Sample ID	Date of Collection	Hospital Area	Sampler Location	Sampling Parameters
	C3	21 January 2021	Nursing area COVID-19	Air sampler placed approximately 1.3 m above the floor and 2 m from a patient bed, in the center of the room	50 L/min, 60 min
	C4	27 January 2021	Respiratory diseases observation room	Air sampler placed approximately 1.3 m above the floor and 2 m from a patient bed, in the center of the room	50 L/min, 60 min
	C5	27 January 2021	Respiratory diseases waiting room	Air sampler placed approximately 1.3 m above the floor in the center of the room	50 L/min, 60 min
	C6	27 January 2021	Clinical decision unit	Air sampler placed approximately 1.3 m above the floor and 2 m from a patient bed, in the center of the room	50 L/min, 60 min
	C7	2 February 2021	COVID-19 testing room	Air sampler placed approximately 1.3 m above the floor in the center of the room	50 L/min, 60 min
	C8	2 February 2021	Non-respiratory diseases waiting room	Air sampler placed approximately 1.3 m above the floor in the center of the room	50 L/min, 60 min
	C9	2 February 2021	Urgency Care (Recovery area)	Air sampler placed approximately 1.3 m above the floor and 2 m from a patient bed, in the center of the room	50 L/min, 60 min
	C10	11 February 2021	Hospital's outside entrance atrium	Air sampler placed approximately 1.3 m above the floor in the center of the room	50 L/min, 60 min
	C11	11 February 2021	Hospital employe's cafeteria	Air sampler placed approximately 1.3 m above the floor in the center of the room	50 L/min, 60 min
Coriolis® μ	M1	21 January 2021	ICU COVID-19	Air sampler placed approximately 1.3 m above the floor and 2 m from a patient bed, in the center of the room	100 L/min, 10 min
	M2	21 January 2021	ICU COVID-19	Air sampler placed approximately 1.3 m above the floor and 2 m from a patient bed, in the center of the room	200 L/min, 10 min

Table 2. Cont.

Device	Sample ID	Date of Collection	Hospital Area	Sampler Location	Sampling Parameters
	M3	21 January 2021	ICU COVID-19	Air sampler placed approximately 1.3 m above the floor and 2 m from a patient bed, in the center of the room	300 L/min, 10 min
	M4	21 January 2021	ICU intermediate COVID-19	Air sampler placed approximately 1.3 m above the floor and 2 m from a patient bed, in the center of the room	100 L/min, 10 min
	M5	21 January 2021	ICU intermediate COVID-19	Air sampler placed approximately 1.3 m above the floor and 2 m from a patient bed, in the center of the room	200 L/min, 10 min
	M6	21 January 2021	ICU intermediate COVID-19	Air sampler placed approximately 1.3 m above the floor and 2 m from a patient bed, in the center of the room	300 L/min, 10 min
	M7	21 January 2021	Nursing area COVID-19	Air sampler placed approximately 1.3 m above the floor and 2 m from a patient bed, in the center of the room	100 L/min, 10 min
	M8	21 January 2021	Nursing area COVID-19	Air sampler placed approximately 1.3 m above the floor and 2 m from a patient bed, in the center of the room	200 L/min, 10 min
	M9	21 January 2021	Nursing area COVID-19	Air sampler placed approximately 1.3 m above the floor and 2 m from a patient bed, in the center of the room	300 L/min, 10 min
	M10	27 January 2021	Respiratory diseases observation room	Air sampler placed approximately 1.3 m above the floor and 2 m from a patient bed, in the center of the room	100 L/min, 10 min
	M11	27 January 2021	Respiratory diseases observation room	Air sampler placed approximately 1.3 m above the floor and 2 m from a patient bed, in the center of the room	200 L/min, 10 min
	M12	27 January 2021	Respiratory diseases observation room	Air sampler placed approximately 1.3 m above the floor and 2 m from a patient bed, in the center of the room	300 L/min, 10 min

Table 2. Cont.

Device	Sample ID	Date of Collection	Hospital Area	Sampler Location	Sampling Parameters
	M13	27 January 2021	Respiratory diseases waiting room	Air sampler placed approximately 1.3 m above the floor in the center of the room	100 L/min, 10 min
	M14	27 January 2021	Respiratory diseases waiting room	Air sampler placed approximately 1.3 m above the floor in the center of the room	200 L/min, 10 min
	M15	27 January 2021	Respiratory diseases waiting room	Air sampler placed approximately 1.3 m above the floor in the center of the room	300 L/min, 10 min
	M16	27 January 2021	Clinical decision unit	Air sampler placed approximately 1.3 m above the floor and 2 m from a patient bed, in the center of the room	100 L/min, 10 min
	M17	27 January 2021	Clinical decision unit	Air sampler placed approximately 1.3 m above the floor and 2 m from a patient bed, in the center of the room	200 L/min, 10 min
	M18	27 January 2021	Clinical decision unit	Air sampler placed approximately 1.3 m above the floor and 2 m from a patient bed, in the center of the room	300 L/min, 10 min
	M19	2 February 2021	COVID-19 testing room	Air sampler placed approximately 1.3 m above the floor in the center of the room	100 L/min, 10 min
	M20	2 February 2021	COVID-19 testing room	Air sampler placed approximately 1.3 m above the floor in the center of the room	200 L/min, 10 min
	M21	2 February 2021	COVID-19 testing room	Air sampler placed approximately 1.3 m above the floor in the center of the room	300 L/min, 10 min
	M22	2 February 2021	Non-respiratory diseases waiting room	Air sampler placed approximately 1.3 m above the floor in the center of the room	100 L/min, 10 min
	M23	2 February 2021	Non-respiratory diseases waiting room	Air sampler placed approximately 1.3 m above the floor in the center of the room	200 L/min, 10 min

Table 2. Cont.

Device	Sample ID	Date of Collection	Hospital Area	Sampler Location	Sampling Parameters
	M24	2 February 2021	Non-respiratory diseases waiting room	Air sampler placed approximately 1.3 m above the floor in the center of the room	300 L/min, 10 min
	M25	2 February 2021	Urgency Care (Recovery area)	Air sampler placed approximately 1.3 m above the floor and 2 m from a patient bed, in the center of the room	100 L/min, 10 min
	M26	2 February 2021	Urgency Care (Recovery area)	Air sampler placed approximately 1.3 m above the floor and 2 m from a patient bed, in the center of the room	200 L/min, 10 min
	M27	2 February 2021	Urgency Care (Recovery area)	Air sampler placed approximately 1.3 m above the floor and 2 m from a patient bed, in the center of the room	300 L/min, 10 min
	M28	11 February 2021	Hospital's outside entrance atrium	Air sampler placed approximately 1.3 m above the floor in the center of the room	100 L/min, 10 min
	M29	11 February 2021	Hospital's outside entrance atrium	Air sampler placed approximately 1.3 m above the floor in the center of the room	200 L/min, 10 min
	M30	11 February 2021	Hospital's outside entrance atrium	Air sampler placed approximately 1.3 m above the floor in the center of the room	300 L/min, 10 min
	M31	11 February 2021	Hospital staff's cafeteria	Air sampler placed approximately 1.3 m above the floor in the center of the room	100 L/min, 10 min
	M32	11 February 2021	Hospital staff's cafeteria	Air sampler placed approximately 1.3 m above the floor in the center of the room	200 L/min, 10 min
	M33	11 February 2021	Hospital staff's cafeteria	Air sampler placed approximately 1.3 m above the floor in the center of the room	300 L/min, 10 min

Collection of air and surface samples

Air samples were collected using two cyclonic microbial air samplers, a Coriolis® µ and a Coriolis® Compact (Bertin Instruments, Montigny-le-Bretonneux, France). Using the Coriolis® µ, three consecutive air samplings were collected from each of the eleven areas of the Hospital for 10 min each with an airflow rate of 100 L/min (total of 1 m^3), 200 L/min (total of 2 m^3) and 300 L/min (total of 3 m^3), respectively. Air samples with the Coriolis® µ were collected on wet medium, with 4 mL of sterile phosphate buffered saline (PBS) added to the collection cones before sampling. With the Coriolis® Compact, one air sampling was performed in the same eleven areas for 60 min, with an airflow rate of 50 L/min (total of 3 m^3). Air samples with Coriolis® Compact were collected on dry medium, with 4 mL of sterile PBS added to the collection cones after sampling. Both Coriolis® samplers were placed side by side at 1.3 m height using a portable table, and the three consecutive Coriolis® μ samplings were performed simultaneously within the 60-min sampling periods of the Coriolis® Compact.

Surface samples were collected on 10 cm × 10 cm surface areas (100 cm^2 area per sampling) using sterile flocked plastic swabs previously wetted on PBS and immediately placed in PBS (4 mL).

All samples were stored at 4 °C before being taken to the laboratory facilities, and were processed within 8 h. Details about the characteristics of the air and surface samples collected are summarized in Tables 2 and 3, respectively.

Table 3. Details of the surface samples' collections for SARS-CoV-2 RNA detection in the Hospital.

Sample ID	Hospital Area	Collection Date	Sample Location
S1	COVID-19 testing room	2 February 2021	Hand sanitizer dispenser
S2			Instruments' counter
S3			Glove box
S4			Wall of a COVID-19 testing booth
S5			Paper dispenser
S6	Non-respiratory disease waiting room	2 February 2021	Faucet handle
S7			Vending machine (buttons)
S8			Bathroom: flush button
S9			Bathroom: inside doorknob
S10			Bathroom: outside doorknob
S11	Hospital's outside outside entrance atrium	11 February 2021	Statue (approx. 3 m away from outside entrance)
S12			ATM (buttons)
S13			Fire extinguisher (approx. 3 m away from outside entrance)
S14	Hospital staff's cafeteria	11 February 2021	Soap dispenser
S15			Faucet handle
S16			Paper dispenser
S17			Table sign on a table *

* Table sign: a sign with precautions to avoid contamination was placed on the table.

RNA extraction and detection of SARS-CoV-2

RNA extraction was performed using the GRS Viral DNA/RNA Purification Kit (GRISP, Porto, Portugal) according to the manufacturer's instructions. RNA extraction was performed on 200 μL of sample suspensions as previously described [19]. A one-step RT-qPCR reaction aimed at two viral gene targets (N1 and N2) using viral target-specific primers and Taqman probe technology based on a previously described protocol [20] was used (Xpert qDetect COVID-19, GRISP, Porto, Portugal). For the CFX Real-Time PCR (qPCR) Detection System (Bio-Rad, Hercules, CA, USA), the Bio-Rad CFX Maestro 1.0 Software version 4.0.2325.0418 was used to control the runs and remotely analyze the data. Each RT-qPCR run included ssDNA targets for both N1 and N2 regions (positive controls) and a no-template control. Reactions were set up and run with initial conditions of 15 min at 45 °C and 2 min at 95 °C, then 45 cycles of 95 °C for 15 sec and 55 °C for 30 sec. A standard curve was constructed using the ssDNA targets for both N1 and N2 regions in a 10-fold serial dilution mixture starting at 200,000 copies/µL, in order to quantify the number of viral gene copies present in each sample from the measured Ct values; the limit of detection (LOD) was 1.3 copies/µL for N1 and 3.2 copies/µL for N2. Air sample results are expressed in copies/m^3, and surface sample results in copies/cm2.

3. Results

Of the 44 air samples collected in eleven different areas of the Hospital, only two (C1 and M1) were positive for SARS-CoV-2 RNA (Table 4). They were both from the same place, the COVID-19 ICU, and were collected at the same time; C1 (viral loads of 6000 and 6575 copies/m^3 for N1 and N2 genes, respectively) was collected during 60 min sampling with the Coriolis® Compact at an airflow rate of 50 L/min (total of 3 m^3), while M1 (viral loads of 6362.5 and 6662.5 copies/m^3 for N1 and N2 genes, respectively) was collected with the Coriolis® µ during the first 10 min of the Coriolis® Compact collection period, at an airflow rate of 100 L/min (total of 1 m^3). The two other Coriolis® µ consecutive samples (M2 and M3) collected within the 60-min time frame of the Coriolis® Compact (air flow rates of 200 L/min and 300 L/min, respectively) were both negative for SARS-CoV-2 RNA.

Table 4. Details of Hospital area, sampling location and viral genome copy numbers of the positive air and surface samples.

	Sample ID	Hospital Area	Sample Location	Copy Number (N1 Gene)	Copy Number (N2 Gene)
Air samples	C1	COVID-19 ICU	Air sampler placed approximately 1.3 m above the floor and 2 m from intubated patients beds, in the center of the room	6000 copies/m^3	6575 copies/m^3
	M1			6362.5 copies/m^3	6662.5 copies/m^3
Surface samples	S4	COVID-19 testing room	Wall of a COVID-19 testing booth	200.6 copies/cm^2	No amplification detected
	S6	Non-respiratory disease patients' waiting room	Faucet handle	179.2 copies/cm^2	No amplification detected
	S8		Bathroom: flush button	No amplification detected	201.7 copies/cm^2

Of the 17 surface samples collected in four different areas of the Hospital, three were positive for SARS-CoV-2 RNA, with viral loads of 200.6 copies/cm^2 (COVID-19 testing room, wall of a testing booth), 179.2 copies/cm^2 (non-respiratory disease waiting room, faucet handle), and 201.7 copies/cm^2 (non-respiratory disease waiting room, bathroom's flush button). The three samples amplified only one of the two target genes (N1, N1 and N2 respectively). Details on the Hospital area, sampling location and viral genome copy numbers of the positive air and surface samples are summarized in Table 4.

4. Discussion

The present study aimed to evaluate SARS-CoV-2 environmental contamination of air and surfaces in a major Hospital in Portugal during the third wave of the COVID-19 pandemic. Eleven different areas of the Hospital were selected to be assessed for air contamination, including four COVID-19 and seven non-COVID-19 areas. SARS-CoV-2 RNA was only detected in the air of the COVID-19 ICU. The viral load of these air samples collected with the Coriolis® Compact and Coriolis® µ ranged from 6000 to 6662.5 copies/m^3. Interestingly, only the first sample of Coriolis® µ, collected during the first 10 min of the 60-min time frame of the Coriolis® Compact, was SARS-CoV-2 RNA positive. The two other consecutive samplings of Coriolis® µ performed within the 60-min time frame of the Coriolis® Compact were negative for SARS-CoV-2 RNA in spite of a higher airflow rate (air flow rates of 200 L/min and 300 L/min, respectively), suggesting a point contamination which could be explained by the fact that, when the sampling period started, a patient had just been intubated. This intubation can explain the presence of aerosols containing virus during the first 10 min of Coriolis® µ, sampling and the negative results in the second and third samples, considering that aerosols containing SARS-CoV-2 may have been removed by the rooms' ventilation system by the time the other two samplings took place.

In this study, we aimed to assess the performance and suitability of both air samplers for SARS-CoV-2 air monitoring. The results of this study suggest that Coriolis® µ and Coriolis® Compact samplers seem robust for SARS-CoV-2 air sampling, as both were able to detect SARS-CoV-2 RNA in the air of the COVID-19 ICU. However, longer collection times are more likely to cover point contaminations, as was seen with the 60-min collection with Coriolis® Compact. During this collection, three consecutive samplings of Coriolis® µ were performed, with only the first providing a positive air sample.

To assess contamination of surfaces, four different areas of the Hospital were selected, one COVID-19 area and three non-COVID-19 areas. SARS-CoV-2 RNA was detected on the wall of one of the testing booths (where patients wait for nasopharyngeal sample collection), which was somewhat expected due to the fact that during sampling there were possibly-infected individuals constantly coming in to collect nasopharyngeal samples for testing, all of them reporting as symptomatic (presenting respiratory symptoms such as coughing or sneezing). Moreover, this is the only room where patients remove their masks, likely increasing the viral load in indoor air. Contamination in this room might have happened through respiratory aerosols or droplets from the infected patients that settled on the surfaces sampled, considering that neither the patients or healthcare staff touch the walls in this area, ruling out the possibility of direct touch contamination in this case. SARS-CoV-2 viral RNA was detected in the non-respiratory disease waiting room as well. This was one of the non-COVID-19 areas sampled, and therefore the presence of viral RNA was not expected. This was a positive pressure room, which ideally prevents unfiltered air from outside the room from coming inside [21]. Nevertheless, viral RNA was detected in two surface samples in this area, namely on a faucet handle located in the middle of the waiting room and on the flush button of a bathroom in this area. As these are frequently-touched surfaces, the most likely explanation for viral RNA presence is direct touch contamination. Nonetheless, SARS-CoV-2 excretion in stools has been described, and the flushing could generate contaminated aerosols that could ultimately deposit on these surfaces [22,23]. These results highlight the importance of hand and general hygiene in public toilets as well as the need for enhanced disinfection protocols in all areas of the Hospital, not only those dedicated to COVID-19 patients.

Airborne transmission of SARS-CoV-2 is now widely accepted as a mode of transmission of SARS-CoV-2 [2,4,8,12]. This route dominates under certain environmental conditions, particularly indoor environments without proper ventilation [24–29], with a recent study demonstrating that some fraction of the RNA-containing aerosols emitted from infected people contain intact, replication-competent virions [30]. On the contrary, current evidence suggests that transmission through contaminated surfaces is rare; however, when it comes to healthcare settings where COVID-19 patients are being treated, especially in ICUs, aerosol-generating medical procedures take place which could potentially exacerbate the contamination of air and surfaces in the surrounding area [31]. To avoid nosocomial infection of healthcare workers, non-COVID-19 patients, and visitors by these virus-laden aerosols as well as to avoid contamination of medical equipment and surfaces, it is imperative that hospital ventilation works properly [4].

COVID-19 patients that need to undergo intubation and extubation are usually placed in negative-pressure isolation rooms, which is considered to be safer [32]. Negative-pressure rooms have a ventilation system in which air flows from the exterior to the interior [21]. This keeps aerosolized viruses from spreading through the heating, ventilation, and air conditioning system. Under these conditions, if an opening exists, air will flow from the surrounding areas into the negatively pressurized space [4]. In the Hospital assessed in this study, the COVID-19 ICU, which was the only negative room sampled, had twelve air changes per hour (ACH), in compliance with the safety rules for these types of rooms [31].

Since the beginning of the pandemic, many articles have been published on detection of SARS-CoV-2 in air samples [24,25,33–35]; however, some inherent problems with air sampling for the detection of viruses have come up, such as the limited diversity of monitored spaces (most studies are done in indoor healthcare facilities), limited number of samples, diversity of methodologies (there is no gold-standard protocol for air sampling of SARS-CoV-2 and other airborne viruses), not all studies performing both surface and air sampling simultaneously, and lastly, the fact that most of these studies were performed during the first wave when little was known about the virus, which could have led to errors in methods and molecular analysis.

This study faced some limitations that are worth highlighting. This was an observational study at a single hospital, which means that the results may not be generalizable to other healthcare facilities. Additionally, no assessment of virus viability was performed, as no BSL3 facility was available to perform such experiments. As a result, the findings in this study, although reflecting the real extent of environmental contamination with SARS-CoV-2 in the Hospital, do not necessarily amount to an infection risk assessment for air and surfaces. Moreover, no surface sampling was performed in the COVID-19 ICU, and we do not have individual data on patients, particularly those who occupied the COVID-19 ICU at the time of sampling. Patients with severe infection influence the viral load in droplets and exhaled aerosols; therefore, it is important that in future studies these individual patient data are acquired in order to allow better interpretation of results. Nevertheless, this study is an important addition to the growing literature on the detection of SARS-CoV-2 RNA in air and on surfaces.

5. Conclusions

The present study showed SARS-CoV-2 hospital environmental contamination both in air and on surfaces in locations where both COVID-19 and non-COVID-19 patients were present. This reinforces the need to remain cautious at all times, not only when in close contact with infected individuals. Hand hygiene and other standard transmission-prevention guidelines should be continuously followed in order to avoid nosocomial COVID-19. Further studies combining air and surface sampling with virus viability assays are still needed to fully elucidate the real risk of air and environmental transmission in healthcare facilities.

Author Contributions: Conceptualization, P.G.d.S., J.R.M., S.I.V.S.; methodology, P.G.d.S., J.R.M. and S.I.V.S.; investigation, P.G.d.S.; resources, J.R.M. and S.I.V.S.; data curation, P.G.d.S.; writing—original draft preparation, P.G.d.S.; writing—review and editing, P.G.d.S., J.R.M., S.I.V.S., M.S.J.N., P.T.B.S.B., R.R.G.S., A.I.B.L., N.A.E., G.E.E.B. and J.G. All authors have read and agreed to the published version of the manuscript.

Funding: This work was financially supported by Base Funding-UIDB/00511/2020 of the Laboratory for Process Engineering, Environment, Biotechnology and Energy–LEPABE–funded by national funds through the FCT/MCTES (PIDDAC).

Institutional Review Board Statement: Not applicable.

Informed Consent Statement: Not applicable.

Data Availability Statement: Not applicable.

Acknowledgments: Priscilla Gomes da Silva thanks the Portuguese Foundation for Science and Technology–FCT for the financial support of her PhD work (2020.07806.BD, CRM: 0026504) contract through the DOCTORATES 4 COVID-19 program. Sofia I.V. Sousa thanks the Portuguese Foundation for Science and Technology (FCT) for the financial support of her work contract through the Scientific Employment Stimulus-Individual Call-CEECIND/02477/2017.

Conflicts of Interest: All the authors certify that they have no affiliations with or involvement in any organization or entity with any financial interest (such as honoraria, educational grants, participation in speakers' bureaus, membership, employment, consultancies, stock ownership, or other equity interest, and expert testimony or patent-licensing arrangements), or non-financial interest (such as personal or professional relationships, affiliations, knowledge or beliefs) in the subject matter or materials discussed in this manuscript.

References

1. Azer, S.A. COVID-19: Pathophysiology, diagnosis, complications and investigational therapeutics. *New Microbes New Infect.* **2020**, *37*, 100738. [CrossRef] [PubMed]
2. WHO. Coronavirus Disease (COVID-19): How Is It Transmitted? Available online: https://www.who.int/news-room/q-a-detail/coronavirus-disease-covid-19-how-is-it-transmitted (accessed on 16 August 2021).
3. Tang, J.W.; Bahnfleth, W.P.; Bluyssen, P.M.; Buonanno, G.; Jimenez, J.L.; Kurnitski, J.; Li, Y.; Miller, S.; Sekhar, C.; Morawska, L.; et al. Dismantling myths on the airborne transmission of severe acute respiratory syndrome coronavirus-2 (SARS-CoV-2). *J. Hosp. Infect.* **2021**, *110*, 89–96. [CrossRef]
4. WHO. Roadmap to Improve and Ensure Good Indoor Ventilation in the Context of COVID-19. Available online: https://www.who.int/publications/i/item/9789240021280 (accessed on 1 June 2021).
5. Fennelly, K.P. Particle sizes of infectious aerosols: Implications for infection control. *Lancet Respir. Med.* **2020**, *8*, 914–924. [CrossRef]
6. Fabian, P.; Brain, J.; Houseman, E.A.; Gern, J.; Milton, D.K. Origin of Exhaled Breath Particles from Healthy and Human Rhinovirus-Infected Subjects. *J. Aerosol Med. Pulm. Drug Deliv.* **2011**, *24*, 137–147. [CrossRef]
7. Zayas, G.; Chiang, M.C.; Wong, E.; MacDonald, F.; Lange, C.F.; Senthilselvan, A.; King, M. Cough aerosol in healthy participants: Fundamental knowledge to optimize droplet-spread infectious respiratory disease management. *BMC Pulm. Med.* **2012**, *12*, 11. [CrossRef] [PubMed]
8. Wang, C.C.; Prather, K.A.; Sznitman, J.; Jimenez, J.L.; Lakdawala, S.S.; Tufekci, Z.; Marr, L.C. Airborne transmission of respiratory viruses. *Science* **2021**, *373*, eabd9149. [CrossRef]
9. United States Environmental Protection Agency. Ventilation and Coronavirus (COVID-19). Available online: https://www.epa.gov/coronavirus/ventilation-and-coronavirus-covid-19 (accessed on 13 September 2021).
10. Hamner, L.; Dubbel, P.; Capron, I.; Ross, A.; Jordan, A.; Lee, J.; Lynn, J.; Ball, A. High SARS-CoV-2 Attack Rate Following Exposure at a Choir Practice. *Morb. Mortal. Wkly. Rep. High* **2020**, *69*, 606–610. [CrossRef]
11. Li, Y.; Qian, H.; Hang, J.; Chen, X.; Cheng, P.; Ling, H.; Wang, S.; Liang, P.; Li, J.; Xiao, S.; et al. Probable airborne transmission of SARS-CoV-2 in a poorly ventilated restaurant. *Build. Environ.* **2021**, *196*, 107788. [CrossRef] [PubMed]
12. Miller, S.L.; Nazaroff, W.W.; Jimenez, J.L.; Boerstra, A.; Buonanno, G.; Dancer, S.J.; Kurnitski, J.; Marr, L.C.; Morawska, L.; Noakes, C. Transmission of SARS-CoV-2 by inhalation of respiratory aerosol in the Skagit Valley Chorale superspreading event. *Indoor Air* **2021**, *31*, 314–323. [CrossRef]
13. Centers for Disease Control and Prevention (CDC). *SARS-CoV-2 Transmission*; CDC: Atlanta, GA, USA, 2021.
14. WHO. Transmission of SARS-CoV-2: Implications for Infection Prevention Precautions. Available online: https://www.who.int/news-room/commentaries/detail/transmission-of-sars-cov-2-implications-for-infection-prevention-precautions (accessed on 28 September 2020).
15. Birgand, G.; Peiffer-Smadja, N.; Fournier, S.; Kerneis, S.; Lescure, F.-X.; Lucet, J.-C. Assessment of Air Contamination by SARS-CoV-2 in Hospital Settings. *JAMA Netw. Open* **2020**, *3*, e2033232. [CrossRef] [PubMed]
16. Centers for Disease Control and Prevention (CDC). *Science Brief: SARS-CoV-2 and Surface (Fomite) Transmission for Indoor Community Environments*; CDC: Atlanta, GA, USA, 2021.
17. Mody, L.; Gibson, K.E.; Mantey, J.; Bautista, L.; Montoya, A.; Neeb, K.; Jenq, G.; Mills, J.P.; Min, L.; Kabeto, M.; et al. Environmental contamination with SARS-CoV-2 in nursing homes. *J. Am. Geriatr. Soc.* **2021**, *8*, S291–S292. [CrossRef]
18. Direção-Geral da Saúde (DGS). *Relatório de Situação*; DGS: Lisboa, Portugal, 2021.
19. Santarpia, J.L.; Rivera, D.N.; Herrera, V.L.; Morwitzer, M.J.; Creager, H.M.; Santarpia, G.W.; Crown, K.K.; Brett-Major, D.M.; Schnaubelt, E.R.; Broadhurst, M.J.; et al. Aerosol and surface contamination of SARS-CoV-2 observed in quarantine and isolation care. *Sci. Rep.* **2020**, *10*, 12732. [CrossRef] [PubMed]

20. Centers for Disease Control and Prevention (CDC). *Real-Time RT-PCR Diagnostic Panel*; CDC: Atlanta, GA, USA, 2021.
21. Al-Benna, S. Negative pressure rooms and COVID-19. *J. Perioper. Pract.* **2021**, *31*, 18–23. [CrossRef]
22. Ding, Z.; Qian, H.; Ph, D.; Xu, B.; Huang, Y.; Miao, T. Toilets dominate environmental detection of SARS-CoV-2 virus in a hospital. *Sci. Total Environ.* **2021**, *753*, 141710. [CrossRef]
23. Peng, L.; Liu, J.; Xu, W.; Luo, Q.; Chen, D.; Lei, Z.; Huang, Z.; Li, X.; Deng, K.; Lin, B.; et al. SARS-CoV-2 can be detected in urine, blood, anal swabs, and oropharyngeal swabs specimens. *J. Med. Virol.* **2020**, *92*, 1676–1680. [CrossRef]
24. Lednicky, J.A.; Lauzard, M.; Fan, Z.H.; Jutla, A.; Tilly, T.B.; Gangwar, M.; Usmani, M.; Shankar, S.N.; Mohamed, K.; Eiguren-Fernandez, A.; et al. Viable SARS-CoV-2 in the air of a hospital room with COVID-19 patients. *Int. J. Infect. Dis.* **2020**, *100*, 476–482. [CrossRef]
25. Ahn, J.Y.; An, S.; Sohn, Y.; Cho, Y.; Hyun, J.H.; Baek, Y.J.; Kim, M.H.; Jeong, S.J.; Kim, J.H.; Ku, N.S.; et al. Environmental contamination in the isolation rooms of COVID-19 patients with severe pneumonia requiring mechanical ventilation or high-flow oxygen therapy. *J. Hosp. Infect.* **2020**, *106*, 570–576. [CrossRef] [PubMed]
26. Liu, Y.; Ning, Z.; Chen, Y.; Guo, M.; Liu, Y.; Gali, N.K.; Sun, L.; Duan, Y.; Cai, J.; Westerdahl, D.; et al. Aerodynamic analysis of SARS-CoV-2 in two Wuhan hospitals. *Nature* **2020**, *582*, 557–560. [CrossRef] [PubMed]
27. Guo, Z.-D.; Wang, Z.-Y.; Zhang, S.-F.; Li, X.; Li, L.; Li, C.; Cui, Y.; Fu, R.-B.; Dong, Y.-Z.; Chi, X.-Y.; et al. Aerosol and Surface Distribution of Severe Acute Respiratory Syndrome Coronavirus 2 in Hospital Wards, Wuhan, China, 2020. *Emerg. Infect. Dis.* **2020**, *26*, 1583–1591. [CrossRef]
28. Morawska, L.; Cao, J. Airborne transmission of SARS-CoV-2: The world should face the reality. *Environ. Int.* **2020**, *139*, 105730. [CrossRef]
29. Morawska, L.; Milton, D.K. It is Time to Address Airborne Transmission of COVID-19. *Clin. Infect. Dis. Off. Publ. Infect. Dis. Soc. Am.* **2020**, *71*, 2311–2313. [CrossRef]
30. Santarpia, J.L.; Herrera, V.L.; Rivera, D.N.; Ratnesar-Shumate, S.; Reid, S.P.; Ackerman, D.N.; Denton, P.W.; Martens, J.W.S.; Fang, Y.; Conoan, N.; et al. The size and culturability of patient-generated SARS-CoV-2 aerosol. *J. Expo. Sci. Environ. Epidemiol.* **2021**, 5–10. [CrossRef] [PubMed]
31. Klompas, M.; Baker, M.; Rhee, C. What Is an Aerosol-Generating Procedure? *JAMA Surg.* **2021**, *156*, 113–114. [CrossRef] [PubMed]
32. Arora, V.; Evans, C.; Langdale, L.; Lee, A. You Need a Plan: A Stepwise Protocol for Operating Room Preparedness During an Infectious Pandemic. *Fed. Pract.* **2020**, *37*, 212–218.
33. Tan, L.; Ma, B.; Lai, X.; Han, L.; Cao, P.; Zhang, J.; Fu, J.; Zhou, Q.; Wei, S.; Wang, Z.; et al. Air and surface contamination by SARS-CoV-2 virus in a tertiary hospital in Wuhan, China. *Int. J. Infect. Dis.* **2020**, *99*, 3–7. [CrossRef] [PubMed]
34. Setti, L.; Passarini, F.; De Gennaro, G.; Barbieri, P.; Perrone, M.G.; Borelli, M.; Palmisani, J.; Di Gilio, A.; Torboli, V.; Fontana, F.; et al. SARS-Cov-2 RNA found on particulate matter of Bergamo in Northern Italy: First evidence. *Environ. Res.* **2020**, *188*, 109754. [CrossRef]
35. Lednicky, J.A.; Shankar, S.N.; Elbadry, M.A.; Gibson, J.C.; Alam, M.M.; Stephenson, C.J.; Eiguren-Fernandez, A.; Glenn Morris, J.; Mavian, C.N.; Salemi, M.; et al. Collection of SARS-CoV-2 virus from the air of a clinic within a university student health care center and analyses of the viral genomic sequence. *Aerosol Air Qual. Res.* **2020**, *20*, 1167–1171. [CrossRef] [PubMed]

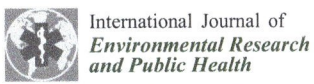

Article

How Does Gender Moderate Customer Intention of Shopping via Live-Streaming Apps during the COVID-19 Pandemic Lockdown Period?

Yuyang Zhao * and Fernando Bacao

NOVA Information Management School (NOVA IMS), Universidade Nova de Lisboa, 1070-312 Lisboa, Portugal; bacao@novaims.unl.pt
* Correspondence: d2015046@novaims.unl.pt; Tel.: +86-156-3993-7262

Abstract: Shopping through Live-Streaming Shopping Apps (LSSAs) as an emerging consumption phenomenon has increased dramatically in recent years, especially during the COVID-19 lockdown period. However, insufficient studies have focused on the psychological processes undergone in different customer demographics while shopping via LSSAs under pandemic conditions. This study integrated the Unified Theory of Acceptance and Use of Technology 2 with Flow Theory into a Stimulus-Organism-Response framework to investigate the psychological processes of different customer demographics during the COVID-19 lockdown period. A total of 374 validated data were analyzed by covariance-based structural equation modelling. The statistical results demonstrated by the proposed model showed a significant discrepancy between different gender groups, in which Flow, as a mediator, representing users' engagement and immersion in shopping via LSSAs, was significantly moderated by gender where connection between stimulus components, hedonic motivation, trust and social influence and response component perceived value are concerned. This study contributed a theoretical development and a practical framework to the explanation of the mental processes of different customer demographics when using an innovative e-commerce technology. Furthermore, the results can support the relevant stakeholders in e-commerce in their comprehensive understanding of customers' behavior, allowing better strategical and managerial development.

Keywords: COVID-19; customer behavior; psychological process; live-streaming shopping apps; stimulus-organism-response framework; Unified Theory of Acceptance and Use of Technology 2; Flow Theory; gender; age

Citation: Zhao, Y.; Bacao, F. How Does Gender Moderate Customer Intention of Shopping via Live-Streaming Apps during the COVID-19 Pandemic Lockdown Period? *Int. J. Environ. Res. Public Health* **2021**, *18*, 13004. https://doi.org/10.3390/ijerph182413004

Academic Editors: Sachiko Kodera, Essam A. Rashed and William Douglas Evans

Received: 6 November 2021
Accepted: 7 December 2021
Published: 9 December 2021

Publisher's Note: MDPI stays neutral with regard to jurisdictional claims in published maps and institutional affiliations.

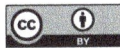

Copyright: © 2021 by the authors. Licensee MDPI, Basel, Switzerland. This article is an open access article distributed under the terms and conditions of the Creative Commons Attribution (CC BY) license (https://creativecommons.org/licenses/by/4.0/).

1. Introduction

Live-streaming commerce, as a burgeoning e-commerce pattern with the unique features of real-time live-streaming demonstration of products and instant interactions among sellers and viewers, provides personalized services for customers remotely [1]. Meanwhile, based on the broad application of telecommunication networks and extensive adoption of mobile devices, live-streaming shopping apps (LSSAs) have provided an immersive experience for viewers [2], which has formulated a new consumption phenomenon, namely, shopping via LSSAs, especially in the Chinese e-commerce industry in recent years. According to a report from iiMedia (2020), live-streaming commerce industry transactions were estimated to exceed 129 billion USD in 2020, up from 61 billion USD in 2019 [3]. In 2019, on the Taobao e-commerce platform alone, over 60,000 live-streaming shows hosted by brands, stores and celebrities attracted more than 400 million consumers [4]. Shopping via LSSAs has established an entertainment environment for customers, facilitating a revolution in commerce. Under the lockdown measures for the defence against COVID-19 transmission especially, interaction and entertainment were in significant demand from individuals. Despite several previous studies demonstrating that the adoption of LSSAs was influenced by the motivations of participants [5,6], technology features [7] and human-computer interaction [2], few studies have focused on the customer's psychological processes when subject to the moderating effects of age and gender in a particular environment. LSSAs are mobile entertainment and commerce applications, and their adoption should take the moderating effects of age and gender into consideration [8].

Consequently, the objective of the current study is to investigate the psychological processes of customers of different ages and genders when shopping via LSSAs during the COVID-19 pandemic lockdown situation. The proposed model embeds the revised Unified Theory of Acceptance and Use of Technology 2 (UTAUT2) as a stimulus, along with Flow Theory as an organism, into the stimulus-organism-response (SOR) framework. In this way, the SOR framework, as the main structural foundation of the research model, explains that customers' behavioral psychological processes are determined by external antecedents as well as internal cognitions [9–12]. UTAUT2, as a theoretical framework, has coordinated consumer-oriented perceptions to predict users' behavioral intentions [13], which is legitimately considered a perceptive process in the explanation of customers' perceptions of LSSAs and the constitution of stimulus components. Flow Theory supports organisms theoretically by representing participants' concentration and engagement in shopping activities via LSSAs [14]. These theoretical frameworks are initially integrated and verified in this study, supporting relevant researchers and stakeholders in order to better understand the behaviors of customers.

The current study comprises eight sections, investigating the psychological processes of customers shopping via LSSAs under pandemic lockdown conditions. Section 2 consists of a literature review regarding the subject of shopping via LSSAs, as well as relevant theoretical frameworks. This section is followed by the research model and hypotheses development, which are presented in Section 3. Section 4 illustrates the method of data collection and the demographic distribution of data. Subsequently, Section 5 presents the results of the data analysis. Section 6 discusses the findings of these results, while Section 7 illustrates their theoretical and practical implications. Finally, limitations and recommendations for future research and conclusion are outlined in Section 8.

2. Theoretical Background
2.1. Live-Streaming Shopping Apps (LSSAs)

The current LSSAs comprise e-commerce functions that are integrated into live-streaming platforms with simultaneous and authentic consumption interactions between vendors and customers [5,6]. Shopping via LSSAs can be divided into two patterns. The first of these patterns is consumption activities on mobile e-commerce apps with extensional live-streaming functions, such as Taobao and AliExpress, while the second is shopping via LSSAs through a third-party e-commerce service, such as Tiktok and LiveMe [6]. Shopping via LSSAs has become a thriving new consumption phenomenon. Off-line consumption activities were restricted, especially under lockdown conditions during the COVID-19 pandemic; shopping via LSSAs supported customers' daily supply and demand requirements and provided a relaxation pattern during the quarantine time, formulating a positive perception among users. Cai et al. (2018) claimed that customers' decisions to shop via live-streaming are not only influenced by utilitarian perceptions of service and production but are also determined by hedonic motivation [5]. According to the entertainment feature of live-streaming, viewers' engagement and gratification significantly affected their shopping activities [15]. Based on LSSA's facilitation of conspicuous human-machine interaction, this affordance of LSSAs and customers' engagement conjointly determine the number of customers purchasing via LSSAs [2].

Meanwhile, previous studies have found that customers' endorsement of, and behavioral responses to LSSAs were observably determined by their intrinsic and extrinsic motivations, social influence, entertainment, perceived flow and emotional engagement [16–18]. Accordingly, customers' mental perceptions, such as trust and perceived value, have significantly influenced their engagement with live-streaming commerce [1]. Moreover, the simultaneity, authenticity, interactivity and customizability characteristics of LSSAs significantly formulate customers' perceptions of this technology, affecting their behavior [7,19]. However, prior literature has insufficiently investigated customers' psychological processes while shopping via LSSAs under specific conditions. Moreover, the moderating effects of age and gender might lead to different results in different market segmentations [20]. Thus, it is meritorious to clarify the role of age and gender in moderating customers' mental processes while shopping via LSSAs in the pandemic lockdown situation.

2.2. Stimulus-Organism-Response (SOR) Framework

The SOR framework demonstrates that external antecedents influence customers' psychological processing, first as a perceptive stimulus, affecting their cognitive and emotional reflections, then as an organism, contributing towards formulating their mental or behavioral traits, and finally as a response, such as an attitude, adoption intention or actual usage [21]. The SOR framework has been modified with external variables to analyze in a qualified way the connections between the stimulus (environmental input), the organism (mental process) and the response (behavioral outputs), in order to explain users' behaviors in various business analysis studies [11,22] as well as works of literature on the adoption of innovative technology [10,12,23], which are demonstrated in Table 1. In their investigation of users' visiting intentions in virtual reality tourism, Kim, Lee and Jung (2020) designated customers' actual experiences as stimuli, their cognition and affection (including enjoyment, emotional involvement and flow) as organisms and their attachment and intention as responses [12]. Zhao, Wang and Sun (2020) proposed that stimuli include interactivity, media richness and sociability, and assumed that virtual experience as an organism would include telepresence, social presence and flow, which in turn determined students' continuing intentions regarding the use of massive open online courses [23]. Moreover, the SOR framework has been applied in an investigation of customers' online shopping intentions, which were significantly influenced by their attitude, which was in turn affected by their internal and external environment [9]. However, compared with traditional online shopping, streaming service quality and promotion campaigns played more significant roles in formulating customers' purchase intentions via mobile shopping apps [22].

Furthermore, the moderating effects of age and gender have rarely been examined in the SOR framework. There have been a few previous studies partially involving the moderators in the SOR model, but their results were presented inconsistently. Wu and Li (2018) found that gender had a significant moderating effect on customers' loyalty in online social commerce [11], against the findings of Islam and Rahman (2017) [24]. Therefore, this study uses the SOR framework as a theoretical foundation to create a research model.

Table 1. Literature review of the SOR framework.

Studies	Topic	Stimulus	Organism	Response
[22]	Mobile shopping	Ubiquity; Ease of use; Information exchange; Discounted price; Scarcity	Impulsive buying tendency; Normative evaluation; Positive affect	Purchase intention
[11]	Social commerce	Structural capital; Cognitive capital; Relational capital; Social identification; Social influence; Social commerce needs; Social commerce risk; Social commerce convivence;	Consumer value	Consumer loyalty
[10]	Mobile payment	Usefulness; Emotion; Security	Flow	Satisfaction; Purchase intention
[12]	Virtual reality tourism	Actual experiences	Enjoyment, Emotional involvement, Flow	Attachment; Visit intention
[23]	Massive open online courses	Interactivity; Media richness; Sociability	Virtual Experience; Telepresence; Social presence; flow	Continuance intention

2.3. Unified Theory of Acceptance and Use of Technology 2 (UTAUT2)

UTAUT2 was developed by Venkatesh, Thong and Xu (2012). As an extension of the UTAUT model, UTAUT2 predicts users' technological perceptions, determining their intention regarding the adoption of a particular technology [13]. Several researchers have modified UTAUT2 in miscellaneous mobile-technology-adoption studies by extending it with additional variables or moderators, for example, trust [25,26], privacy [27] and Hofstede's cultural values [28,29]. Some studies have incorporated UTAUT2 into other theoretical frameworks, such as diffusion of innovation [30] and the expectation-confirmation model [31,32], in investigating customers' behaviors while using mobile technology. Furthermore, UTAUT2 involves the use of age, gender and experience as moderators to explain individual differences in adoption intention [13]. Moreover, UTAUT2 was applied to the adoption of mobile shopping applications by Tak and Panwar (2017), who found that hedonic motivation was the most significant antecedent, which corresponds with the recognition of the current study that LSSAs are entertaining mobile shopping applications [33]. Therefore, UTAUT2 is considered the appropriate theoretical foundation for investigating users' perceptions as a stimulus in the proposed model.

2.4. Flow Theory

Flow Theory was initially proposed by Csikszentmihalyi (1975) as a way to predict individuals' mental engagement in a certain activity [14]. Subsequently, Flow Theory's applicability has been extended into the human-computer interaction domain to describe users' absorption in technology [34]. Specifically, flow represents users' holistic, immersive consciousness when they concentrate entirely on a particular activity or technology; their involvement will be self-reinforced by constitutional enjoyment and engaging interactivity, and, in turn, their self-consciousness will become indistinct in order to ignore irrelevant interruptions [35]. Flow has been applied as a mediator in various technology adoption studies to describe customers' cognition and engagement for predicting users' adoption intention [10,36,37], especially in the fields of entertaining technologies, such as live-streaming [16] and mobile shopping [38]. Flow is significantly influenced by users' technological perceptions [37,39], as well as mental determinants such as emotion [10], trust [38] and enjoyment [16]. Meanwhile, the combination of Flow Theory with other frameworks, such as the Information Systems Success Model [37,38] and the Stimulus-Organism-Response framework [10], also reasonably illustrated users' adoption intention. Thus, Flow Theory is considered a theoretical foundation for the representation of users' shopping engagement via LSSAs during the pandemic lockdown period, acting as the organism in the proposed model.

2.5. Moderating Effects of Age and Gender

According to the current research objectives, age and gender are proposed as moderating variables involved in the analysis process. Venkatesh, Thong and Xu (2012) initially confirmed that age and gender have moderating effects on the UTAUT2 constructs affecting users' adoption intention [13]. Moreover, other works of literature have integrated age and gender as moderators within various frameworks (UTAUT, Technology Acceptance Model (TAM), Diffusion of Innovation (DOI) Theory) and have confirmed that age and gender significantly moderate constructs in different contexts [20,40–44]. However, based on the differences in research objectives, sample targets and involved variables in various scenarios, the moderating effects of age and gender have been diverse in different literature. Venkatesh and Zhang (2010) validated the idea that performance expectancy in the behavioral intention of information technology was significantly moderated by younger male users, and effort expectancy was strongly moderated by older female customers [40], which is contrary to the findings of Riskinanto, Kelana and Hilmawan (2017), who claimed that stated age had insignificant effects on perceived usefulness and ease of use regarding the intention of adoption of E-payment technology [43]. On the other hand, Liébana-Cabanillas, Sánchez-Fernández and Muñoz-Leiva (2014) complementarily illustrated that social influence bore a strong influence on users above 35 years old, and that trust was more affected by younger groups in the adoption of mobile payments [41]. Moreover, Shao et al. (2018) claimed that males had a stronger moderating effect on mobility and reputation in the trust-formation process of mobile payments, while females moderated customization and security of trust more [44]. Likewise, Pascual-Miguel, Agudo-Peregrina and Chaparro-Peláez (2015) found that the moderating effects of female customers on effort expectancy and social influence were significantly stronger than male customers on online purchase intention [45]. In order to analyse the moderating effects of age and gender on all constructs in the proposed research model, a multi-group analysis is applied in this research, which is widely applied in previous studies for multi-group comparisons [20,44,45].

3. Development of Research Model and Hypotheses

Based on the previous literature reviews, the integration of the SOR framework with UTAUT2 and Flow Theory is considered a theoretical foundation on which to propose a comprehensive model for the investigation. Specifically, according to previous paradigms of the SOR framework application, this research extends the SOR framework by integrating variables from the revised UTAUT2 model, which are proposed as stimulus components, roused by technological perceptions of LSSAs during the pandemic lockdown period (performance expectancy, effort expectance) [22,24], namely, social influence [11], hedonic motivation [12] and trust [12]. These variables reflect users' external and internal perceptions towards inciting their further psychological cognition. On the other hand, due to the popularization of smartphones, proficiency in using various mobile applications and the absence of monetary cost in the operation of LSSAs, original variables such as facilitating conditions, habit and price value are excluded from the UTAUT2 model, which is in accordance with previous findings [25,26,28,31,32]. Flow Theory provides theoretical support to the reflection of customers' mental, cognitive and affective intermediary states during shopping via LSSAs in the COVID-19 pandemic lockdown period, which it is appropriate to consider as an organism in the SOR framework [10,12,23]. Moreover, this study proposes that perceived value and adoption intention reflects customers' psychological reactions and behaviors, constituting the response elements of the SOR framework [10,12]. In addition, age and gender are considered moderators of the theoretical model comparing the different effects of antecedents on customers' adoption intention regarding LSSAs in each subgroup. The proposed research model is generalized and presented in Figure 1 with the relevant hypotheses relations.

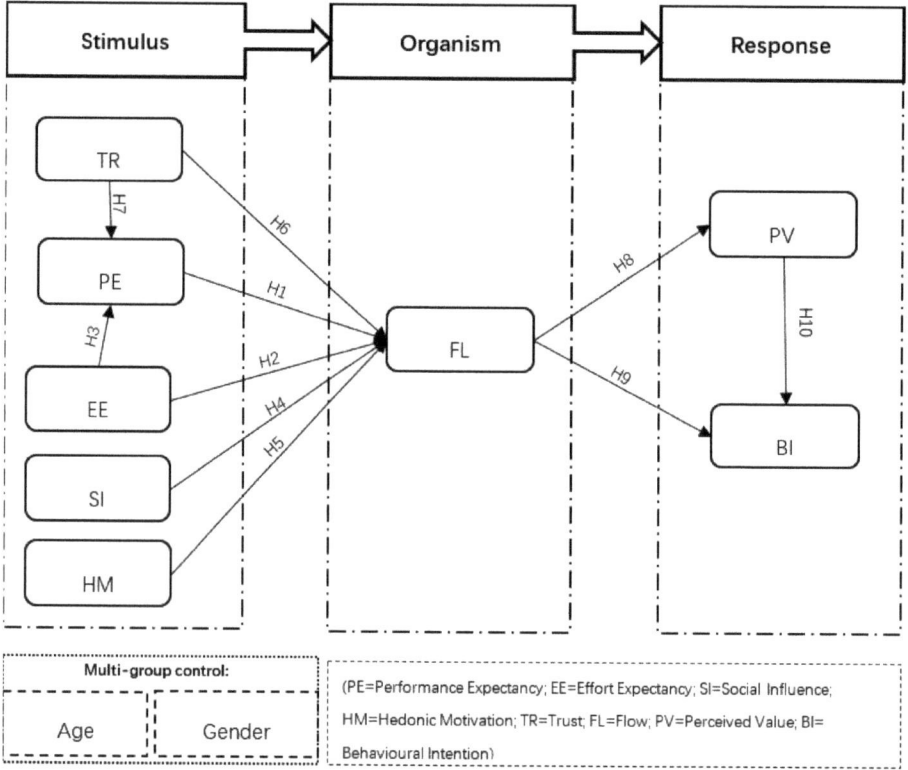

Figure 1. Proposed research model.

3.1. Stimulus Components: Variables from the Revised UTAUT2 Model

Performance expectancy (PE), as a technological perception, represents the perceived usefulness of a certain technology in the eyes of a user, and its potential to optimize their experience of a specific technology or to reinforce their performance in particular activities [13]. Moreover, the technological features which users perceive, such as compatibility, service quality, information quality and system quality, can be generalized as perceived usability of technology, represented as PE [37,46,47]. Related to technology adoption, PE significantly formulates users' mental responses, such as attitude, adoption intention and continued usage intention, which are confirmed by prior literature [30,48,49]. Accordingly, customers' psychological cognitions are formulated by their perceptions of satisfying usability, which indicates that PE significantly influences customers' perceived flow when they intend to adopt new technology [10,39]. Therefore, the hypothesis can be generalized as follows:

Hypothesis 1 (H1). *Customers' performance expectancy (PE) as a stimulus positively determines the organism flow (FL) when shopping via LSSAs during the pandemic lockdown period.*

Effort expectancy (EE), as a technological perception, expresses the idea that users acquire feelings of easiness from understanding, operating and interacting with a specific information technology [13]. A variety of literature has verified EE's considerable effect on customers' attitude and behavioral intention in technology adoption research [43,47,48]. Consequently, customers' engagement and flow experience are formulated by understandability, operability and intractability [36,39]. Moreover, the influence of EE has been confirmed by Kim et al. (2013) as not only affecting flow but also performance expectancy when users adopt entertainment technology [39]. When customers recognize that a technology is easy to access, they will tend to confirm its usability. This phenomenon has been validated in various technology adoption works of literature, such as live-streaming [19], mobile banking [26,46,49] and mobile payment [41,47]. Thus, the hypotheses related to EE are proposed as follows:

Hypothesis 2 (H2). *Customers' effort expectancy (EE) as a stimulus positively determines the organism flow (FL) when shopping via LSSAs during the pandemic lockdown period.*

Hypothesis 3 (H3). *Customers' effort expectancy (EE) as a stimulus positively determines performance expectancy (PE) when shopping via LSSAs during the pandemic lockdown period.*

Social influence (SI), as an environmental perception, represents customers perceiving an influence from people particularly relevant to them, such as close friends, family members and colleagues, who recommend and support them in using a certain technology [13]. Customers' anxiety is derived from the uncertainty of new technology, which can be decreased by the influence of their close social network [25]. Various technology adoption studies have involved SI in theoretical frameworks and have confirmed SI as an essential antecedent in determining customers' attitudes and behaviors [27,29,42,50]. Moreover, Chen and Lin (2018) claimed that the effect of SI was to dramatically formulate users' mental awareness of engagement when using live-streaming [16]. Accordingly, interacting with relevant people on a specific information technology can facilitate users' flow experience [23]. Hence, the current study proposes that users' flow experience of LSSAs is positively determined by SI, which formulated the following hypothesis:

Hypothesis 4 (H4). *Social influence (SI) as a stimulus positively determines the organism flow (FL) when shopping via LSSAs during the pandemic lockdown period.*

Hedonic motivation (HM) was initially adapted in UTAUT2 by Venkatesh, Thong and Xu (2012), which is defined as the internal emotional perception of enjoyment and pleasure descend from a user's expectation or experience of a certain information technology [13]. The directly positive effect of HM on adoption intention has been confirmed by prior researchers who applied UTAUT2 on mobile technology adoption, e.g., mobile payment [27] and mobile banking [26,28]. Meanwhile, HM has been recognised as an antecedent which also has a significant indirect effect on customers' behavioral intention. Yeo, Goh and Rezaei (2017) claimed that HM formulated attitude via convenience motivation and post-usage usefulness when customers adopt online food delivery services [51]. Likewise, engagement, as the main characteristic of users' flow experience, is formulated by enjoyment, curiosity and concentration [52,53].

Consequently, Wongkitrungrueng and Assarut (2018) validated HM directly and indirectly (through trust), formulating users' engagement in live-streaming commerce [1]. Furthermore, Chen and Lin (2018) illustrated that live-streaming's entertainment features formulated viewers' HM, which positively determined their mental perception of value, which in turn affected their final behavioral intention [16]. Thus, the current study assumes that HM positively affects customers' engagement and affection in Hypothesis 5.

Hypothesis 5 (H5). *Customers' hedonic motivation (HM) as a stimulus positively determines the organism flow (FL) when shopping via LSSAs during the pandemic lockdown period.*

Gefen (2000) defined trust (TR) as describing users' subjective awareness of believing a particular technology can fulfil obligations and positively guarantee a qualified performance to meet their expectations [54]. Specifically, under the lockdown measures of the COVID-19 pandemic, trust reflected users' perceptions of technological characteristics such as mobility, security, etc., which correspond with perceived security against perceived risk and uncertainty conditions [44]. LSSAs' contactless online consumption functions, a beneficial feature in the lockdown situation during the COVID-19 pandemic, formulated customers' perceived trust and positively influenced enjoyable and practical cognitions [42]. Accordingly, trust as an essential variable in the investigation of users' behavioral intention has been integrated into various adoption models, such as UTAUT2 [25], TAM [46] and the IS success model [37]. Moreover, from the participation aspect, the interaction between customers and vendors on live-streaming commerce platforms facilitated users' perceived trust in sellers and products, which in turn optimized engagement [1]. Therefore, this paper proposes that trust formulates users' engagement and cognitive acceptance, positively influencing flow [37,38]. Meanwhile, as an antecedent of users' utilitarian perceptions, trust positively facilitates customers' performance expectancy stimulus [26,46]. Hence, the following hypotheses are addressed:

Hypothesis 6 (H6). *Trust (TR) as a stimulus positively determines the organism flow (FL) when shopping via LSSAs during the pandemic lockdown period.*

Hypothesis 7 (H7). *Trust (TR) as a stimulus positively determines performance expectancy (PE) when shopping via LSSAs during the pandemic lockdown period.*

3.2. Organism Component: Flow (FL)

Csikszentmihalyi (1975) defined flow as an individual's feeling of intrinsic absorption in a particular activity or technology [14]. Flow experience of technology was described as users' temporary unawareness caused by their internal enjoyment of, pleasure in and engagement and interaction with a certain technology [16,38]. Moreover, lockdown measures provided an appropriate environment for the enhancement of an individual's immersive shopping experience via LSSAs at home. Various technology adoption studies have validated the idea that flow is significantly formulated by users' technological perceptions regarding their behavioral intention of adoption or continued usage [18,37,38]. Consequently, flow is in accordance with the conception of an organism, which is assumed as a mediator connecting technological and environmental stimuli and responses in shopping via LSSAs.

Flow has been examined by previous researchers as also having an indirect effect on users' final responses, such as adoption intention, actual usage and continuance intention, via users' mental reflection variables, such as perceived value, satisfaction and attitude [16,39,55]. Meanwhile, the effects of flow and mental reflections has been validated as a way in which to determine customers' behavioral intentions conjointly in various pieces of literature [10,37,38]. Chen and Lin (2018) claimed that flow positively affected perceived value regarding the formulation of customers' intention to use live-streaming [16]. Therefore, the following hypotheses are proposed:

Hypothesis 8 (H8). *Customers' flow (FL) as an organism positively determines the response perceived value (PV) when shopping via LSSAs during the pandemic lockdown period.*

Hypothesis 9 (H9). *Customers' flow (FL) as an organism positively determines the response behavioral intention (BI) when shopping via LSSAs during the pandemic lockdown period.*

3.3. Response Components: Perceived Value (PV) and Behavioral Intention (BI)

Perceived value (PV), as defined by Zeithaml (1988), represents customers' universal assessments of a service or technology. PV is determined by users' perceptions of acquisition and investment [56]. Sweeney and Soutar (2001) extended the dimensions of perceived value, including quality and price of production, customers' emotional responses and social influence [57]. Meanwhile, Petrick (2002) modified behavioral price, monetary price, emotional response, quality and reputation, all of which emerged as other dimensions of PV [58]. PV also represents customers' perceived multi-dimensional benefits, including those from utilitarian, hedonic and social perspectives [50,59]. Specifically, in this study, perceived value represents the customers' general mental responses to shopping via LSSAs during the COVID-19 pandemic lockdown period. Perceived value has been assumed as a cognitive variable in various adoption models, such as the Expectation Confirmation Model [36], the Value-based Adoption Model [60] and the Mobile user Engagement Model [59], which positively determines customers' behaviors. On the other hand, Chen and Lin (2018) confirmed that perceived value, as a conative factor, was determined by flow and, in turn, formulated users' behaviors [16]. Therefore, this study proposes that perceived value, which, in a customer, would be a conational response, constitutes one component amongst a variety of responses, which is demonstrated in the following hypothesis:

Hypothesis 10 (H10). *Customers' perceived value (PV) positively determines behavioral intention (BI) when shopping via LSSAs during the pandemic lockdown period.*

3.4. Moderation Hypotheses

Gender and age moderators were incorporated within the UTAUT2 model to investigate information technology adoption [13]. Various studies involved gender and age moderators in different adoption models, and validated gender and age as moderating constructs in different scenarios respectively [13,20,40–45]. As shown in Figure 1, gender and age moderators are assumed to be multi-group controls, which should optimize the predictive validity of the proposed model in the explanation of any conflicting results [42]. Meanwhile, due to the way in which the proposed model was initially developed, the moderation hypotheses are established by the exploratory approach in this study, which was common in previous studies [42]. The moderating effect will be assessed by subgroup analysis after the general model evaluation. Therefore, the following hypotheses are proposed in investigation of the different moderating effects of age and gender on customers' psychological processes experienced while shopping via LSSAs.

Hypothesis 11 (H11). *Gender moderates the relations among all constructs of the proposed model.*

Hypothesis 12 (H12). *Age moderates the relations among all constructs of the proposed model.*

4. Methodology and Data Demographic Distribution
4.1. Measurement

A quantitative methodology was applied in this study to evaluate the proposed model. An online questionnaire survey was conducted to collect data in China, which comprised two parts. The first part requested demographic information (consisting of gender, age and frequency of using LSSAs during the COVID-19 pandemic lockdown period) of participants, using dichotomous, bounded continuous and ordinal-polytomous close-ended questions; the second part consisted of a seven-point Likert scale (from strongly disagree = "1" to strongly agree = "7"), comprising structural questions which evaluated performance expectancy (PE), effort expectancy (EE), social influence (SI), hedonic motivation (HM), trust (TR), flow (FL), perceived value (PV) and behavioral intention (BI), with 34 measurement items taken from previous literature, shown in Table A1 in Appendix A.

The questionnaire was designed and managed in English, before being translated into the Chinese language by language experts to avoid the biases of language and culture (the target population of the survey was smartphone users in China). Afterwards, according to the translation-back translation method, it was reverse-translated into the English language. In order to minimize the non-response rate, a short introduction and respondent-friendly survey questionnaire techniques were applied in the survey [61].

4.2. Data Collection

The online questionnaire was designed via Wenjuan.com (a Chinese online survey platform). According to the formulae from Westland (2010) and the numbers of 34 observed indicators and eight latent variables in the proposed model, the recommended minimum sample size for the model structure was 91 [62]. The questionnaires were distributed online and via WeChat (a Chinese mobile social media application) on 9 August 2020 for data collection. After four weeks of data collection, 400 empirical data were collected on 6 September 2020, of which 138 were derived from online responses and 262 via WeChat. After filtering out the responses with missing values in a scrutinizing process, 374 valid data were accepted for data analysis, which obtained a 93.5% final response rate. The Kolmogorov-Smirnov test was applied to examine the early respondents' group with 100 participants and the late respondents with 274 participants. This test confirmed no statistical difference between the two independent groups [63]. Meanwhile, the Shapiro-Wilk test of the demographic data, age, gender and frequency of those shopping via LSSAs were 0.636, 0.862 and 0.918, respectively, and all showed a significant level of 0.000, which indicated the data was non-normally distributed.

4.3. Data Demographic Characteristics

The data was collected online and via WeChat randomly, and the geographical distribution of respondents consisted of 43.5%, 13.1% and 3.5% located in Henan, Guangdong and Shandong provinces, respectively, which are the three largest Chinese provinces in terms of population. This represented general smartphone users in China. 51.87% female and 48.13% male smartphone users participated in the survey. The largest age group was adults between 21 and 35, at 27.01%, while the age range of participants younger than 36 comprised 51.07%, with the group over 35 years old being 48.93%. These figures are consistent with the QusetMobile report (2020) that users between 19 and 35 years old were the leading group of shoppers via LSSAs in China [64]. Moreover, 24.06% of participants used LSSAs at least once per week. More than 39% of respondents shopped via LSSAs every week. Table 2 presents the specific demographic distribution of participants.

Table 2. Demographic distribution of participants.

Measure	Item	N	%
Gender	Male	180	48.13%
	Female	194	51.87%
Age	<20	90	24.06%
	21–35	101	27.01%
	36–50	96	25.67%
	>51	87	23.26%
Frequency of using LSSAs during the COVID-19 pandemic lockdown period	At least 1 time per 1 day	59	15.78%
	At least 1 time per 1 week	90	24.06%
	At least 1 time per 2 weeks	81	21.66%
	At least 1 time per 1 month	55	14.71%
	At least 1 time per 3 months	41	10.96%
	At least 1 time per 6 months	29	7.75%
	Never used during the pandemic lockdown period	19	5.08%

5. Data Analysis

As the proposed model was generated based on a solid theoretical foundation, structural equation modelling is appropriate to operationalizing the hypothesized latent constructs and associated indicators for theory development [65]. Besides minimizing the difference between the observed and estimated covariance matrices, covariance-based structural equation modelling (CB-SEM) applies a maximum likelihood procedure to assess correlations among all constructs and their interactive effects simultaneously [66,67]. Meanwhile, the proposed model in this study consists of mediating variables and moderators. The CB-SEM approach is well suited to the assessment of models involving mediation and moderating effects [65,67]. CB-SEM performs very accurately, with sum scores higher than both PLS-SEM and regression in a small sample size [68]. Meanwhile, CB-SEM presents more accurately than PLS-SEM for non-normally distributed data with a sample size over 50 [69]. CB-SEM provides optimal coefficient estimates and more accurate model analyses in the evaluation of research models [70]. Moreover, the two-step approach, consisting of the measurement model assessment and structural model evaluation [71], is applied in this study. Specifically, the CB-SEM technique is conducted for confirmatory factor analysis (CFA), to assess the convergent and discriminant validity for each construct in the measurement model assessment, and to evaluate the path coefficient to test hypotheses with a comparison of differences between age (<36 VS >35) and gender (Male VS Female) sub-samples in the structural model evaluation by AMOS.

Before implementing the two-step approach, The Exploratory Factor Analysis (EFA) was applied by SPSS to evaluate the dataset adequacy. The Kaiser criterion and scree plot were applied in order to identify the number of underlying extractive factors. The Kaiser test obtained an eight-factor solution with eigenvalues larger than 1, and the first inflexion point was located at the 9th point in the scree plot. The results indicate that eight factors can be extracted, which is aligned with the proposed model [72].

5.1. Measurement Model

Firstly, the reliability and validity of the measurement model was assessed by the following criteria: Construct reliability was confirmed by Cronbach's alpha (CA). The CAs of all constructs exceeded 0.70 [73], and convergent validity was validated by factor loadings above 0.7 [74]; Composite Reliability (CR) exceeded 0.7; Average Variance Extracted (AVE) exceeded 0.5 [75]; discriminant validity was qualified by the square root of AVE of each latent construct exceeding any two pairs of its inter-construct correlation [75] and the AVE was higher than the maximum shared squared variance (MSV) of each construct [66]. The constructs' CA, CR, AVE, MSV, and factor loading of items results are presented in Table 3.

Table 4 displays the results of the square root of AVE, which are bigger than the correlations of each latent construct. The values of the results reached the relevant recommended threshold of each criterion. Therefore, the reliability and validity of the measurement model were confirmed for further assessment.

Moreover, the model-fit of measurement model shown in Table 5 was validated by the goodness-of-fit results meeting the standards of each index [70]. Namely, the ratio of chi-square to degrees-of-freedom ($X^2/df < 3$), comparative fit index (CFI > 0.9), the goodness of fit index (GFI > 0.8) [76], adjusted goodness-of-fit index (AGFI > 0.8) [70], normalized fit index (NFI > 0.9), Tucker-Lewis index (TLI > 0.9) and root mean square error of approximation (RMSEA < 0.08) [77].

Furthermore, the potential common method bias of this study was evaluated by Harman's one-factor test and the fitness of a single-factor model. The result of Harman's one-factor test is 49.63%, which meets the criteria proposed by Podsakoff et al. (2003) that the largest variance of one factor should be below 50% in order to confirm that a single factor cannot explain the majority of the variance [78]. The fitness results of a single-factor model are shown in Table 5, which illustrates the unqualified model fit of a single-factor model.

Based on the previous assessments, the measurement model is eligible for further structural model evaluation.

Table 3. Latent constructs' CA, CR, AVE, MSV, and items' factor loading.

Factors	CA	CR	AVE	MSV	Items	Loadings
Performance expectancy (PE)	0.943	0.943	0.807	0.510	PE1	0.875
					PE2	0.912
					PE3	0.905
					PE4	0.899
Effort expectancy (EE)	0.935	0.932	0.820	0.326	EE1	0.896
					EE2	0.874
					EE3	0.916
					EE4	0.858
Social influence (SI)	0.949	0.936	0.785	0.264	SI1	0.896
					SI2	0.904
					SI3	0.925
					SI4	0.902
Hedonic motivation (HM)	0.946	0.949	0.822	0.416	HM1	0.868
					HM2	0.89
					HM3	0.909
					HM4	0.869
					HM5	0.869
Trust (TR)	0.948	0.946	0.776	0.412	TR1	0.905
					TR2	0.883
					TR3	0.873
					TR4	0.898
					TR5	0.873
Flow (FL)	0.965	0.948	0.786	0.446	FL1	0.911
					FL2	0.923
					FL3	0.930
					FL4	0.910
					FL5	0.927
Perceived value (PV)	0.943	0.965	0.847	0.510	PV1	0.882
					PV2	0.901
					PV3	0.909
					PV4	0.900
Behavioral Intention (BI)	0.923	0.923	0.800	0.394	BI1	0.892
					BI2	0.892
					BI3	0.899

(CA = Cronbach's alpha; CR = Composite Reliability; AVE = Average Variance Extracted; MSV = maximum shared squared variance).

Table 4. Latent constructs' square root of AVE and correlation.

	PV	PE	EE	SI	HM	TR	FL	BI
PV	**0.898**							
PE	0.571	**0.905**						
EE	0.514	0.416	**0.886**					
SI	0.645	0.408	0.427	**0.907**				
HM	0.642	0.422	0.463	0.551	**0.881**			
TR	0.668	0.506	0.460	0.565	0.535	**0.886**		
FL	0.714	0.523	0.470	0.599	0.592	0.635	**0.920**	
BI	0.608	0.494	0.486	0.538	0.541	0.600	0.628	**0.894**

(Number in **Bold**: Latent constructs' square root of AVE).

Table 5. The Model-fit of each model.

	X^2/df	CFI	GFI	AGFI	NFI	TLI	RMSEA
Recommend Value	<3	>0.9	>0.8	>0.8	>0.9	>0.9	<0.08
Single-Factor Model	12.471	0.526	0.398	0.360	0.505	0.525	0.175
Measurement Model	1.166	0.994	0.918	0.902	0.959	0.993	0.021
Original Structural Model	1.477	0.982	0.899	0.882	0.947	0.980	0.036
Model with Age Subgroups	1.433	0.968	0.825	0.796	0.902	0.965	0.034
Model with Gender Subgroups	1.371	0.972	0.829	0.801	0.906	0.970	0.032

5.2. Structural Model

According to the research objectives and proposed hypotheses, the structural equation model was created by AMOS and developed into two versions with age and gender subgroups, respectively.

Firstly, the model-fits of structural models (including the original structural model and two structural models with age and gender subgroups) were assessed consistently as the previous evaluation process of model-fit of the measurement model. The results met all thresholds of goodness-of-fit as presented in Table 5, which demonstrates that all structural models have eligible goodness-of-fit.

Moreover, the R^2 values of endogenous variables were assessed to evaluate the structural models' explanatory powers. The R^2 values of endogenous variables in the three structural models are presented in Table 6. Specifically, the model with gender subgroups has the highest R^2 values of performance expectancy ($R^2 = 0.35$), flow ($R^2 = 0.70$) and behavioral intention ($R^2 = 0.45$). The model with age subgroups has the highest R^2 value of perceived value ($R^2 = 0.55$).

Table 6. R^2 values of endogenous variables in different models.

Endogenous Variables	R^2		
	Original Structural Model	Model with Age Subgroups	Model with Gender Subgroups
PE	0.30	0.30	0.35
FL	0.58	0.58	0.70
PV	0.53	0.55	0.52
BI	0.45	0.42	0.45

Furthermore, the testing of the hypotheses was evaluated by the coefficient of each path. The results are depicted in Table 7. Specifically, except for H2 (EE → FL) being rejected (ß = 0.078, p = 0.068), all the other hypotheses were supported in the original structural model and sorted by the significance from high to low, shown as follows: H8 (FL → PV, ß = 0.732, p < 0.001), H9 (FL → BI, ß = 0.44, p < 0.001), H7 (TR → PE, ß = 0.38,

$p < 0.001$), H10 (PV → BI, ß = 0.308, $p < 0.001$), H6 (TR → FL, ß = 0.275, $p < 0.001$), H5 (HM → FL, ß = 0.232, $p < 0.001$), H3 (EE → PE, ß = 0.209, $p < 0.001$), H4 (SI → FL, ß = 0.205, $p < 0.001$) and H1 (PE → FL, ß = 0.187, $p < 0.001$).

Table 7. Hypotheses testing of the original structural model.

			Original Model			
H	Relations	Estimate	S.E.	T	P	Decisions
H1	PE→FL	0.187	0.047	3.958	***	Supported
H2	EE→FL	0.078	0.043	1.825	0.068	Rejected
H3	EE→PE	0.209	0.048	4.319	***	Supported
H4	SI→FL	0.205	0.044	4.642	***	Supported
H5	HM→FL	0.232	0.052	4.485	***	Supported
H6	TR→FL	0.275	0.053	5.196	***	Supported
H7	TR→PE	0.38	0.052	7.323	***	Supported
H8	FL→PV	0.732	0.046	15.799	***	Supported
H9	FL→BI	0.44	0.069	6.38	***	Supported
H10	PV→BI	0.308	0.069	4.469	***	Supported

(Est. = estimate; S.E. = standard error; T = t-value; P = p-value; ***: p-value < 0.01).

Moreover, based on the evaluation of path coefficients of each subgroup in Table 8, the model performed variously. With regards to moderation hypotheses, H11 and H12 were confirmed partially. Five out of ten paths were significantly different when comparing the gender groups. However, only one out of ten hypotheses were significantly different for age groups. The effect of flow on perceived values (H8) was validated, having the most significantly positive influence in all four subgroups. Meanwhile, the effect of flow on behavioral intention (H9) was verified with the second largest coefficient in the male subgroup (ß = 0.555, $p < 0.001$) and the over-35 subgroup (ß = 0.51, $p < 0.001$), respectively. The male subgroup significantly moderated effort expectancy on flow (ß = 0.162, $p = 0.003$). However, H2 (EE → FL) was rejected in the model with the female group (ß = 0.038, $p = 0.55$), the group with age below and equal to 35 (ß = 0.076, $p = 0.18$) and the group with age higher than 35 (ß = 0.084, $p = 0.207$). Meanwhile, relations between hedonic motivation and flow, and perceived value and behavioral intention, were significantly moderated by the female moderator. Hypotheses H5 (HM → FL, ß = 0.07, $p = 0.248$) and H10 (PV → BI, ß = 0.179, $p = 0.083$) were rejected in the model with the male subgroup. Likewise, the male subgroup moderated the effects of social influence and trust on flow. H4 (SI → FL, ß = 0.124, $p = 0.062$) and H6 (TR → FL, ß = 0.12, $p = 0.155$) were found with insignificant effects in the female subgroup. On the other hand, the age moderator only caused a significant difference in hedonic motivation as part of flow in two age groups, the younger age group having a more significant moderating effect on hedonic motivation as part of flow than the older age group.

In addition, the model invariances were evaluated by comparing the chi-square of two subgroup models to evaluate the moderating effects of gender and age, and to assess the H11 and H12; see the results presented in Table 9. H11 was supported by the results of the model, which demonstrated a variance under the moderating effect of gender. However, there were insignificant differences at the level of the model with different age groups, and thus H12 should be interpreted cautiously. Specifically, to illustrate the differences of the path effect in each subgroup, the critical ratio was assessed to test the hypotheses, and the z-score was tested to evaluate the data. As shown in Table 8, the results demonstrate the effects of hedonic motivation, trust and social influence on flow, as well as the effects of perceived values on behavioral intention, both of which were significantly variant between male and female groups. Meanwhile, only the flow path to perceived value significantly differed between younger and older age groups.

Table 8. Hypotheses testing of the subgroups.

		Model with Gender Subgroups										
		Male					Female					
H	Relations	Est.	S.E.	T	P	Dec.	Est.	S.E.	T	P	Dec.	Z-Score
H1	PE→FL	0.146	0.061	2.401	0.016	Sup.	0.186	0.068	2.73	0.006	Sup.	0.446
H2	EE→FL	0.162	0.054	3.014	0.003	Sup.	0.038	0.064	0.598	0.55	Rej.	−1.485
H3	EE→PE	0.265	0.066	4.009	***	Sup.	0.151	0.07	2.151	0.031	Sup.	−1.173
H4	SI→FL	0.283	0.056	5.075	***	Sup.	0.124	0.067	1.866	0.062	Rej	−1.83 *
H5	HM→FL	0.07	0.061	1.154	0.248	Rej.	0.465	0.088	5.297	***	Sup.	3.699 ***
H6	TR→FL	0.367	0.064	5.697	***	Sup.	0.12	0.084	1.421	0.155	Rej.	−2.331 **
H7	TR→PE	0.385	0.071	5.447	***	Sup.	0.389	0.076	5.145	***	Sup.	0.035
H8	FL→PV	0.681	0.066	10.293	***	Sup.	0.771	0.065	11.902	***	Sup.	0.973
H9	FL→BI	0.555	0.099	5.609	***	Sup.	0.337	0.096	3.526	***	Sup.	−1.583
H10	PV→BI	0.179	0.103	1.734	0.083	Rej.	0.409	0.092	4.46	***	Sup.	1.664 *
		Model with Age Subgroups										
		≤35					>35					
H	Relations	Est.	S.E.	T	P	Dec.	Est.	S.E.	T	P	Dec.	Z-Score
H1	PE→FL	0.196	0.063	3.106	0.002	Sup.	0.182	0.071	2.57	0.01	Sup.	1.431
H2	EE→FL	0.076	0.056	1.341	0.18	Rej.	0.084	0.067	1.263	0.207	Rej.	−0.153
H3	EE→PE	0.145	0.068	2.131	0.033	Sup.	0.285	0.07	4.097	***	Sup.	−0.411
H4	SI→FL	0.21	0.063	3.319	***	Sup.	0.205	0.062	3.295	***	Sup.	0.096
H5	HM→FL	0.287	0.066	4.383	***	Sup.	0.155	0.082	1.892	0.058	Rej	−0.058
H6	TR→FL	0.204	0.076	2.666	0.008	Sup.	0.342	0.075	4.58	***	Sup.	−1.259
H7	TR→PE	0.479	0.074	6.512	***	Sup.	0.277	0.073	3.773	***	Sup.	1.293
H8	FL→PV	0.744	0.065	11.37	***	Sup.	0.72	0.065	10.995	***	Sup.	−1.947 *
H9	FL→BI	0.352	0.099	3.566	***	Sup.	0.51	0.096	5.308	***	Sup.	−0.268
H10	PV→BI	0.341	0.1	3.405	***	Sup.	0.284	0.095	2.983	0.003	Sup.	1.15

(Est. = estimate; S.E. = standard error; T = t-value; P = p-value; Dec.= decision; Sup. = Supported; Rej. = Rejected; ***: p-value < 0.01; **: p-value < 0.05; *: p-value < 0.1).

Table 9. Comparison between the models of gender and age subgroups.

	Model with Gender Subgroups			Model with Age Subgroups		
	Chi-Square	df	p-Value	Chi-Square	df	p-Value
Unconstrained	1401.159	1022		1464.315	1022	
Fully Constrained	1451.548	1058		1496.514	1058	
Number of Groups		2			2	
Difference	50.389	36	0.056	32.199	36	0.650
Model Invariant		NO			YES	

6. Discussion

Based on the key objectives of this research, as well as the data analysis results, the findings are discussed in the sequence of the stimulus-organism-response of customers' psychological shopping processes via LSSAs under lockdown measures during the COVID-19 pandemic. Specifically, the significant determinants of each subgroup's stimulus-organism-response components were summarized in Table 10.

Table 10. The significant determinants of each subgroup.

Mediator	Subgroup	Stimulus	Organism	Response
Gender	Male	Performance expectancy; Effort expectancy; Social influence; Trust	Flow	Behavioral Intention
	Female	Performance expectancy; Hedonic motivation;	Flow	Perceived value; Behavioral Intention
Age	≤35	Performance expectancy; Social influence; Hedonic motivation; Trust	Flow	Perceived value; Behavioral Intention
	>35	Performance expectancy; Social influence; Trust	Flow	Perceived value; Behavioral Intention

The variables from the revised UTAUT2 model, as the stimulus in users' psychological processing, demonstrated variance in different sub-models. Specifically, except for performance expectancy, which had significant effects on flow in all subgroups, the other path effects of antecedences of flow presented differently in different subgroups. Effort expectancy only significantly affected flow in the male subgroup, contrary to the previous findings [45]. This study found that male customers' engagement and immersion were more determined regarding the understandability, accessibility and operability of LSSAs. On the other hand, effort expectancy had a positive influence on performance expectancy in all subgroups, which was consistent with previous findings that when customers perceive the ease of using LSSAs, they will feel using an LSSA is a useful and efficient way to shop online [26,43,79]. LSSA providers should maintain applications with easily understandable interfaces and functions to increase the accessibility of LSSAs.

Meanwhile, social influence had a significant effect on flow in all subgroups except for female customers, which was consistent with the findings of Liébana-Cabanillas, Sánchez-Fernández and Muñoz-Leiva [41], but contrary to the results of Pascual-Miguel, Agudo-Peregrina and Chaparro-Peláez's study [45]. The results of this study validated that female customers are more influenced with more difficulty by other relevant people when they purchase through LSSAs during the COVID-19 pandemic lockdown period. However, recommendations and support from relevant important people significantly formulate users' mental cognition in the male subgroup and both age subgroups, which means they would feel less anxiety and uncertainty if provided with the support of important, relevant people when using LSSAs during the pandemic lockdown period [25,80]. When customers' close friends or families are engaged in LSSAs, they are more inclined to participate and interact with sellers on LSSAs [16]. Therefore, word-of-mouth marketing is an efficient and reliable way to establish the excellent reputation of LSSAs, to increase male customers' engagement and to increase enjoyment when shopping via LSSAs during the pandemic lockdown period.

Moreover, hedonic motivation had more significant influences on the younger female group when they were shopping via LSSAs during the pandemic lockdown period. Therefore, the enjoyment of live-streaming content, as well as its entertainment features, are essential to optimize users' experience and increase engagement, especially for younger female customers. Furthermore, trust had a significant impact on flow in all age subgroups and the male group. Specifically, male customers paid more attention to the trustworthiness and security of LSSAs [44]. On the other hand, trust was an essential antecedent of flow in all age ranges, which was opposite to the findings of Liébana-Cabanillas, Sánchez-Fernández and Muñoz-Leiva (2014), where trust was more affected by younger groups [41]. Under the situation of social commerce lockdown, live-streaming production demonstration increased customers' perceived trust by providing reliable control, which positively influenced consumers' shopping experiences during the pandemic lockdown period [38]. Likewise, trust had a significant influence on performance expectancy in all subgroups. When users perceive a higher sense of trust in shopping via LSSAs under the pandemic lockdown measures, their holistic mental perceptions of the utility of technology will increase accordingly [80]. Therefore, information accuracy, information security and customers' privacy should be guaranteed by LSSA providers, especially for male customers [39].

Furthermore, flow, as an organism of users' psychological processing, had the most significant effects on perceived value and behavioral intention in all subgroup models, which is consistent with previous findings, which suggest that engagement and an immersive experience can significantly formulate users' mental and physical reactions to shopping via LSSAs during the pandemic lockdown period [16,38,39]. Specifically, flow as mediator in the proposed model performed diversely in each subgroup, the proportion of the variance for flow in gender subgroup model and age subgroup model being 0.70 and 0.58, respectively, which demonstrates the higher explanatory power in the model with the gender subgroup than the model with the age subgroup. Meanwhile, comparing the coefficients of flow with other variables between four subgroup models, flow has the most significant relations with effort expectancy, social influence, trust and behavioral intention in the male subgroup, while flow has the strongest relations with hedonic motivation and perceived value in the female group. Performance expectancy has the most significant effect on flow in the young age subgroup. The result indicates that functional and environmental factors affect young male customers' immersive experience more, while the entertainment factor influences female users' flow experience more. When customers are immersed in live-streaming shopping, they tend to escape from the pandemic situation and forget about time and problems, which irrelevant things do not easily disturb [10]. Therefore, optimizing customer engagement and interaction in live-streaming demonstrations is necessary to increase users' immersive shopping experiences via LSSAs in the pandemic lockdown situation [38].

In addition, in response components, perceived value significantly determined customers' behavioral intention regarding the use of LSSAs in all subgroups except male customers. When customers feel pleasure when purchasing through LSSAs during the pandemic lockdown period, they will perceive higher multi-dimensional benefits of LSSAs, including utilitarian, hedonic and social benefits, which in turn significantly determine customers' usage intention [16,50,59]. Male customers' holistic perceptions of the benefits of LSSAs might be indirectly influenced by their perceptions of technology [9]. Therefore, it is necessary to optimize the interfaces and functions of LSSA-services for improving the practicability, usability and creditability of LSSAs, to attract male customers' engagement. These methods can increase users' enjoyment, recognition and satisfaction when shopping through LSSAs, contributing towards formulating their actual usages.

7. Theoretical and Practical Implications

7.1. Theoretical Implications

As shopping via live-streaming is becoming an immensely popular social and commercial phenomenon, the factors determining customers' intentions regarding shopping via live-streaming apps have attracted increasing attention in recent years. Current research has demonstrated novel insights into explaining customers' psychological shopping processes via LSSAs during the COVID-19 pandemic lockdown period. This study contributes three theoretical implications. Firstly, this study bridges a gap in the existing literature by initially evaluating the moderating effects of gender and age on the determinants of customers' psychological processing in the use of LSSAs, which enriches the literature of relevant fields and verifies previous findings regarding the moderating effects of gender and age. Comparing the influences of different moderators, especially gender and age, on each path provides a better understanding of the effects of customers' demographic characteristics on LSSA adoption. Secondly, this study contributes to theoretical development by extending the SOR framework with UTAUT2 and Flow Theory. Notably, this study integrates the variables from the revised UTAUT2 model as the stimulus component of the SOR framework, and Flow Theory supports the organism in the SOR framework as a mediator of the adoption model. The comprehensive model was validated in this study to support the understanding of applying the SOR framework in the LSSA adoption context. Thirdly, the current study successfully explains that customers' psychological processes experienced while shopping via LSSAs under the pandemic lockdown condition are induced by perceived technological perceptions (performance expectancy, effort expectance, hedonic motivation) and environmental perceptions (social influence, trust), mediated by mental cognition (flow) and demonstrated by actual responses (perceived value and behavioral intention). This finding generates new insights for future research to assess various connections, interactions, and relationships among the variables between or within different components in the SOR framework for different technology adoption studies.

7.2. Practical Implications

This study's results are essential for LSSA-service providers, LSSA sellers, streamers and relevant stakeholders interested in the live-streaming commerce industry. The current study supports stakeholders relevant to LSSAs in understanding the behaviors of different customer demographics influenced by the moderating effects of gender and age. In particular, hedonic motivation, trust and social influence had the most significant differences in male and female groups. This study provides insights for LSSA stakeholders, encouraging them to consider gender differences affecting various antecedents at different stages of psychological processes experienced by customers while shopping via LSSAs, helping them to create or manage a better strategy for their target customers in the future. For example, LSSA providers and vendors should focus on maintaining a relaxing and comfortable live-streaming environment and guaranteeing the originality and fascination of the live-streaming context to optimize entertainment for attracting female customers.

Moreover, this study helps LSSA-platform providers, streamers and LSSA sellers, acting as a guidebook to understanding each component in the mental processes undergone by customer when using LSSAs for shopping during the pandemic lockdown period. Based on the findings, flow had both significant effects on perceived value and behavioral intention. LSSA-platform providers should emphasize user-centered principles to guarantee the reliability, convenience and efficiency of LSSA-services to meet customers' expectations and requirements, helping to formulate an immersive environment for customers to improve their engagement and optimize their mental cognition of shopping through LSSAs. Streamers and LSSA sellers should ensure entertainment, instantaneity and accuracy of interactions with customers to formulate a pleasant and enjoyable environment for optimizing their shopping experience when using LSSAs. Furthermore, the current research contributes a framework for the investigation of customers' mental processes under a specific environmental condition. This study proposed a critical procedure (technological and environmental perceptions → engagement and mental cognition → reaction) to evaluate customers' psychological processes. Meanwhile, the assessment and evaluation of the moderating effects of gender and age applied in this study provide a reference with which to analyze demographically different customers' behaviors. Relevant stakeholders can generate particular strategies for their different customers based on the variation of the moderating effects of gender and age on different determinants.

8. Conclusions

Shopping via live-streaming is booming after the lockdown measures of the COVID-19 pandemic. This study investigated the psychological processes undergone by customer shopping via LSSAs during the COVID-19 pandemic lockdown period in China. The proposed model extended the SOR framework with UTUAT2 and Flow Theory and was tested by CB-SEM with 374 valid data, with four subgroups divided by age and gender.

8.1. Result of the Study

The empirical results demonstrate that flow as a mediator had the most significant influence on users' responses. Technological and environmental perceptions significantly formulate customers' engagement and immersive experience, which determine their behaviors. This study validates that gender has significant moderating effects on effect expectancy, hedonic motivation, trust, social influence and perceived value. Specifically, effect expectancy, social influence and trust had significant effects on flow in the male group. On the other hand, hedonic motivation and perceived value were found to significantly affect female customers' psychological processes when shopping via LSSAs. Moreover, hedonic motivation has a more significant effect on flow in younger customers than in older customers.

The current research provides a better understanding of customers' psychological processes under a particular condition, namely, the COVID-19 lockdown situation. The current study contributes a theoretical development, helping to integrate psychological framework with technological adoption models, and provides a practical guideline on investigating the psychological processes experienced by customer who shopped via LSSAs under the pandemic lockdown situation. This helps by supporting relevant researchers and stakeholders in understanding customers' behaviors under a specific condition.

8.2. Limitations and Future Research

Although the current study proposed a rigorous framework of psychological processing on behalf of customers to adopt LSSAs, four limitations are summarized as follows with correspondent recommendations for future research. First, this study's target location was China, which indicates the limited generalizability of results in different cultures, regions and countries. Therefore, future researchers are recommended to pay more attention to investigating relevant studies in various regions and cultural backgrounds, as well as to make comparisons between locations with different cultures. Second, moderators analyzed in this study only consisted of the participants' basic demographic characteristics, namely, gender and age. Various moderators can contribute different moderating effects to different constructs in the model. Thus, future research is recommended to investigate users' behaviors under various moderating effects, such as experience, educational background, Hofstede's cultural values, etc. Third, this research did not distinguish the types of LSSAs in the study. The different types of LSSAs may lead to different results [6]. Consequently, future research is recommended to distinguish the differences between various technologies and platforms. Last, this study conducted a four-week data collection during the COVID-19 pandemic lockdown period, indicating the limitation of a short investigation period for generalizing an overall analysis in different scenarios. Thus, a long-term approach, as well as a comparison between customers' different stages of shopping experiences via LSSAs and under different situations might be several meritorious directions for future research.

Author Contributions: Conceptualization, Y.Z. and F.B.; methodology, Y.Z.; software, Y.Z.; validation, Y.Z.; formal analysis, Y.Z.; investigation, Y.Z.; resources, Y.Z.; data curation, Y.Z.; writing—original draft preparation, Y.Z.; writing—review and editing, Y.Z.; visualization, Y.Z.; supervision, F.B.; project administration, Y.Z. All authors have read and agreed to the published version of the manuscript.

Funding: This research received no external funding.

Institutional Review Board Statement: Not applicable.

Informed Consent Statement: Informed consent was obtained from all subjects involved in the study.

Data Availability Statement: Data available on request due to restrictions eg privacy or ethical.

Conflicts of Interest: The authors declare no conflict of interest.

Appendix A

Table A1. Online questionnaire.

Dear participant:

Thank you for taking a few minutes to participate in this questionnaire! The purpose of this questionnaire is to collect the factors of shopping via live-streaming shopping app. (i.e., Douyin app, Kuaishou app, Taobao live, etc.). The questionnaire is anonymous. The data obtained is only for academic research. Please feel free to fill in the questionnaire according to your personal situation.

Thank you for your support!

Part 1–Demographic Information	
Measure	**Item**
Gender	Male
	Female
Age	<20
	21–35
	36–50
	>51
Frequency of using LSSAs during lockdown period	At least 1 time per 1 day
	At least 1 time per 1 week
	At least 1 time per 2 weeks
	At least 1 time per 1 month
	At least 1 time per 3 months
	At least 1 time per 6 months
	Never used during lockdown period

Part 2–Structural Evaluation		
Construct	**Items**	**References**
Performance expectancy (PE)	PE1: I feel using LSSA is a useful way of shopping during lockdown period. PE2: Using LSSAs makes purchasing easier during lockdown period. PE3: Using LSSAs improves my shopping efficiency during lockdown period. PE4: Using LSSAs makes shopping more convenient during lockdown period.	[13]
Effort expectancy (EE)	EE1: Learning how to use LSSAs is easy. EE2: It is easy to follow all the functions of LSSAs. EE3: It is easy to become skillful at using LSSAs. EE4: Interaction with LSSAs is clear and comprehensible.	[13]
Social influence (SI)	SI1: People who are important to me (e.g., family members, close friends, and colleagues) recommend I use LSSAs for shopping during lockdown period. SI2: People who are important to me view LSSA as beneficial way for shopping during lockdown period. SI3: People who are important to me think it is a good idea to use LSSAs for shopping during lockdown period. SI4: People who are important to me support my use of LSSAs.	[13]
Hedonic motivation (HM)	HM1: Shopping via LSSAs is entertaining during lockdown period. HM2: Shopping via LSSAs relaxes me during lockdown period. HM3: Shopping via LSSAs gives me pleasure during lockdown period. HM4: Activities (e.g., flash sales, freebies) on LSSAs make me excited. HM5: I enjoy shopping via LSSAs during lockdown period.	[1,13]

Table A1. *Cont.*

Dear participant:
Thank you for taking a few minutes to participate in this questionnaire! The purpose of this questionnaire is to collect the factors of shopping via live-streaming shopping app. (i.e., Douyin app, Kuaishou app, Taobao live, etc.). The questionnaire is anonymous. The data obtained is only for academic research. Please feel free to fill in the questionnaire according to your personal situation.
Thank you for your support!

Part 2–Structural Evaluation		
Construct	Items	References
Trust (TR)	TR1: I believe LSSAs are competent and effective in handling customers' shopping activities. TR2: I believe LSSAs keep customers' interests in mind. TR3: I trust the product demonstration from high-reputation sellers on LSSAs. TR4: I believe that the products I purchase from LSSAs will be the same as those demonstrated on LSSAs. TR5: Overall, I believe LSSAs are trustworthy way for shopping during lockdown period.	[1,13]
Flow (FL)	FL1: When using LSSAs, my attention is focused on the shopping activities. FL2: When shopping via LSSAs, I do not realize how time passes. FL3: Using LSSAs gives me a temporary escape from the real-world pandemic situation. FL4: While shopping through LSSAs, I am able to forget my problems. FL5: When shopping via LSSAs, I often forget the work I should do.	[16,38]
Perceived value (PV)	PV1: Using LSSAs makes shopping more efficient and safer during lockdown period. PV2: Shopping via LSSAs would allow me to take advantage of additional promotions during live-streaming. PV3: Shopping via LSSAs provides me with a lot of enjoyment, or gives me happiness during lockdown period. PV4: Given the time I need to spend doing it during lockdown period, shopping via LSSAs is worthwhile to me.	[50]
Behavioral intention (BI)	BI1: Shopping via LSSAs had become one of consumption and entertainment patterns for me. BI2: Given the opportunity, I will continuously shop via LSSAs in future. BI3: I would like to recommend others to use LSSAs for shopping during lockdown period.	[13]

References

1. Wongkitrungrueng, A.; Assarut, N. The role of live streaming in building consumer trust and engagement with social commerce sellers. *J. Bus. Res.* **2018**, *117*, 543–556. [CrossRef]
2. Sun, Y.; Shao, X.; Li, X.; Guo, Y.; Nie, K. How live streaming influences purchase intentions in social commerce: An IT affordance perspective. *Electron. Commer. Res. Appl.* **2019**, *37*, 100886. [CrossRef]
3. iiMedia. Big Data Analysis and Trend Research Report of China's Live-Streaming E-Commerce Industry Operation in 2020–2021. 2020. Available online: https://www.iimedia.cn/c400/68945.html (accessed on 9 October 2021).
4. Taobangdan. 2019 Taobao Live Streaming Ecological Development Report. 2019. Available online: http://www.199it.com/archives/855530.html (accessed on 9 July 2021).
5. Cai, J.; Wohn, D.Y.; Mittal, A.; Sureshbabu, D. Utilitarian and hedonic motivations for live streaming shopping. In Proceedings of the 2018 ACM International Conference on Interactive Experiences for TV and Online Video, Seoul, Korea, 26–28 June 2018; pp. 81–88. [CrossRef]
6. Cai, J.; Wohn, D.Y. Live Streaming Commerce: Uses and Gratifications Approach to Understanding Consumers' Motivations. In Proceedings of the 52nd Hawaii International Conference on System Sciences, Maui, HI, USA, 8–11 January 2019. [CrossRef]
7. Wu, B. Research on Influencing Factors of Users' Continuance Intention toward Taobao Live Streaming. *E-Commer. Lett.* **2017**, *6*, 44–53. [CrossRef]
8. Yu, E.; Jung, C.; Kim, H.; Jung, J. Impact of viewer engagement on gift-giving in live video streaming. *Telemat. Inform.* **2018**, *35*, 1450–1460. [CrossRef]
9. Peng, C.; Kim, Y.G. Application of the Stimuli-Organism- Response (S-O-R) Framework to Online Shopping Behavior. *J. Internet Commer.* **2014**, *13*, 159–176. [CrossRef]

10. Hossain, M.S.; Zhou, X. Impact of m-payments on purchase intention and customer satisfaction: Perceived flow as mediator. *Int. J. Sci. Bus.* **2018**, *2*, 503–517. [CrossRef]
11. Wu, Y.; Li, E.Y. Marketing mix, customer value, and customer loyalty in social commerce: A stimulus-organism-response perspective. *Internet Res.* **2018**, *28*, 74–104. [CrossRef]
12. Kim, M.J.; Lee, C.; Jung, T. Exploring Consumer Behavior in Virtual Reality Tourism Using an Extended Stimulus-Organism-Response Model. *J. Travel Res.* **2020**, *59*, 9–89. [CrossRef]
13. Venkatesh, V.; Thong, J.Y.L.; Xu, X. Consumer acceptance and user of information technology: Extending the unified theory of acceptance and use of technology. *MIS* **2012**, *36*, 157–178.
14. Csikszentmihalyi, M. *Beyond Boredom and Anxiety: Experiencing Flow in Work and Play*; Jossey-Bass Publishers: San Francisco, CA, USA, 1975.
15. Sjöblom, M.; Hamari, J. Why do people watch others play video games? An empirical study on the motivations of Twitch users. *Comput. Hum. Behav.* **2017**, *75*, 985–996. [CrossRef]
16. Chen, C.C.; Lin, Y.C. What drives live-stream usage intention? The perspectives of flow, entertainment, social interaction, and endorsement. *Telemat. Inform.* **2018**, *35*, 293–303. [CrossRef]
17. Zhao, Q.; Chen, C.; Cheng, H.; Wang, J. Determinants of live streamers' continuance broadcasting intentions on Twitch: A self-determination theory perspective. *Telemat. Inform.* **2018**, *35*, 406–420. [CrossRef]
18. Lim, J.S.; Choe, M.; Zhang, J.; Noh, G. The role of wishful identification, emotional engagement, and parasocial relationships in repeated viewing of live-streaming games: A social cognitive theory perspective. *Comput. Hum. Behav.* **2020**, *108*, 106327. [CrossRef]
19. Ho, C.T.; Yang, C.H. A study on behavior intention to use live streaming video platform based on TAM model. In Proceedings of the Asian Conference on Psychology and Behavioral Sciences 2015, Osaka, Japan, 26–29 March 2015. [CrossRef]
20. Marinković, V.; Đorđević, A.; Kalinić, Z. The moderating effects of gender on customer satisfaction and continuance intention in mobile commerce: A UTAUT-based perspective. *Technol. Anal. Strateg. Manag.* **2020**, *32*, 306–318. [CrossRef]
21. Mehrabian, A.; Russell, J. *An Approach to Environmental Psychology*; MIT Press: Cambridge, UK, 1974.
22. Chen, C.; Yao, J. What drives impulse buying behaviors in a mobile auction? The perspective of the Stimulus-Organism-Response model. *Telemat. Inform.* **2018**, *35*, 1249–1262. [CrossRef]
23. Zhao, Y.; Wang, A.; Sun, Y. Technological environment, virtual experience and MOOC continuance: A stimulus—Organism—Response perspective. *Comput. Educ.* **2020**, *144*, 103721. [CrossRef]
24. Islam, J.U.; Rahman, Z. The impact of online brand community characteristics on customer engagement: An application of Stimulus-Organism-Response paradigm. *Telemat. Inform.* **2017**, *34*, 96–109. [CrossRef]
25. Slade, E.; Williams, M.; Dwivedi, Y.; Piercy, N. Exploring consumer adoption of proximity mobile payments. *J. Strateg. Mark.* **2015**, *23*, 209–223. [CrossRef]
26. Alalwan, A.A.; Dwivedi, Y.K.; Rana, N.P. Factors influencing adoption of mobile banking by Jordanian bank customers: Extending UTAUT2 with trust. *Int. J. Inf. Manag.* **2017**, *37*, 99–110. [CrossRef]
27. Morosan, C.; DeFranco, A. It's about time: Revisiting UTAUT2 to examine consumers' intentions to use NFC mobile payments in hotels. *Int. J. Hosp. Manag.* **2016**, *53*, 17–29. [CrossRef]
28. Baptista, G.; Oliveira, T. Understanding mobile banking: The unified theory of acceptance and use of technology combined with cultural moderators. *Comput. Hum. Behav.* **2015**, *50*, 418–430. [CrossRef]
29. Chopdar, P.K.; Sivakumar, V.J. Understanding continuance usage of mobile shopping applications in India: The role of espoused cultural values and perceived risk. *Behav. Inf. Technol.* **2019**, *38*, 42–64. [CrossRef]
30. Oliveira, T.; Thomas, M.; Baptista, G.; Campos, F. Mobile payment: Understanding the determinants of customer adoption and intention to recommend the technology. *Comput. Hum. Behav.* **2016**, *61*, 404–414. [CrossRef]
31. Tam, C.; Santos, D.; Oliveira, T. Exploring the influential factors of continuance intention to use mobile Apps: Extending the expectation confirmation model. *Inf. Syst. Front.* **2020**, *22*, 243–257. [CrossRef]
32. Zhao, Y.; Bacao, F. What factors determining customer continuingly using food delivery apps during 2019 novel coronavirus pandemic period? *Int. J. Hosp. Manag.* **2020**, *91*, 102683. [CrossRef] [PubMed]
33. Tak, P.; Panwar, S. Using UTAUT 2 Model to Predict Mobile App Based Shopping: Evidences from India. *J. Indian Bus. Res.* **2017**, *9*, 248–264. [CrossRef]
34. Webster, J.; Trevino, L.K.; Ryan, L. The dimensionality and correlates of flow in human-computer interactions. *Comput. Hum. Behav.* **1993**, *9*, 411–426. [CrossRef]
35. Csikszentmihalyi, M.; Csikszentmihalyi, I.S. *Optimal Experience: Psychological Studies of Flow in Consciousness*; Cambridge University Press: Cambridge, UK, 1988.
36. Hsu, C.L.; Lu, H.P. Why do people play online games? An extended TAM with social influences and flow experience. *Inf. Manag.* **2004**, *41*, 853–868. [CrossRef]
37. Zhou, T. An empirical examination of continuance intention of mobile payment services. *Decis. Support Syst.* **2013**, *54*, 1085–1091. [CrossRef]
38. Gao, L.; Waechter, K.A.; Bai, X. Understanding consumers' continuance intention towards mobile purchase: A theoretical framework and empirical study—A case of China. *Comput. Hum. Behav.* **2015**, *53*, 249–262. [CrossRef]

39. Kim, G.; Choe, D.; Lee, J.; Park, S.; Jun, S.; Jang, D. The Technology Acceptance Model for Playing Console Game in Korea. *Int. J. Comput. Sci. Netw. Secur.* **2013**, *13*, 9–12.
40. Venkatesh, V.; Zhang, X. Unified theory of acceptance and use of technology: U.S. vs. China. *J. Glob. Inf. Technol. Manag.* **2010**, *13*, 5–27. [CrossRef]
41. Liébana-Cabanillas, F.; Sánchez-Fernández, J.; Muñoz-Leiva, F. Antecedents of the adoption of the new mobile payment systems: The moderating effect of age. *Comput. Hum. Behav.* **2014**, *35*, 464–478. [CrossRef]
42. Khalilzadeh, J.; Ozturk, A.B.; Bilgihan, A. Security-related factors in extended UTAUT model for NFC based mobile payment in the restaurant industry. *Comput. Hum. Behav.* **2017**, *70*, 460–474. [CrossRef]
43. Riskinanto, A.; Kelana, B.; Hilmawan, D.R. The Moderation Effect of Age on Adopting E-Payment Technology. *Comput. Sci.* **2017**, *124*, 536–543. [CrossRef]
44. Shao, Z.; Zhang, L.; Li, X.; Guo, Y. Antecedents of Trust and Continuance Intention in Mobile Payment Platforms: The Moderating Effect of Gender. *Electron. Commer. Res. Appl.* **2018**, *33*, 100823. [CrossRef]
45. Pascual-Miguel, F.J.; Agudo-Peregrina, Á.F.; Chaparro-Peláez, J. Influences of gender and product type on online purchasing. *J. Bus. Res.* **2015**, *68*, 1550–1556. [CrossRef]
46. Gu, J.C.; Lee, S.C.; Suh, Y.H. Determinants of behavioral intention to mobile banking. *Expert Syst. Appl.* **2009**, *36*, 11605–11616. [CrossRef]
47. Di Pietro, L.; Guglielmetti Mugion, R.; Mattia, G.; Renzi, M.F.; Toni, M. The Integrated Model on Mobile Payment Acceptance (IMMPA): An empirical application to public transport. *Transp. Res. Part C Emerg. Technol.* **2015**, *56*, 463–479. [CrossRef]
48. Suh, B.; Han, I. Effect of trust on customer acceptance of Internet banking. *Electron. Commer. Res. Appl.* **2002**, *1*, 247–263. [CrossRef]
49. Yuan, S.; Liu, Y.; Yao, R.; Liu, J. An investigation of users' continuance intention towards mobile banking in China. *Inf. Dev.* **2016**, *32*, 20–34. [CrossRef]
50. Kerviler, G.; Demoulin, N.T.M.; Zidda, P. Adoption of in-store mobile payment: Are perceived risk and convenience the only drivers? *J. Retail. Consum. Serv.* **2016**, *31*, 334–344. [CrossRef]
51. Yeo, V.C.S.; Goh, S.K.; Rezaei, S. Consumer experiences, attitude and behavioral intention toward online food delivery (OFD) services. *J. Retail. Consum. Serv.* **2017**, *35*, 150–162. [CrossRef]
52. Ghani, J.A.; Deshpande, S.P. Task characteristics and the experience of optimal flow in human-computer interaction. *J. Psychol.* **1994**, *128*, 381–391. [CrossRef]
53. Moon, J.W.; Kim, Y.G. Extending the TAM for the world wide web context. *Inf. Manag.* **2001**, *38*, 217–230. [CrossRef]
54. Gefen, D. E-commerce: The role of familiarity and trust. *Omega* **2000**, *28*, 725–737. [CrossRef]
55. Hung, S.Y.; Tsai, J.C.; Chou, S.T. Decomposing perceived playfulness: A contextual examination of two social networking sites. *Inf. Manag.* **2016**, *53*, 698–716. [CrossRef]
56. Zeithaml, V.A. Consumer Perceptions of Price, Quality and Value: A Means-End Model and Synthesis of Evidence. *J. Mark.* **1988**, *52*, 2–22. [CrossRef]
57. Sweeney, J.C.; Soutar, G.N. Customer perceived value: The development of a multiple item scale. *J. Retail.* **2001**, *77*, 203–220. [CrossRef]
58. Petrick, J.F. Development of a multi-dimensional scale for measuring the perceived value of a service. *J. Leis. Res.* **2002**, *34*, 119–134. [CrossRef]
59. Kim, Y.H.; Kim, D.J.; Wachter, K. A study of mobile user engagement (MoEN): Engagement motivations, perceived value, satisfaction, and continued engagement intention. *Decis. Support Syst.* **2013**, *56*, 361–370. [CrossRef]
60. Kim, H.; Chan, H.C.; Gupta, S. Value-based Adoption of Mobile Internet: An empirical investigation. *Decis. Support Syst.* **2007**, *43*, 111–126. [CrossRef]
61. Lynn, P. The problem of non-respons. In *International Handbook of Survey Methodology*; De Leeuw, E.D., Hox, J., Dillman, D., Eds.; Erlbaum: Mahwah, NJ, USA, 2008; Chapter 3; pp. 35–55.
62. Westland, J.C. Lower Bounds on Sample Size in Structural Equation Modeling. *Electron. Commer. Res. Appl.* **2010**, *9*, 476–487. [CrossRef]
63. Ryans, A.B. Estimating consumer preferences for a new durable brand in an established product class. *J. Mark. Res.* **1974**, *11*, 434–443. [CrossRef]
64. QusetMobile. 2020 Double 11 E-Commerce Insight. 2020. Available online: https://www.questmobile.com.cn/research/report-new/132 (accessed on 20 December 2020).
65. Hair, J.F.; Gabriel, M.L.D.S.; Patel, V.K. AMOS Covariance-Based Structural Equation Modeling (CB-SEM): Guidelines on its Application as a Marketing Research Tool. *Braz. J. Mark.* **2014**, *13*, 44–55.
66. Hair, J.F.; Black, W.C.; Babin, B.J.; Anderson, R.E. *Multivariate Data Analysis*, 7th ed.; Prentice-Hall, Inc.: Upper Saddle River, NJ, USA, 2010.
67. Bagozzi, R.; Yi, Y. Specification, evaluation, and interpretation of structural equation models. *J. Acad. Mark. Sci.* **2012**, *40*, 8–34. [CrossRef]
68. Goodhue, D.L.; Lewis, W.; Thompson, R. Does PLS Have Advantages for Small Sample Size or Non-Normal Data? *MIS Q.* **2012**, *36*, 981–1001. [CrossRef]

69. Jannoo, Z.; Yap, B.W.; Auchoybur, N.; Lazim, M.A. The Effect of Nonnormality on CB-SEM and PLS-SEM Path Estimates. *Int. Sch. Sci. Res. Innov.* **2014**, *8*, 285–291.
70. Gefen, D.; Straub, D.; Boudreau, M.-C. Structural Equation Modeling and Regression: Guidelines for Research Practice. *Commun. Assoc. Inf. Syst.* **2000**, *4*, 7. [CrossRef]
71. Anderson, J.C.; Gerbing, D.W. Structural equation modeling in practice: A review and recommended two-step approach. *Psychol. Bull.* **1988**, *103*, 411–423. [CrossRef]
72. Cattell, R.B. The scree test for the number of factors. *Multivariate Behav. Res.* **1966**, *1*, 245–276. [CrossRef] [PubMed]
73. Nunnally, J.C.; Bernstein, I.H. The assessment of reliability. *Psychom. Theory* **1994**, *3*, 248–292.
74. Henseler, J.; Ringle, C.M.; Sarstedt, M. A new criterion for assessing discriminant validity in variance-based structural equation modeling. *J. Acad. Mark. Sci.* **2014**, *43*, 115–135. [CrossRef]
75. Fornell, C.G.; Larcker, D.F. Evaluating structural equation models with unobservable variables and measurement error. *J. Mark. Res.* **1981**, *18*, 39–50. [CrossRef]
76. Doll, W.; Xia, W.; Torkzadeh, G. A Confirmatory Factor Analysis of the End-User Computing Satisfaction Instrument. *MIS Q.* **1994**, *18*, 453–461. [CrossRef]
77. Bollen, K.A. *Structural Equations with Latent Variables*; Wiley: New York, NY, USA, 1989.
78. Podsakoff, P.M.; MacKenzie, S.B.; Lee, J.Y.; Podsakoff, N.P. Common method biases in behavioral research: A critical review of the literature and recommended remedies. *J. Appl. Psychol.* **2003**, *88*, 879–903. [CrossRef]
79. de Luna, I.R.; Liébana-Cabanillas, F.; Sánchez-Fernández, J.; Muñoz-Leiva, F. Mobile payment is not all the same: The adoption of mobile payment systems depending on the technology applied. *Technol. Forecast. Soc. Chang.* **2018**, *146*, 931–944. [CrossRef]
80. Park, J.; Ahn, J.; Thavisaya, T.; Ren, T. Examining the role of anxiety and social influence in multi-benefits of mobile payment service. *J. Retail. Consum. Serv.* **2018**, *47*, 140–149. [CrossRef]

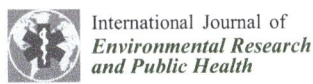

Article

Facilitators and Reducers of Korean Travelers' Avoidance/Hesitation Behaviors toward China in the Case of COVID-19

Heesup Han [1], Chen Che [2] and Sanghyeop Lee [3,*]

1. College of Hospitality and Tourism Management, Sejong University, Seoul 143-747, Korea; heesup.han@gmail.com
2. College of History and Tourism Culture, Inner Mongolia University, Hohhot 010021, China; cecencan@naver.com
3. Major in Tourism Management, College of Business Administration, Keimyung University, Daegu 42601, Korea
* Correspondence: leesanghyeop@kmu.ac.kr

Abstract: Given that little is known about overseas travelers' responses and behaviors toward China after the outbreak of COVID-19, this study aimed to uncover risk perception factors and investigate its role in Korean travelers' avoidance/hesitation behaviors toward China as an international tourism destination in the case of the COVID-19 pandemic. To explore the relationship with risk perception, anticipated emotion and avoidance/hesitation behavior, a quantitative method along with an online survey was employed. This focus was on Korean tourists who had traveled to China at least once. Findings revealed that risk perception and negative anticipated emotion are vital facilitators of avoidance/hesitation behaviors, and that positive anticipated emotion reduces such behaviors. The efficacy of a higher-order structure of risk perception, which encompasses six dimensions, was also demonstrated. In addition, destination attachment lowered the influence of risk perception on the formation of avoidance/hesitation behaviors. Overall, our results will help tourism researchers and practitioners understand what factors drive and reduce international travelers' avoidance/hesitation behaviors toward China in the post-pandemic world. Implications for theory and practice are offered.

Keywords: risk perception; China as an international tourism destination; anticipated emotions; destination attachment; post-pandemic

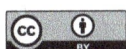

1. Introduction

The impact of a coronavirus diseases 19 (COVID-19) on the entire world is substantial [1–3]. The pathogenic influence of COVID-19 has been drastically increased since China reported the first confirmed case in late 2019 [4,5]. This virus fast became a huge threat to human health [6]. Moreover, ever since the detection of the COVID-19, this disease has considerably affected human mobility [7]. COVID-19 had a huge adverse effect on the tourism sector [1,8]. Particularly, the international tourism industry has been massively reduced due to border closing, lockdowns, and bans on traveling [3,5]. The COVID-19 characteristics of high prevalence, broad distribution, and geographical variables made this situation worse for the tourism industry [3,4,7].

Until 11 November 2021, the World Health Organization (WHO) reported that there had been 25.127 million confirmed cases of COVID-19 in the world, including 0.507 million deaths [9]. In China, there have been 3283 confirmed cases of COVID-19 [10]. Most overseas travelers have inevitably restrained themselves from visiting international tourism destinations until the pandemic is entirely under control [1,8]. COVID-19 has also blocked international tourists' visit to China. The global concern for human health derived from the pandemic significantly reduced international tourism demand throughout the world. According to Chen et al. [11], there is a high possibility that another new type of coronavirus will emerge in the future because of rapid climate change, ecological problems, fast-increasing flows of human populations, and increase in human–animal interactions. Indeed, many countries are shifting to the with-corona era.

Irrefutably, there exists a critical association between COVID-19 and tourist responses/behavior [7,8]. Yet scant research has uncovered the possible influence of perceived risk pertinent to the disease on overseas travelers' anticipated emotions and avoidance responses to traveling to China. Especially, very little is known about Korean international travelers' responses and behaviors toward traveling to China since the emergence of COVID-19. For Korean travelers, China is one of the preferred destination countries. Indeed, the statistics of the Korea Tourism Organization [12] showed that about 4,346,567 Koreans visited China in 2019 before the outbreak of the pandemic. They traveled to China for diverse purposes (wellness, sightseeing, reputation/image of local destinations, low price, shopping, leisure, and foods) [12]. Undoubtedly, the image and popularity of China as a tourism destination has been considerably influenced by COVID-19. Exploring Korean international tourists' perception of traveling to China in the post-pandemic world is vital to better understand their emotional tendencies and behaviors.

The objectives of this study were therefore to identify Korean travelers' perception regarding possible risks of traveling to China in the post-pandemic world and to explore the influence of such risk perception and its dimensions (i.e., human crowding risk, spatial crowding risk, quality risk, psychological risk, health and safety risk, and financial risk) on the formation of avoidance/hesitation behaviors. In addition, this research aimed to uncover the efficacy of a higher-order structure of risk perception. Moreover, this study was designed to unearth the moderating impact of destination attachment and to investigate the mediating effect of positive and negative anticipated emotions. Lastly, this research assessed the impact of Korean travelers' avoidance/hesitation behaviors in the COVID-19 era.

2. Literature Review

2.1. Risk Perception and Its Role

The criticality of risk perception has long been emphasized in various sectors due to its considerable influence on individuals' behaviors [13–15]. Particularly in the hospitality/tourism literature, risk perception and its importance are extensively stressed [13,16,17]. Undoubtedly, risk perception that has multiple dimensional characteristics is the major constituent of traveler approach/avoidance decision formation [17,18]. The vital facet of risk perception in tourism as well as in consumer behavior and psychology is uncertainty and an individual's apprehension of it [15,19]. Such uncertainty is negatively linked to anticipated responses from individuals [19]. The critical aspects of risk perception in an unsafe consumption environment (e.g., the pandemic world) can be crowding risk (human and spatial), quality risk, psychological risk, health and safety risk, and financial risk [15,16,18,20]. Given this, the concept of risk perception in the present research indicates travelers' uncertainty about tourism-destination performances and their cognitive anxiety regarding the disparity between such performances and travelers' expectations.

An extensive amount of the extant literature has assessed the possible effect of risk perception on individuals' approach/avoidance responses and behaviors [14,17,21]. Olya and Altinay [22] explored how risk perception influences traveler post-purchase behaviors either in a positive or negative way. In their investigation on international travelers' behaviors, Al-Ansi et al. [13] found risk perception as a vital contributor to behavioral intention generation. More interesting in this research is how to manage consumers' perceived risk to improve their satisfaction and trust. Law [23] examined travelers' decision formation for overseas destination choices when there is any probability of the occurrences of virus infection, terrorist attack, and natural disasters. He found that ones' international tourism decision is significantly affected by risk perception level. Scholars in recent research have also revealed that risks related to crowdedness, quality/performance, mental health/personal psychology, physical health/safety, and money are of importance as such risks elicit positive and negative emotional evaluations and avoidance/hesitation behaviors [16,17,20]. Olya and Al-Anish [16] examined how health risk, quality risk, and psychological risk positively influence tourist satisfaction, and financial risk significantly affected tourist behavioral intention. Yu et al. [17] point out the risk perception (psychological and financial risk) of COVID-19, which strongly negatively influences tourist behavioral intention. The studies discussed above support the possible linkages among risk perception, anticipated emotional responses, and avoidance/hesitation behaviors. In addition, the finding of a recent study evidenced the efficacy of a second-order structure of risk perception in the tourism context [13]. Therefore, we developed hypotheses as follows:

Hypothesis 1 (H1). *Risk perception has a significant influence on positive anticipated emotion.*

Hypothesis 2 (H2). *Risk perception has a significant influence on negative anticipated emotion.*

Hypothesis 3 (H3). *Risk perception has a significant influence on avoidance/hesitation behavior.*

2.2. Anticipated Emotions

For the last few decades, anticipated emotions have been an important concept in customer behavior and tourism [24,25]. Anticipated emotions are described as anticipated affective process. Perugini and Bagozzi [26] indicate the prospect of feeling favorable or unfavorable affects when conducting or not conducting a particular action [27]. This conceptualization is in line with Han [28] who described these anticipated emotions are one's expected positive/negative feelings after performing or not performing a specific action. In general, researchers agree that anticipated emotions have two dimensions (positive and negative) [28–30]. These positive and negative forms of anticipated affective responses are believed to be important determinants of consumer behaviors [25].

There has been a significant improvement in extant socio-psychological theories/models of anticipated emotion, such as the theory of planned behavior, norm activation theory, and the value-belief-norm model [24,26,30]. Rosenthal and Ho [24] found that personal norms have a mediating effect on anticipated negative emotions and awareness of consequences. According to their two studies, Perugini and Bagozzi [26] demonstrated that anticipated emotions are an essential factor of desire. Lu et al. [30] distinguish anticipated guilt and anticipated pride in analyzing employees' pro-environment behavior. Indeed, theoretical/conceptual frameworks encompassing positive and negative forms of anticipated emotion, which were designed for self-interest/pro-social consumer behaviors, have benefited from the increase in prediction power for consumer approach/avoidance responses and behaviors [26,28]. The inclusion of positive and negative anticipated emotions often increases the ability of a theoretical model in explicating individuals' behaviors in a product-purchase or consumption situation [29,31]. Findings of the existing studies in the extant literature have also revealed that positive and negative anticipated emotions play a crucial role in inducing avoidance or approach behaviors for products/services [24,31]. Therefore, we developed hypotheses as follows:

Hypothesis 4 (H4). *Positive anticipated emotion has a significant influence on avoidance/hesitation behavior.*

Hypothesis 5 (H5). *Negative anticipated emotion has a significant influence on avoidance/hesitation behavior.*

2.3. Destination Attachment

Destination attachment has received increasing attention from tourism marketers and academics since it contributes considerably to enhancing travelers' favorable decisions/behaviors regarding a tourism destination (retention, loyalty behaviors, protection behaviors, word-of-mouth, sustainable actions at a destination) [24,32–34]. Destination attachment is a concept that describes the emotional tie between visitors and place [35]. Similarly, Rosenthal and Ho [24] described destination attachment as an affective bond between the place and its visitors. This concept is often an alternative for terms such as sense of belonging and involvement [28].

Sohn and Yoon [36] identified five characteristics of risk perception (social, physical, financial, health and psychological risk). They argued that destination attachment had a moderate influence on risk perception (physical and health) and destination image. Pangaribuan et al. [37] demonstrated that risk perception had a moderate effect on destination attachment and voluntary behavior. In general, risk perception is important for tourist avoidance/hesitation behavior [38]. According to Pradhananga and Davenport [34] and Fournier and Lee [32], a traveler with a strong attachment to a certain destination will more actively practice loyalty and citizenship behaviors regarding that destination (e.g., volunteering, repeat visit, recommendation). Indeed, when visitors' level of destination attachment is high, they are likely to show positive emotional responses, feel involvement, and show approach behaviors towards the destination [28,32,34,35]. Undoubtedly, destination attachment is a significant contributor influencing the formation of emotional reactions and behavioral responses [24]. The contributing role of attachment/involvement as a moderator is evident in consumer behavior and tourism [32,33]. Accordingly, the following hypotheses were developed:

Hypothesis 6a (H6a). *Destination attachment has a moderating influence on relation between risk perception and positive anticipated emotion.*

Hypothesis 6b (H6b). *Destination attachment has a moderating influence on relation between risk perception and negative anticipated emotion.*

Hypothesis 6c (H6c). *Destination attachment has a moderating influence on relation between risk perception and avoidance/hesitation behavior.*

2.4. Theoretical Model

The research model is exhibited in Figure 1. Our proposed framework contains risk perception and anticipated emotions (positive and negative) as predictors of traveler avoidance/hesitation behaviors and encompasses destination attachment as a moderator. Human crowding risk, spatial crowding risk, quality risk, psychology risk, health and safety risk, and financial risk are incorporated as the first-order factors of risk perception. In addition, the model includes six research hypotheses within its theoretical framework.

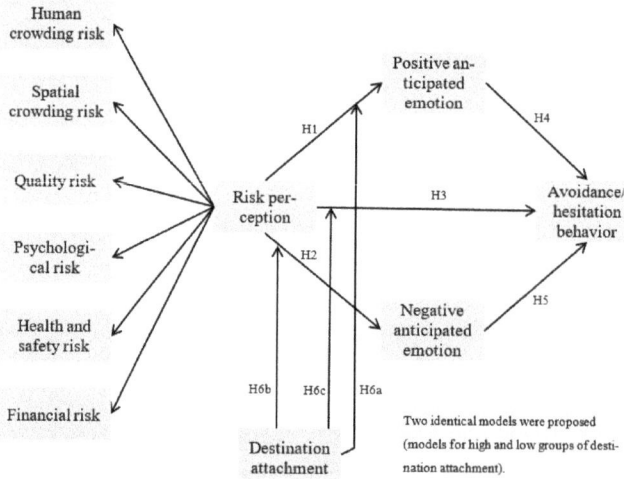

Figure 1. The proposed model.

3. Methods

3.1. Measurement Development

The measures of risk perception and its dimensions are generated based on a thorough review of the literature [13,15,39–41]. Additionally, several measurement items were added on the basis of qualitative interviews (i.e., "The flow of people in the tourist areas of China is slow because of too many people", "Hotels/restaurants/shopping places are in general not spacious enough", "I am worried that the quality of tourism products in China will be lower after the COVID-19 pandemic ends in the near future", and "The thought of traveling to China causes me to experience unnecessary tension although the COVID-19 pandemic may end in the near future"). The person-to-person interviews were conducted with actual Korean travelers who often visited China for international tourism before the outbreak of the pandemic. Overall, three items were utilized to measure human crowding risk (i.e., "Too many people are in tourist sites in China", "Because of the huge number of tourists, visitors feel crowded in many tourist sites in China", "The flow of people in the tourist areas of China is slow because of too many people"), and three items were employed to assess spatial crowding risk (i.e., Because of spatial crowdedness, visitors often feel stuffy in many tourist sites in China", "Due to little space, moving around is not easy in many of the tourist sites of China", "Hotels/restaurants/shopping places are in general not spacious enough". Additionally, two items and three items were utilized to measure quality risk (i.e., "I am concerned with the lower quality of tourism products in China after the COVID-19 pandemic ends in the near future", "I am worried that the quality of tourism products in China will become lower after the COVID-19 pandemic ends in the near future". and psychological risk (i.e., "The thought of traveling to China makes me feel anxious although the COVID-19 pandemic may end in the near future.", "The thought of traveling to China makes me feel psychologically uncomfortable although the COVID-19 pandemic may end in the near future", "The thought of traveling to China causes me to experience unnecessary tension although the COVID-19 pandemic may end in the near future"), respectively. Health and safety risk (i.e., "Traveling to China, although the COVID-19 pandemic may end in the near future, is still unsafe", "Traveling to China, although the COVID-19 pandemic may end in the near future, is still unhealthy", "Traveling to China, although the COVID-19 pandemic may end in the near future, is still risky") and financial risk (i.e., "I am afraid there will be considerable extra expenses in many tourist sites in China after the COVID-19 pandemic ends in the near future", "I worry that visiting China will involve unexpected extra expenses after the COVID-19 pandemic ends in the near future") were measured with three items and two items, respectively.

The measures for other constructs were taken from the existing studies [26,31,32,42,43]. Specifically, destination attachment was assessed with three items. Four items were used to measure positive anticipated emotions whereas three items were used to evaluate negative anticipated emotions. Moreover, avoidance/hesitation behavior was measured with five items. That is, multiple measures with a seven-point Likert-scale for all constructs were used in the present research.

3.2. Data Collection Procedure and Sample Characteristics

To test the proposed hypothesized framework, this study employed a Web-based survey method. Using an online market research firm's system, the survey link was generated. Afterwards, using social media (e.g., kakaotalk, Instagram), this was frequently used by Korean people to send this link to potential survey participants who had traveled to China at least once. Before sending the questionnaire link, respondents were asked about their willingness to participate and their experience of visiting China. The qualified survey participants were asked to read thoroughly the study description and questions when filling out the questionnaire. To complete this survey, the participants had to answer all inquiries in the questionnaire. A total of 450 survey questionnaires was collected. Among them 429 usable responses were gathered through this process. These cases were used for data analysis.

Among 429 survey participants, 50.6% were male travelers whereas 49.4% were female travelers. The participants' age fell between 20–73 years old with a mean age of 40.1 years. Specifically, about 23.3% were less than 29 years old; 25.6% were between 30–39 years old; 24.7% were between 40–49 years old; and 26.3% were above 50 years old. About 94.6% of the participants reported that they had visited China within the last three years. All respondents had visited to China within the last 5 years. Regarding education level, 69.2% were college graduates, followed by graduate-degree holders (16.8%), high-school graduates (9.3%), and others (4.7%). About 56.9% of the survey participants reported that they were married whereas 43.1% reported other forms of marital status. In terms of annual income level, about 38.9% indicated an income between 30,000–50,000 USD, followed by less than 30,000 USD (28.0%), 50,000–80,000 USD (23.3%), and over 80,000 USD (9.8%).

4. Results

4.1. Reliability and Validity Assessment

A confirmatory factor analysis was performed to create a measurement model. The model assessment revealed that a satisfactory model fit (χ^2 = 969.977, df = 387, p < 0.001, χ^2/df = 2.506, RMSEA = 0.059, CFI = 0.963, IFI = 0.963, TLI = 0.956). All items were loaded to their relevant latent factor in a significant manner (p < 0.01). As shown in Table 1, all composite reliability values (human crowding = 0.925; spatial crowding = 0.831; quality risk = 0.955; psychological risk = 0.946; health and safety risk = 0.959; financial risk = 0.914; positive anticipated emotion = 0.957; negative anticipated emotion = 0.885; destination attachment = 0.969; and avoidance/hesitation behavior = 0.967) exceeded the suggested threshold of 0.70 [44]. This result evidenced internal consistency of the multiple-item measures. Average variance extracted values were calculated. All values (human crowding = 0.804; spatial crowding = 0.622; quality risk = 0.913; psychological risk = 0.853; health and safety risk = 0.886; financial risk = 0.841; positive anticipated emotion = 0.846; negative anticipated emotion = 0.720; destination attachment = 0.913; and avoidance/hesitation behavior = 0.853) exceeded the recommended threshold of 0.50 [44]. In addition, the values were greater than between-construct correlations (squared), as evidenced in Table 1. This evidenced the convergent and discriminant validity of the multiple-construct measures.

4.2. Structural Model Assessment and Hypothesis Testing

A structural equation modeling was conducted with the use of Maximum likelihood estimation (see Table 2). The result demonstrated a satisfactory model fit (χ^2 = 1079.063, df = 337, p < 0.001, χ^2/df = 3.202, RMSEA = 0.072, CFI = 0.946, IFI = 0.946, TLI = 0.939) (see Figure 2). The second-order model for risk perception indicates that the global higher-order factor is significantly related to the six first-order variables (human crowding, spatial crowding, quality risk, psychological risk, health and safety risk, and financial risk). The coefficients were 0.419 (p < 0.01) for human crowding risk, 0.457 (p < 0.01) for spatial crowding risk, 0.405 (p < 0.01) for quality risk, 0.961 (p < 0.01) for psychological risk, 0.987 (p < 0.01) for health and safety risk, and 0.531 (p < 0.01) for financial risk, respectively. The higher-order latent variable accounted for about 17.6%, 20.9%, 16.4%, 92.4%, 97.5%, and 28.2% of the total variance for human crowding, spatial crowding, quality risk, psychological risk, health and safety risk, and financial risk, respectively. This evidenced the adequacy and effectiveness of the higher-order structure of risk perception within the proposed theoretical framework.

Table 1. Measurement model and data quality assessment results (n = 429).

Constructs	(1)	(2)	(3)	(4)	(5)	(6)	(7)	(8)	(9)	(10)
(1) Human crowding risk	1.000	–	–	–	–	–	–	–	–	–
(2) Spatial crowding risk	0.523 [a] (0.274) [b]	1.000	–	–	–	–	–	–	–	–
(3) Quality risk	0.223 (0.050)	0.363 (0.132)	1.000	–	–	–	–	–	–	–
(4) Psychological risk	0.403 (0.162)	0.412 (0.170)	0.380 (0.144)	1.000	–	–	–	–	–	–
(5) Health and safety risk	0.378 (0.143)	0.431 (0.186)	0.375 (0.141)	0.905 (0.819)	1.000	–	–	–	–	–
(6) Financial risk	0.235 (0.055)	0.375 (0.141)	0.415 (0.172)	0.456 (0.208)	0.501 (0.251)	1.000	–	–	–	–
(7) Positive anticipated emotion	−0.269 (0.072)	−0.246 (0.061)	−0.145 (0.021)	−0.564 (0.318)	−0.569 (0.324)	−0.217 (0.047)	1.000	–	–	–
(8) Negative anticipated emotion	0.159 (0.025)	0.251 (0.063)	0.209 (0.044)	0.528 (0.279)	0.573 (0.328)	0.336 (0.113)	−0.649 (0.421)	1.000	–	–
(9) Destination attachment	−0.262 (0.069)	−0.207 (0.043)	−0.080 (0.006)	−0.533 (0.284)	−0.532 (0.283)	−0.180 (0.032)	0.743 (0.552)	−0.482 (0.232)	1.000	–
(10) Avoidance/Hesitation behavior	0.363 (0.132)	0.338 (0.114)	0.238 (0.057)	0.751 (0.564)	0.780 (0.608)	0.317 (0.100)	−0.674 (0.454)	0.642 (0.412)	−0.631 (0.398)	1.000
Mean	5.664	5.117	4.622	5.677	5.601	4.944	3.385	4.759	3.045	5.509
Standard deviation	1.147	1.170	1.624	1.269	1.290	1.423	1.539	1.383	1.603	1.367
CR	0.925	0.831	0.955	0.946	0.959	0.914	0.957	0.885	0.969	0.967
AVE	0.804	0.622	0.913	0.853	0.886	0.841	0.846	0.720	0.913	0.853

Note1: [a] Correlations between variables are below the diagonal. Note2: [b] Squared correlations between variables are within parentheses.
Note3: Goodness-of-fit statistics: χ^2 = 969.977, df = 387, $p < 0.001$, χ^2/df = 2.506, RMSEA = 0.059, CFI = 0.963, IFI = 0.963, TLI = 0.956.

The hypothesized influence of risk perception on anticipated emotions and avoidance/hesitation behavior was tested. Our findings showed that risk perception exerted a significant influence on positive anticipated emotion (β = −0.614, $p < 0.01$) and negative anticipated emotion (β = 0.635, $p < 0.01$). Additionally, risk perception affected avoidance/hesitation behavior significantly (β = 0.555, $p < 0.01$). Hypotheses 1, 2, and 3 were hence supported. The proposed effect of anticipated emotions was assessed. Results revealed that both positive anticipated emotion (β = −0.237, $p < 0.01$) and negative anticipated emotion (β = 0.202, $p < 0.01$) had a significant impact on avoidance/hesitation behavior. Therefore, Hypotheses 4 and 5 were supported. About 37.8% and 40.3% of the variance in positive and negative anticipated emotions were accounted for by risk perception. In addition, these variables explained 74.5% of the total variance in avoidance/hesitation behavior. A close examination of indirect relationship showed that risk perception contained a significant indirect influence on avoidance/hesitation behavior through positive and negative anticipated emotions (β = 0.274, $p < 0.01$). The total impact of risk perception on avoidance/hesitation behavior (β = 0.828, $p < 0.01$) was the greatest among study variables. Overall, these results indicate that risk perception (e.g., human crowding risk, spatial crowding risk, quality risk, psychological risk, health and safety risk, financial risk) has a positive relationship with anticipated emotions (positive and negative anticipated emotion) and avoidance/hesitation behavior.

Table 2. Structural equation modeling results and hypothesis testing ($n = 429$).

	Hypothesized Paths			Standardized Estimates	t-Values
H1	Risk perception	→	Positive anticipated emotion	−0.614 **	−7.430
H2	Risk perception	→	Negative anticipated emotion	0.635 **	7.327
H3	Risk perception	→	Avoidance/hesitation behavior	0.555 **	7.253
H4	Positive anticipated emotion	→	Avoidance/hesitation behavior	−0.237 **	−5.659
H5	Negative anticipated emotion	→	Avoidance/hesitation behavior	0.202 **	4.494
	Risk perception	→	Human crowding risk	0.419 **	-
	Risk perception	→	Spatial crowding risk	0.457 **	6.198
	Risk perception	→	Quality risk	0.405 **	6.145
	Risk perception	→	Psychological risk	0.961 **	8.451
	Risk perception	→	Health and safety risk	0.987 **	8.463
	Risk perception	→	Financial risk	0.531 **	6.861
Total Variance Explained:			**Indirect Impact on Retention:**	**Total Impact on RI:**	
R^2 for avoidance/hesitation behavior = 0.745 R^2 for positive anticipated emotion = 0.378 R^2 for negative anticipated emotion = 0.403 R^2 for human crowding risk = 0.176 R^2 for spatial crowding risk = 0.209 R^2 for quality risk = 0.164 R^2 for psychological risk = 0.924 R^2 for health and safety risk = 0.975 R^2 for financial risk = 0.282			$\beta_{\text{risk perception} \rightarrow \text{positive \& negative anticipated emotions}}$ $\rightarrow$ avoidance/hesitation behavior $= 0.274$ **	$\beta_{\text{risk perception}} = 0.828$ ** $\beta_{\text{positive anticipated emotion}} = -0.237$ ** $\beta_{\text{negative anticipated emotion}} = 0.202$ **	

Note1. Goodness-of-fit statistics for the structural model (higher-order framework): $\chi^2 = 1079.063$, $df = 337$, $p < 0.001$, $\chi^2/df = 3.202$, RMSEA = 0.072, CFI = 0.946, IFI = 0.946, TLI = 0.939. Note2. ** $p < 0.01$.

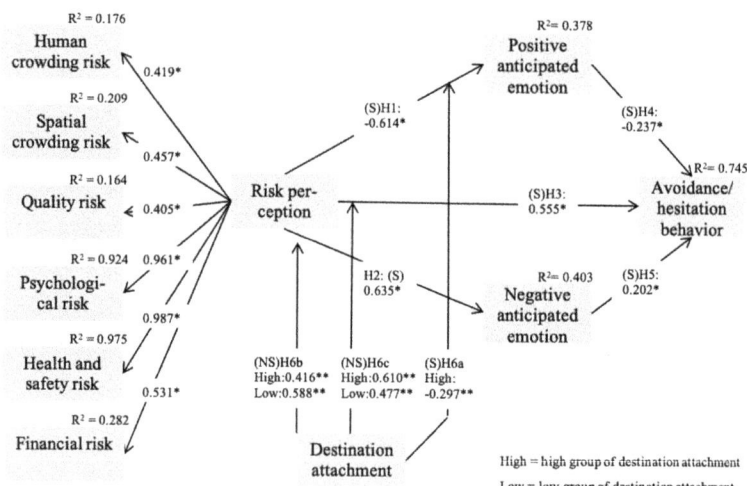

Figure 2. Structural model and invariance model results. Note1. Goodness-of-fit statistics for the structural model (higher-order model $\chi^2 = 1079.063$, $df = 337$, $p < 0.001$, $\chi^2/df = 3.202$, RMSEA = 0.072, CFI = 0.946, IFI = 0.946, TLI = 0.939. Note2. Goodness-of-fit statistics for the baseline model: $\chi^2 = 1567.221$, $df = 693$, $p < 0.001$, $\chi^2/df = 2.262$, RMSEA = 0.054, CFI = 0.925, IFI = 0.925, TLI = 0.918. Note3. * $p < 0.05$, ** $p < 0.01$. Note4. Two identical models were proposed (models for high and low groups of destination attachment).

4.3. Baseline Model and Test for Metric Invariance

A baseline model was created to evaluate the hypothesized moderating influence of destination attachment. A total of 429 responses gathered through the survey were divided into high destination attachment group ($n = 198$) and low destination attachment group ($n = 231$). We utilized a k-means cluster analysis for the grouping process. Findings showed that this baseline model contained a satisfactory model fit ($\chi^2 = 1567.221$, $df = 693$, $p < 0.001$, $\chi^2/df = 2.262$, RMSEA = 0.054, CFI = 0.925, IFI = 0.925, TLI = 0.918). The baseline model results are shown in Table 3.

The generated baseline model was compared to the nested models, where a particular link of interest was constrained equivalently across high and low destination attachment groups. The results of a Chi-square test indicated that the linkage from risk perception to positive anticipated emotion significantly differed across groups ($\Delta\chi^2 (1) = 3.888$, $p < 0.05$). Therefore, Hypothesis 6a was supported. Yet findings revealed that the paths from risk perception to negative anticipated emotion ($\Delta\chi^2 (1) = 2.712$, $p > 0.05$) and to avoidance/hesitation behavior ($\Delta\chi^2 (1) = 0.772$, $p > 0.05$) were not significantly dissimilar between destination attachment groups. Accordingly, Hypotheses 6b and 6c were not supported. In summary, these results indicate that destination attachment has positive moderating effect on risk perception and avoidance/hesitation behavior. Conversely, the destination attachment was not a moderating effect on risk perception and anticipated emotions (positive and negative anticipated emotion).

Table 3. Baseline and invariance model assessment results.

Paths	High Group of Destination Attachment ($n = 198$)		Low Group of Destination Attachment ($n = 231$)		Baseline Model (Freely Estimated)	Nested Model (Constrained to Be Equal)
	β	t-Values	β	t-Values		
Risk perception → Positive anticipated emotion	−0.297 **	−3.014	−0.481 **	−3.729	$\chi^2 (693) = 1567.221$	$\chi^2 (694) = 1571.109$ a
Risk perception → Negative anticipated emotion	0.416 **	3.536	0.588 **	3.883	$\chi^2 (693) = 1567.221$	$\chi^2 (694) = 1569.933$ b
Risk perception → avoidance/ hesitation behavior	0.610 **	4.186	0.477 **	3.741	$\chi^2 (693) = 1567.221$	$\chi^2 (694) = 1567.993$ c
Chi-square Difference Test:						
a $\Delta\chi^2 (1) = 3.888$, $p < 0.05$ (H6a—supported)						
b $\Delta\chi^2 (1) = 2.712$, $p > 0.05$ (H6b—not supported)						
c $\Delta\chi^2 (1) = 0.772$, $p > 0.05$ (H6c—not supported)						

Note1. Goodness-of-fit statistics for the baseline model: $\chi^2 = 1567.221$, $df = 693$, $p < 0.001$, $\chi^2/df = 2.262$, RMSEA = 0.054, CFI = 0.925, IFI = 0.925, TLI = 0.918; Note2. ** $p < 0.01$.

5. Discussion

This study provides a meaningful theorization related to tourist international behaviors in the with-corona era. The present research is one of few studies that have built a theoretical framework by risk perception factors as core variables and considered their influence on international travelers' avoidance behavior through anticipated emotions. This research aimed to integrate the moderating impact of overseas travelers' destination attachment with the formation of their anticipated emotional responses and hesitation behaviors. In sum, the findings of the present research help us to comprehend more explicitly the role of risk perception, which increases international travelers' negative anticipated emotion, decreases their positive anticipated emotion, and ultimately enhances their avoidance actions regarding travel to China. In addition, our findings help us to clearly understand the criticality of attachment and how it moderates the risk perception and positive anticipated emotion relationship. Given that international tourism toward China can be one of the most critical issues in the global tourism industry in the with-corona era, the findings of the present research are of utmost importance in helping international tourism practitioners and researchers in Korea enhance their knowledge about outbound travelers' decision-making processes and behaviors in relation to China in the with-corona era.

It is indisputable that there exists a significant relation between disease outbreak and tourist behaviors. Nevertheless, little research has yet uncovered the possible effect of perceived risk related to COVID-19 on Korean travelers' destination choices in the outbound tourism sector. Filling this void, this is the first empirical study that identifies the possible risks of traveling to China after the outbreak of COVID-19 and explores the influence of various risk factors on Korean travelers' avoidance behaviors/responses toward traveling to China. Our result therefore enriches the literature on international tourism and can be used as a basic framework for future research about disease outbreak and tourist behavior.

Al-Ansi [13] determined the risk perception dimension of health risk, psychological risk, environmental risk, social risk, quality risk, financial risk, and time-loss risk and found that, except for time-loss risk, risk perception significantly influenced tourist behavioral intention. In the current research, a particular meaningful point is the second-order framework of risk perception. It was apparent that the six first-order dimensions (human crowding risk, spatial crowding risk, quality risk, psychological risk, health and safety risk, and financial risk) belong to the global latent factor of risk perception. In other words, the commonality underlying the six dimensions was fully extracted by its second-order variable. This empirical result enriches the extant literature by providing a higher-order approach, which clearly captures risk perception pertinent to international tourism in China. Moreover, the parsimonious framework of this hierarchical structure enlightens academics and destination marketers regarding the effectiveness of theorizing intricate risk perception factors more succinctly in the with-corona era of the international tourism sector. For sector can ensure social distancing in tourism destinations to avoid human crowding and spatial crowding risk. Zhang et al. [45] suggested that destination managers should weigh up destination measures and tourist health risk perception, and that destination anti-epidemic measures positively influence destination image. Combined with this research, tourism departments need to improve this destination management measure.

In a previous study on the relationship between health risk and tourist protective behavior, worry played a crucial role in health risk perceptions [17,46]. A prior study confirmed the relationship between financial and quality risk and tourist behavioral intention [11,16]. In this research health and safety risk were two prominent factors of risk perception. Therefore, for tourism practitioners in China, improving unhealthy, unsafe, and uncomfortable tourism environments can be crucial to minimize risk perception of Korean international travelers regarding China.

Financial risk and quality risk were also uncovered as vital dimensions of risk perception. In addition, human crowding risk and spatial crowing risk were unearthed as significant dimensions of risk perception. Hence, lowering financial and quality risks in tourist sites in China, as well as minimizing human and spatial crowding risks, are critical. The facilitators and inhibitors of tourist avoidance behaviors relating to international tourism are weakly researched and understood in the with-corona era. Employing an empirical approach, this research successfully provides evidence that risk perception and its constituents are fundamental sources for helping tourism academics/practitioners in Korea and China in understanding outbound and inbound travelers' responses/behaviors, respectively.

According to prior research, tourists' destination attachment strongly influences destination loyalty and positive emotional response [32,34,35]. The findings of our research from metric-invariance assessment evidenced that destination attachment significantly moderates the relation between risk perception and positive anticipated emotion. Particularly, the risk perception→positive emotion relationship was weaker in the high group of destination attachment ($\beta_{\text{risk perception} \to \text{positive anticipated emotion}} = -0.297, p < 0.01$) as compared to the low group ($\beta_{\text{risk perception} \to \text{positive anticipated emotion}} = -0.481, p > 0.05$). Our result indicates that Korean overseas travelers' risk perception is less likely to reduce their positive anticipated emotion when they feel a strong attachment to China as an international tourism destination. Sohn and Yoon [36] reported that destination attachment has a moderate effect on risk perception and destination image. The result of this research evidence provides theoretically important information that the risk perception and positive anticipated emotion link significantly depends on the level of destination attachment. The use of this moderator concept can hence be hence for a better grasp of understanding Korean tourists' avoidance responses when considering China for international tourism. Practically, our result offers critical insights as it reports that strong bonding between a destination and its visitors reduces the detrimental influence of risk perception on otherwise positive anticipated emotional responses.

6. Conclusions

Our investigation of the indirect influence of research constructs evidenced that positive and negative anticipated emotions are crucial mediators within the hypothesized conceptual framework. Two main influential factors mediated the impact of their proximal antecedent to their outcome construct. The result indicates that for a clear understanding of the role of risk perception in overseas travelers' behaviors, dealing with positive and negative anticipated emotions is a fundamental requisite. Based on this finding, tourism practitioners need to boost anticipated positive emotion and lower anticipated negative emotion pertinent to international traveling as this effort minimizes the impact of the predictor on international-tourism avoidance behavior. This research contains a few limitations. First, the present study includes an issue of high correlation. Although the between-construct correlations in this study are not at the problematic level, some correlations are still high. Future research should minimize this issue by effective design of the measurement framework. Second, this research centers on the role of risk perception in eliciting emotional and behavioral responses among international travelers. Yet, according to recent destination studies in tourism, many crucial factors influence such affective and behavioral processes (e.g., satisfaction, image, destination performance, attributes, trust, value, travel experience) [1,47–49]. Future research should expand the proposed theoretical framework to better account for the total variance of avoidance/hesitation behavior. Such effort would enhance the comprehensiveness of the conceptual framework and its prediction power.

Author Contributions: Conceptualization, H.H.; methodology, H.H.; Writing—original draft preparation, H.H.; writing—review and editing, C.C. and S.L.; visualization, C.C.; supervision, S.L.; project administration, S.L.; funding acquisition, H.H. and S.L. All authors have read and agreed to the published version of the manuscript.

Funding: This work was supported by the Ministry of Education of the Republic of Korea and the National Research Foundation of Korea (NRF-2020S1A5A2A01046684).

Institutional Review Board Statement: Not applicable.

Informed Consent Statement: Informed consent was obtained from all subjects involved in the study.

Data Availability Statement: The dataset used in this research are available upon request from the corresponding author. The data are not publicly available due to restrictions, i.e., privacy or ethics.

Conflicts of Interest: The authors declare no conflict of interest.

References

1. Chan, C.-S. Developing a conceptual model for the post-COVID-19 pandemic changing tourism risk perception. *Int. J. Environ. Res. Public Health* **2021**, *18*, 9824. [CrossRef] [PubMed]

2. Cortellis Disease Briefing: Coronaviruses. Clarivate Analytics. 2020. Available online: https://clarivate.com/wp-content/uploads/dlm_uploads/2020/01/CORONAVIRUS-REPORT-1.30.2020.pdf?utm_campaign=EM2_Coronavirus_complimentary_resources_science_APAC_Korea_2020_Limited&utm_medium=email&utm_source=Eloqua (accessed on 23 June 2021).
3. Volgger, M.; Taplin, R.; Aebli, A. Recovery of domestic tourism during the COVID-19 pandemic: An experimental comparison of interventions. *J. Hosp. Tour. Manag.* 2021, *48*, 428–440. [CrossRef]
4. Han, H.; Lee, S.; Kim, J.; Ryu, H. Coronavirus disease (COVID-19), traveler behaviors, and international tourism businesses: Impact of the corporate social responsibility (CSR), knowledge, psychological distress, attitude, and ascribed responsibility. *Sustainability* 2020, *12*, 8338. [CrossRef]
5. Kim, J.; Lee, J. Effect of COVID-19 on preference for private dining facilities in restaurants. *J. Hosp. Tour. Res.* 2020, *45*, 67–70. [CrossRef]
6. Hui, D.S.I.; Azhar, E.; Madani, T.A. The continuing 2019-nCoV epidemic threat of novel coronaviruses to global health—The latest 2019 novel coronavirus outbreak in Wuhan, China. *Int. J. Infect. Dis.* 2020, *91*, 264. [CrossRef]
7. Gössling, S.; Scott, D.; Hall, C. Pandemics, tourism and global change: A rapid assessment of COVID-19. *J. Sustain. Tour.* 2021, *29*, 1–20. [CrossRef]
8. Bhalla, R.; Chowdhary, N.; Ranjan, A. Spiritual tourism for psychotherapeutic healing post COVID-19. *J. Travel Tour. Mark.* 2021, *38*, 769–781. [CrossRef]
9. World Health Organization (WHO). WHO Coronavirus (COVID-19) Dashboard. 2021. Available online: https://covid19.who.int (accessed on 12 November 2021).
10. National Health Commission of the People's Republic of China (NHCPRC). The Latest COVID-19 Situation on 11 November. 2021. Available online: http://www.nhc.gov.cn/xcs/yqfkdt/202111/0d0aff2098494e5c96fd08d00ca9202c.shtml (accessed on 12 November 2021).
11. Chen, Y.; Liu, Q.; Guo, D. Emerging coronaviruses: Genome structure, replication, and pathogenesis. *J. Med. Virol.* 2020, *92*, 418–423. [CrossRef]
12. Korea Tourism Organization (KTO) Tourism Statistics. 2020. Available online: https://datalab.visitkorea.or.kr/site/portal/ex/bbs/View.do;ksessionid=RgYOeHAhXnkJkKFAf9vFiN5WrdyLsIULqbzRu81N.wiws01?cbIdx=1129&bcIdx=297486&cateCont=tlt02&searchKey=&searchKey2=&tgtTypeCd= (accessed on 23 June 2021).
13. Al-Ansi, A.; Olya, H.G.T.; Han, H. Effect of general risk on trust, satisfaction, and recommendation intention for halal food. *Int. J. Hosp. Manag.* 2019, *83*, 210–219. [CrossRef]
14. Cahyanto, I.; Liu-Lastres, B. Risk perception, media exposure, and visitor's behavior responses to Florida red tide. *J. Travel Tour. Mark.* 2020, *37*, 447–459. [CrossRef]
15. Simpson, P.M.; Siguaw, J.A. Perceived travel risks: The traveler perspective and manageability. *Int. J. Tour. Res.* 2008, *10*, 315–327. [CrossRef]
16. Olya, H.G.T.; Al-Ansi, A. Risk assessment of halal products and services: Implication for tourism industry. *Tour. Manag.* 2018, *65*, 279–291. [CrossRef]
17. Yu, J.; Lee, K.; Hyun, S. Understanding the influence of the perceived risk of the coronavirus disease (COVID-19) on the post-traumatic stress disorder and revisit intention of hotel guests. *J. Hosp. Tour. Manag.* 2021, *46*, 327–335. [CrossRef]
18. Olya, H.G.T.; Han, H. Antecedents of space traveler behavioral intention. *J. Travel Res.* 2020, *59*, 528–544. [CrossRef]
19. Bauer, R.A. Consumer behaviour as risk taking. In Proceedings of the 43rd Conference of the American Marketing Association, Chicago, IL, USA, 15–17 June 1960; Hancock, R.F., Ed.; American Marketing Association: Chicago, IL, USA, 1960; pp. 389–398.
20. Quan, W.; Al-Ansi, A.; Han, H. Spatial and human crowdedness, time pressure, and Chinese traveler word-of-mouth behaviors for Korean restaurants. *Int. J. Hosp. Manag.* 2021, *94*, 1–10. [CrossRef]
21. Huifeng, P.; Ha, H.; Lee, J. Perceived risks and restaurant visit intentions in China: Do online customer reviews matter? *J. Hosp. Tour. Manag.* 2020, *43*, 179–189. [CrossRef]
22. Olya, H.G.T.; Altinay, L. Asymmetric modeling of intention to purchase weather insurance and loyalty. *J. Bus. Res.* 2016, *69*, 2791–2800. [CrossRef]
23. Law, R. The perceived impact of risks on travel decisions. *Int. J. Tour. Res.* 2006, *8*, 289–300. [CrossRef]
24. Rosental, S.; Ho, K.L. Minding other people's business: Community attachment and anticipated negative emotion in an extended norm activation model. *J. Environ. Psychol.* 2020, *69*, 1–12. [CrossRef]
25. Zhang, Y.; Wong, I.A.; Duan, X.; Chen, Y.V. Craving better health? Influence of socio-political conformity and health consciousness on goal-directed rural-eco tourism. *J. Travel Tour. Mark.* 2021, *38*, 511–526. [CrossRef]
26. Perugini, M.; Bagozzi, R.P. The role of desires and anticipated emotions in goal-directed behaviors: Broadening and deepening the theory of planned behavior. *Br. J. Soc. Psychol.* 2001, *40*, 79–98. [CrossRef]
27. Rivis, A.; Sheeran, P.; Armitage, C.J. Expanding the affective and normative components of the theory of planned behavior: A meta-analysis of anticipated affect and moral norms. *J. Appl. Soc. Psychol.* 2009, *39*, 2985–3019. [CrossRef]
28. Han, H. Consumer behavior and environmental sustainability in tourism and hospitality: A review of theories, concepts, and latest research. *J. Sustain. Tour.* 2021, *29*, 1021–1042. [CrossRef]
29. Bagozzi, R.P.; Dholakia, U.M. Antecedents and purchase consequences of customer participation in small group brand communities. *Int. J. Res. Mar.* 2006, *23*, 45–61. [CrossRef]

30. Lu, H.; Zou, J.; Chen, H.; Long, R. Promotion or inhibition? Moral norms, anticipated emotion and employee's pro-environmental behavior. *J. Clean. Prod.* **2020**, *258*, 1–10. [CrossRef]
31. Odou, P.; Schill, M. How anticipated emotions shape behavioral intentions to flight climate change. *J. Bus. Res.* **2020**, *121*, 243–253. [CrossRef]
32. Fournier, S.; Lee, L. Getting brand communities right. *Harv. Bus. Rev.* **2009**, *4*, 1–10.
33. Kaufmann, H.R.; Petrovici, D.A.; Filho, C.G.; Ayres, A. Identifying moderators of brand attachment for driving customer purchase intention of original vs. counterfeits of luxury brands. *J. Bus. Res.* **2016**, *69*, 5735–5747. [CrossRef]
34. Pradhananga, A.K.; Davenport, M.A. Community attachment, beliefs and residents' civic engagement in stormwater management. *Landsc. Urban Plan.* **2017**, *168*, 1–8. [CrossRef]
35. Scannell, L.; Gifford, R. Defining place attachment: A tripartite organizing framework. *J. Environ. Psychol.* **2010**, *30*, 1–10. [CrossRef]
36. Sohn, H.K.; Yoon, Y.S. Verification of destination attachment and moderating effects in the relationship between the perception of and satisfaction with tourism destinations: A focus on Japanese tourists. *J. Travel Tour. Mark.* **2016**, *33*, 757–769. [CrossRef]
37. Çetinsöz, B.C.; Ege, Z. Impacts of perceived risks on tourists' revisit intentions. *Anatolia* **2013**, *24*, 173–187. [CrossRef]
38. Imboden, A. Between risk and comfort: Representations of adventure tourism in Sweden and Switzerland. *Scand. J. Hosp. Tour.* **2012**, *12*, 310–323. [CrossRef]
39. Reisinger, Y.; Mavondo, F. Cultural differences in travel risk perception. *J. Travel Tour. Mark.* **2006**, *20*, 13–31. [CrossRef]
40. Wei, Q.; Han, H. How crowdedness affects Chinese customer satisfaction at Korean restaurants? *Korean J. Hosp. Tour.* **2019**, *28*, 161–177.
41. Yin, J.; Cheng, Y.; Bi, Y.; Ni, Y. Tourists perceived crowding and destination attractiveness: The moderating effects of perceived risk and experience quality. *J. Dest. Mark. Manag.* **2020**, *18*, 100489. [CrossRef]
42. Assaker, G.; Hallak, R. Moderating effects of tourists' novelty-seeking tendencies on destination image, visitor satisfaction, and short-and long-term revisit intentions. *J. Travel Res.* **2013**, *52*, 600–613. [CrossRef]
43. Wong, J.-Y.; Yeh, C. Tourist hesitation in destination decision making. *Ann. Tour. Res.* **2009**, *36*, 6–23. [CrossRef]
44. Hair, J.F.; Black, W.C.; Babin, B.J.; Anderson, R.E. *Multivariate Data Analysis*, 7th ed.; Prentice-Hall: Upper Saddle River, NJ, USA, 2010; pp. 600–638.
45. Zhang, H.; Zhuang, M.; Cao, Y.; Pan, J.; Zhang, X.; Zhang, J.; Zhang, H. Social Distancing in Tourism Destination Management during the COVID-19 Pandemic in China: A Moderated Mediation Model. *Int. J. Environ. Res. Public Health* **2021**, *18*, 11223. [CrossRef]
46. Chien, P.M.; Sharifpour, M.; Ritchie, B.W.; Watson, B. Travelers' health risk perceptions and protective behavior: A psychological approach. *J. Travel. Res.* **2017**, *56*, 744–759. [CrossRef]
47. Che, C.; Koo, B.; Wang, J.; Ariza-Montes, A.; Vega-Munoz, A.; Han, H. Promoting rural tourism in Inner Mongolia: Attributes, satisfaction, and behaviors among sustainable tourists. *Int. J. Environ. Res. Public Health* **2021**, *18*, 3788. [CrossRef] [PubMed]
48. Oliver, R.L. *Satisfaction: A Behavioral Perspective on the Consumer*, 2nd ed.; Routledge: New York, NY, USA, 2010.
49. Pai, C.; Lee, T.; Kang, S. Examining the role of service quality, perceived value, and trust in Macau food festival. *Int. J. Environ. Res. Public Health* **2021**, *18*, 9214. [CrossRef] [PubMed]

MDPI
St. Alban-Anlage 66
4052 Basel
Switzerland
Tel. +41 61 683 77 34
Fax +41 61 302 89 18
www.mdpi.com

International Journal of Environmental Research and Public Health Editorial Office
E-mail: ijerph@mdpi.com
www.mdpi.com/journal/ijerph

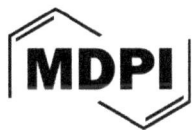

www.ingramcontent.com/pod-product-compliance
Lightning Source LLC
LaVergne TN
LVHW070145100526
838202LV00015B/1896